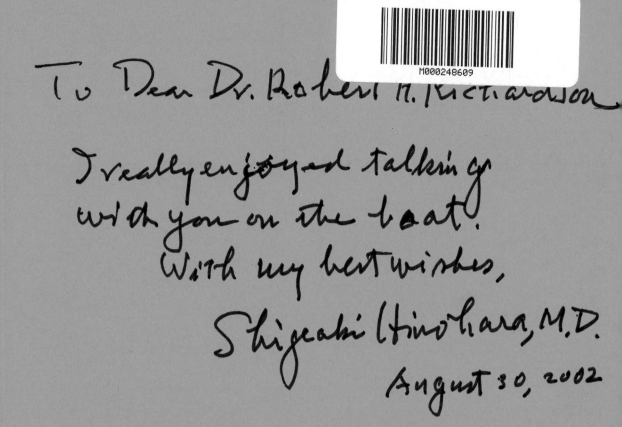

To Dear Dr. Robert H. Richardson

I really enjoyed talking
with you on the boat!
With my best wishes,
Shigeaki Hinohara, M.D.
August 30, 2002

Osler's
"A Way of Life"
and Other Addresses,
with Commentary and
Annotations

OSLER'S "A WAY OF LIFE" AND OTHER ADDRESSES, WITH COMMENTARY AND ANNOTATIONS

Sir William Osler

Shigeaki Hinohara, M.D., and Hisae Niki, M.A.

with a Foreword by John P. McGovern, M.D.

DUKE UNIVERSITY PRESS

DURHAM & LONDON

2001

© 2001 Duke University Press
All rights reserved
Printed in the United States of America on acid-free paper ∞
Designed by Mary Mendell
Typeset in Aldus by Tseng Information Systems, Inc.
Library of Congress Cataloging-in-Publication Data appear
on the last printed page of this book.

TO
THE LATE DR. WARNER F. BOWERS,
THE LATE DR. GRANT TAYLOR,
AND TO
DR. JOHN P. MCGOVERN

CONTENTS

FOREWORD

MORE THAN A century and a half after his birth and eighty years after his death, Sir William Osler (1849–1919) continues to be an icon for the medical profession. He followed a career of accelerating excellence, after his graduation from McGill University, first in Canada, then in the United States, and finally in Great Britain. In particular, at Johns Hopkins University in Baltimore his medical expertise made him a leader of the profession and the most sought-after consultant in North America. He and his colleagues there perfected methods of medical education that continue to be the working model more than a century later. Dr. Hinohara's brief chronology of Osler's career succinctly epitomizes his remarkable life. Osler's influence spread rapidly through his many writings, innovative teaching, and way of life. His medical text, *The Principles and Practice of Medicine* (first edition, 1892), became the standard for the English-speaking world and, through translations, far beyond. It was this first edition that inspired the creation of the Rockefeller Institute for Medical Research. But today it is his nonscientific books and articles that continue to be read, enjoyed, and ofttimes to inspire: his message is the practical art of living. One of his cardinal messages is the primacy of being humane, in one's life and one's patient-centered medical practice. The practical, everyday utility of his insight and example reaches beyond the practice of medicine and holds value for all who investigate his words. And it is Osler's essays that this book celebrates. It does so by presenting them anew to the reading public. But much more than that, it also clarifies the numerous literary allusions and metaphors that, a century and more after they were written, may be unclear to a public that is less at home with the classics of all ages than was the case then.

Although this collection of Osler's essays, with comments and annotations, is timeless, its publication could hardly be more timely. Finding one's way in the world of medicine today is a daunting challenge for health care providers as well as the recipients of their care. The profession of medicine presently is under severe pressure of a nature rarely if ever before witnessed, while the image of the physician is increasingly called into question. In addition to rapid technological growth and the massive accumulation of scientific data that physicians must understand, assimilate, and use on an ongoing basis, other profound forces have been shaping medicine and surgery at an accelerating rate during the past twenty years. Among the shifting influences on the contemporary practice of medicine are the recent healthcare reform programs, which greatly influence rationing of professional time; those caregivers whose time is excessively restricted may well lose altogether the interlude necessary to develop the trust that in turn empowers patients to enter into their own healing process.

There always has been societal pressure on the practice of medicine. Today, medical services are more in demand than ever before, at a time that people are less happy with the medical profession. This is true despite the fact that modern medicine empowers its practitioners to offer their patients more than ever before in the way of prevention, treatment, and cures to avoid or alter the course of disease. They have at their disposal precise technologies for diagnosis and for monitoring treatment, and exponentially more effective drugs than in Osler's day, and physicians are much better equipped than their forebears to relieve the agonies of constant pain and physical handicap. Nevertheless, doctors today are less trusted and respected than in years past. Could it be that in spite of the modern medical armamentarium an essential ingredient in medical care has been attenuated or neglected, and if so, what would it be?

There is today much debate as to whether the practice of medicine is a science, an art, a trade, a business, a profession, or some combination thereof. Here is what Osler stated in "The Master-Word in Medicine": "The practice of medicine is an art, not a trade; a calling, not a business; a calling in which your heart will be exercised equally with your head." At the time of that quote (1903) there was precious little science, and the technology of medicine has advanced to a degree beyond imagination in his day. Today, one could speculate that Osler might say: "The practice of medicine is an art *based on science; a profession not a trade;* a calling, not a business; a calling in which your heart must always be exercised along with your head." As technology and science advanced, Osler clearly would still have realized that a physician would always not be treating just a disease, but rather a *unique, living, feeling human being* with disease. The "heart" then signified compassion, empathy, and deep caring, as it still does. That is the essential ingredient that seems to many patients to be neglected today. Far too often I hear such remarks as: "He/she doesn't seem to really listen to me; to answer my questions; to explain anything; always appears to be in a hurry; I just feel that they don't really care—I'm just a number."

An inordinate overemphasis on science can easily tip the balance away from the art, the caring and compassionate side of medicine. Thus, between the science and the art, the rapid changes in healthcare delivery systems are challenging medical schools throughout the country to find and teach the relevance of that balance. Osler's cogent observations and insight reflected in these essays give much timeless good guidance toward the resolution of this imbalance.

Osler insisted that for physicians to be properly educated to practice their art, knowledge of the science of medicine (limited as it was) must be supplemented by familiarity with the humanities. He believed firmly that the humanities were the leaven in the dough of caring, compassion, and empathy. "Twin berries on one stem, grievous damage has been done to both in regarding the Humanities and Science in any other light than complemental" ("The Old Humanities and the New Science"). His own command of the humanities shines through in these essays, and lights the way not only toward the practice of "head and heart" medicine, but a way of life for anyone.

What a burden a physician takes on: to be knowledgeable and up to date in medical science, versed in the humanities, and caring at every level of the struggle of the patient. This calls for one additional necessary attribute of a physician, a philosophy of life that enables him to carry and manage that burden, one that is clearly laid out in the first Osler essay, "A Way of Life." In it he said that he owed much of his success to a simple habit, cultivated early in his life—one of "living in day-tight compartments." He emphasized the wisdom of not dwelling morbidly on the mistakes and cares of yesterday or of anticipating with anxiety and fear what tomorrow might bring. Instead he urged that all of one's resources be brought to bear on today, because "the load of tomorrow, added to that of yesterday, carried today makes the strongest falter." Such an approach is also appropriate for the anxious patient or one in great pain. Pain is easier to bear if it is seen as just for today.

Even with the rapidly changing medical delivery system and the dominance of technological and scientific discoveries that occur at an accelerating pace, Osler's ethics, principles, and practices portrayed herein, in concert with increasing efforts in our medical and nursing schools, could help transform and energize academic teaching and the delivery of quality care. Practicing physicians and nurses, as well as paramedics, physical therapists, and other invaluable members of the healthcare team must all persevere as compassionate scientific healers.

Though there have been several other collations of Osler's addresses, no other exists with cogent comments before each essay, nor especially with comprehensive annotations, making each essay much more lucid for modern readers. We all owe a deep debt of gratitude to co-editor Professor Hisae Niki, for her expertise and devoted and persevering work for more than twenty years in making this book possible.

In a more personal vein, from my own lifetime experience as a teacher, clinician, and Oslerian, I am convinced that these annotations add clarity to the many metaphorical expressions, citations, and allusions, and thus an increased insight into these important Osler essays—thereby providing an invaluable resource not readily available prior to this publication. My great regret is that these outstanding annotations were unavailable to me many years earlier as they will be a tremendous asset for the serious reader. I strongly believe that all who thoughtfully read and digest the messages of the life and calling in this book will find enhanced satisfaction—even joy—in their demanding work. An understanding of Osler's patient-centered approach will especially help the healthcare provider participate in finding solutions to the pressing problems in our current healthcare delivery systems and to be better able to practice "head and heart" service to the ill who come to them in need; and who, in turn, will be much more satisfied with their care.

It is important not to forget that the messages of Osler are truly messages of life with practical insight about daily living and human potential that reach beyond the healthcare professional to all whom venture to turn these pages. No matter what one's occupation or calling, we all share in common a continual need to sharpen our skills at daily living. A gifted physician and teacher, Osler never ceased in his own quest for self-improvement as both a physician and a citizen. To that end, these essays represent a real treasure that extends the reach of his essays from the archives of medical history to our contemporary world of the new millennia.

About the Editor

Dr. Shigeaki Hinohara is an indefatigable, peripatetic international medical ambassador and renowned Oslerian. As an internist and educator, Dr. Hinohara has devoted more than sixty years to medicine and medical science, in his home country of Japan and internationally. He has developed and maintained a lifelong affiliation with St. Luke's International Hospital in Tokyo, where he is currently the chairman of its board. In addition, he also serves as the chairman of the board of St. Luke's College of Nursing and maintains a number of consultative positions in medical schools in Japan.

Dr. Hinohara received his M.D. degree from Kyoto University Medical School in 1938. There he also was awarded a Ph.D. for his study on atrial heart sounds, detected through the esophagus by a tiny microphone that he devised. Later, he undertook advanced studies in general internal medicine and residency training programs under Professor Paul Beeson at the Emory University School of Medicine.

Dr. Hinohara's affiliation with St. Luke's International Hospital dates back to 1941, when he joined the medical staff in the Department of Internal Medicine. In 1951, he became Chief Physician of that department, a position he held for a quarter century. During this period in his career, his principal medical interests were in the fields of cardiology, psychosomatic medicine, water and electrolyte metabolism, and preventive medicine.

From 1971 to 1989, Hinohara served on a number of governmental committees established by the Japanese Ministries of Education and Health and Welfare. His responsibilities included serving as chairman of the Council on Graduate Medical Education and chairman of the Council of Accreditation of Specialties Board.

Dr. Hinohara is a member of a number of Japanese medical organizations, including the Society of Medical Education and the Medical Society of Primary Care. Internationally, his memberships include fellowship in the American College of Cardiology and honorary fellowship in the American College of Physicians. He is past president of the International Society of Internal Medicine and the International Health Evaluation Association. Lately, his writings have focused on aging and hospice care and on alternative approaches in healing such as music therapy.

Among the plethora of awards that Dr. Hinohara has received over his extensive career are the Japanese Medical Association Supreme Award for Scientific Achievement (1982), the Japan-United States Visiting Medical Scientist, The College of Physicians of Philadelphia (1985), and the Japanese-American Award of Merit, from the Foundation of Thanatology, Columbia Presbyterian Medical Center, USA (1992). In 1993 he received the Order of the Secret Treasure, Gold and Silver Star from the Japanese Emperor Akihito. In 1998 he was elected as one of two honorary citizens of Tokyo Metropolitan and also in that year received a Doctor of Humane Letters at the 174th Commencement from Jefferson Medical College, Thomas Jefferson University. On November 3, 1999, the Memorial Day of Culture in Japan, Dr. Hinohara was named by Ministry of Education, Science, Sports, and Culture a Person of Cultural Merit, the only physician so honored.

Dr. Hinohara is known as a great Oslerian who has spread Osler's principles and ideals throughout the world. He has conducted extensive studies and published articles and books about the life and works of Sir William Osler. He founded the Japan Osler Society in 1983 and still serves as its President; he was elected an honorary member of both the American Osler Society (1983), and the Osler Club of London (1984). Significant articles published in English relative to his Oslerian interests include "Osler's Peregrinations in Asia—A Report on an Unusual Event," *American Diseases of Children*, vol. 24, September, 1972, "Osler in Japan," *Osler Library Newsletter*, no. 45, February 1984, and "Sir William Osler's Philosophy on Death," *Annals of Internal Medicine*, 118:8, 13 April, 1993.

John P. McGovern, M.D.

PREFACE

WILLIAM OSLER (1849–1919) dedicated his life to practice, education, research, and social concerns in medicine. He was active in Canada, the United States, and Britain during the latter half of the nineteenth century and the early twentieth century. This book is a collection of some of his nonclinical lectures, with added commentaries and bibliographical annotations that clarify the citations and metaphorical expressions he used.

Osler wrote 1,158 medical publications, and 182 literary papers and essays in his lifetime, of which we have chosen twenty. In 1905 he published a collection of his essays entitled *Aequanimitas with Other Addresses to Medical Students, Nurses and Practitioners of Medicine.*

"Aequanimitas," the first essay in the volume, is the farewell lecture he gave when he resigned his position of Professor of Internal Medicine at the University of Pennsylvania. In it he emphasized that "aequanimitas" (serenity) of the mind is the most important quality for a physician, no matter what crises he might face. Subsequently, Osler gave twenty-two nonclinical addresses up to 1905, as Professor of Medicine at Johns Hopkins University. They were addressed to medical students, nurses, medical practitioners and teachers at various medical schools, medical associations, nursing schools, and medical-science institutions.

In 1941, I started working as a hospital physician at St. Luke's International Hospital, Tokyo, Japan. Immediately after World War II, in August 1945, St. Luke's was requisitioned by the Supreme Commander for the Allied Forces as one of their army general hospitals. As I stood witnessing the hand-over ceremony, the head of this army general hospital, Dr. Warner Bowers, gave me a copy of *Aequanimitas with Other Addresses to Medical Students, Nurses, and Prac-*

titioners of Medicine. Ever since, the book has been my "comes viae vitaeque," companion on the journey. Dr. Bowers himself admired Osler; I was told that the book was given to him by Eli Lilly and Company when he graduated from medical school, and even during the war he read it on the hospital ship.

With deepest appreciation I read this gift from Dr. Bowers. I then resolved, although the text was rather difficult, that one day I would translate it into Japanese for Japanese medical students. My plan was to select sixteen lectures out of the twenty-two, which are still applicable to contemporary medical personnel, and add four splendid lectures, ones that Osler gave after he moved to Britain in 1905 to become Regius Professor of Medicine at Oxford University. Those four are: "Sir Thomas Browne," given in 1905 at Guy's Hospital in London, which introduces this man, whom Osler greatly admired; "Man's Redemption of Man," a lay sermon delivered at a Sunday service for the students of the University of Edinburgh in 1910; "A Way of Life," to the Yale students given in 1913 the day before he delivered the annual Silliman Lectures at Yale University; and "The Old Humanities and the New Science," his Presidential Address delivered before the Classical Association at Oxford, May 1919, the year of Osler's death.

In November 1980, Professor Hisae Niki of Meikai University (who was then a professor at St. Luke's College of Nursing and a Shakespearean scholar) and I started translating the lectures into Japanese. By 1983, we had added over 800 annotations to the text, and published it through the medical publisher Igaku-Shoin Ltd. The book was widely read by the Japanese general public, not only by Japanese medical students, physicians, nursing staff, and other medical personnel. At the end of March 2001 more than 27,000 copies had been sold. In his lectures relating to medicine, Osler referred frequently to the literary and philosophical passages of ancient and contemporary authors, philosophers, and educators. But he lived in an age when people wrote allusively, making extensive references to literature and the Bible without citing chapter and verse, because all readers, sharing a common classical education, were expected to recognize the sources. Graceful allusion to those texts was the mark of a learned and distinguished writer. But Japanese readers are generally outside that common education of the English-speaking world, and thus our detailed commentaries and annotations must have enhanced the comprehension of the original difficult lectures for Japanese readers. That might be why more than twenty-seven thousand copies of the Japanese translation were sold.

Then the idea came to us that we might publish the original lectures with our commentaries and annotations in English. Such a book would help contemporary medical students and medical personnel in the English-speaking world to better understand Osler's thoughts and spirit, for no longer was the "classical" education the prevalent academic curriculum as in Osler's day.

For this purpose, Professor Niki visited many libraries in the United States, Canada, and Britain to work further on the annotations. After more than twenty years, with assistance from Professor Niki's friends such as Jane Kuwana of the United States and other scholars in the United States, Canada, and Britain, we completed the project.

Finally, I wish to express my warm and sincere gratitude to my friend and colleague Dr. John P. McGovern, founder of the American Osler Society, for his great efforts in helping structure and edit parts of this book, writing its foreword and in helping guide it to publication. I would also like to voice appreciation to Mr. Yuu Kanahara, president of Igaku-Shoin Ltd, for his expert technical help and support.

Shigeaki Hinohara, M.D.

TO THE READER

THE PRESENT TEXT is a collection of Osler's addresses aimed at sharing the importance and relevance of his ideas to modern times, in particular those writings that deal with ethics in the medical profession. The essays were originally published in *The Collected Essays of Sir William Osler,* ed. by John P. McGovern and Charles G. Roland (Birmingham: The Classics of Medicine Library, 1985); *Aequanimitas: With other Addresses to Medical Students, Nurses and Practitioners of Medicine,* 3d ed. (New York: McGraw-Hill, 1961); *Selected Writings of Sir William Osler* (London: Oxford University Press, 1951), and *Man's Redemption of Man* (New York: Paul B. Hoeber, Inc., 1913). The date when each address was originally delivered or printed is stated at the beginning of the chapter.

Osler's writings abound in references, the range of which is very extensive, to all literature from the classics down to the works of his contemporaries. The notes not only give definitions of words that may be unfamiliar to medical students and the general public but also clarify references—classical, historical, literary, theological, and medical (especially the names of Osler's contemporaries). Some explanatory notes have also been added to help elucidate the text. Obviously, medical schools have greatly changed, and Osler would certainly be waging different campaigns now; this book is not meant to propound his arguments for more laboratories nor his very Victorian views of women. However, we have decided to leave these issues intact for their historical interest and hope that the reader will focus on those things that do not change. Examples of these are the physician's need for perspective and equanimity; the relationship among physicians and between physician and patient; and the complementary but still understressed roles of the humanities and the sciences. Although his writings are primarily directed to medical students, we hope they will give enjoyment and inspiration to many others, including physicians, nurses, librarians, and laypeople, and that they will add richness to each reader's life.

Since this project has occupied me for over twenty years, my indebtness to colleagues and other scholars is correspondingly extensive. Directly and indirectly I am indebted to the work of many preceding editors and scholars. I also owe much to the staff of several libraries: especially, the Osler Library (McGill University), the Bodleian Library (Oxford University), the Library of the University of Illinois, the Library of Johns Hopkins University, the Library of Iowa State University, the Library of the University of Toronto, and many other institutions. My thanks are especially due to Dr. Faith Wallis and Mrs. June Schachter, Osler Library, for having facilitated my work.

I am most grateful and deeply indebted to Jane Kuwana for preparing the introductory notes before each address. In the preparation of the manuscript and in proofreading, I had the assistance of Sylvia Garfield, Alicia Andre, Megumi Kishino, and Kiyoshi Nanao (Igaku-Shoin Ltd.), to all of whom I express my sincere thanks.

Dr. Miriam Skey, on the staff of the Records of Early English Drama at the University of Toronto, was very encouraging and helpful in looking over some of my chapters. Also, I owe special gratitude to Dr. William Cooke, now an independent scholar in Toronto, for his editorial assistance, in reading all the chapters in manuscript and making many valuable suggestions.

Last of all, I would like to thank Dr. Hinohara and Dr. McGovern. This book would never have been conceived nor brought to publication without their steadfast guidance and support of my efforts.

Hisae Niki, M.A.

CHRONOLOGY OF
SIR WILLIAM OSLER'S LIFE

1849 (July 12) Born in Bond Head, Upper Canada (later Canada West, now the Province of Ontario), youngest son of Rev. Featherstone Lake Osler and Ellen Free (Pickton).

1857 (March) Family moves to Dundas, the very western tip of Lake Ontario.

1866 (January) Enters Trinity College School, an independent school for boys, then in Weston and now in Port Hope. Meets Rev. W. A. Johnson, founder and warden of Trinity College School and Dr. James Bovell, medical director appointed by the bishop. Both men had a great influence upon the young Osler.

1867 (autumn) Enters Trinity College, Toronto, with the idea of becoming a clergyman. Later, he abandons the idea to become a physician.

1868 (autumn) Enrolls in Toronto School of Medicine.

1869 (February) "Christmas and the Microscope" published in *Hardwicke's Science-Gossip*, his first published paper.

1870 (autumn) Enters the McGill Medical Faculty in Montreal because of the better clinical opportunities it had to offer. Meets Dr. Robert Palmer Howard, his mentor.

1872 (spring) Graduates from McGill.

1872–1874 Spends two years studying in Europe visiting clinics in London, Berlin, and Vienna.

1874 (July) Receives an offer to lecture upon the Institutes of Medicine at the McGill Medical Faculty.

1875 (April) Upon the death of Dr. M. Drake, he is officially appointed professor of medicine at the McGill Medical Faculty.

1878 (summer) Visits Britain (London and Edinburgh) with George Ross to take his membership of the Royal College of Physicians and to work in clinical medicine.

1879 (May–July) Starts teaching clinical medicine at the Montreal General Hospital. During the following five years he teaches physiology and pathology in the winter season and clinical medicine in the summer.

1884 (spring) Spends time in Europe (London, Berlin, Leipzig) and accepts an appointment as professor of clinical medicine at the University of Pennsylvania.

(October) Appointed professor of clinical medicine at the University of Pennsylvania. This is the beginning of a twenty-one-year period of work and residence in the United States.

1888 (September) Appointed professor of medicine and physician in chief at the new Johns Hopkins Medical School and Hospital in Baltimore, Maryland.

1889 (May) "Aequanimitas," a valedictory address, delivered to the graduates in medicine of the University of Pennsylvania.

1891 (June) "Doctor and Nurse" delivered to the first class of graduates from the Training School for Nurses at the Johns Hopkins Hospital.

1892 (February) *Principles and Practices of Medicine* published.

(May) Marries Grace Linzee (Revere), widow of Dr. Samuel W. Gross of Philadelphia.

(October) "Teacher and Student" delivered at the opening of the new medical buildings of the University of Minnesota.

(December) "Physic and Physicians as Depicted in Plato" delivered at the meeting of the Johns Hopkins Hospital Historical Club.

1894 (May) "The Leaven of Science" delivered at the opening of the Wistar Institute of Anatomy and Biology at the University of Pennsylvania.

1895 (January) "Teaching and Thinking—The Two Functions of a Medical School" delivered at the opening of the new building at the McGill Medical Faculty.

(December 28) His son, Edward Revere Osler, born.

1897 (February, June) "Nurse and Patient" delivered in February at the commencement exercises of the Training School for Nurses at the Philadelphia Hospital, and again in June at the commencement exercises of the Training School for Nurses at the Johns Hopkins Hospital.

1899 (September) "After Twenty-Five Years" delivered before the faculty and students of the Medical Faculty, McGill University.

1901 (January) "Books and Men" delivered at the opening of the new building of the Boston Medical Library.

1902 (September) "Chauvinism in Medicine" delivered before the Canadian Medical Association.

1903 (October) "The Mater-Word in Medicine" delivered at the opening of the new laboratories for physiology and pathology of the University of Toronto, thirty-five years after he studied there.

(December) "The Hospital as a College" delivered at the Academy of Medicine, New York.

1904 (August) Accepts the offer of the Regius Chair of Medicine at Oxford University.

1905 (February) "The Fixed Period," a farewell address, delivered at the commencement exercises before the alumni, faculty, and students of Johns Hopkins University. (April) "The Student Life," a farewell address to Canadian and American medical students, delivered at McGill University, and later the same month at the University of Pennsylvania. (April) "Unity, Peace, and Concord," a farewell address to leaders of the medical profession of the United States, delivered at the annual meeting of the Medical and Chirurgical Faculty of Maryland, Baltimore. (May) "L'Envoi," a speech at a farewell dinner in New York, delivered before leaders of the medical profession of Canada and the United States. (June) The Oslers move to Oxford. Appointed regius professor of medicine at Oxford University.

(October) "Sir Thomas Browne" delivered at the Physical Society of Guy's Hospital, London.

1910 (July) "Man's Redemption of Man: A Lay Sermon" delivered at McEwan Hall, Edinburgh.

1911 (June) Baronetcy conferred by King George V.

1913 (April) "A Way of Life" delivered to Yale students. His last visit to the United States.

1917 (August) The Oslers' son Revere killed in Belgium while on active service as an officer in the Royal Field Artillery.

1919 (May) "The Old Humanities and the New Science" delivered before the Classical Association of Oxford. Osler was president of the Association.
  (July) Has a sharp attack of bronchial pneumonia.
  (December 29) Dies aged 70.

1920 (January 1) A simple service at Christ Church Cathedral in Oxford held for "one of the most greatly beloved physicians of all time" (Cushing).

References

Cushing, Harvey. *The Life of Sir William Osler* (1925). Reprint. New York: Oxford University Press, 1977.

Golden, Richard L., and Charles G. Roland eds. *Sir William Osler, An Annotated Bibliography with Illustrations.* San Francisco: Jeremy Norman and Co., 1988.

Nation, Earl F., Charles G. Roland, and John P. McGovern. *An Annotated Checklist of Osleriana.* Kent, Ohio: Kent State University Press, 1976.

OSLER'S
"A WAY OF LIFE"
AND OTHER ADDRESSES,
WITH COMMENTARY AND
ANNOTATIONS

1

A WAY OF LIFE

What each day needs that shalt thou ask,
Each day will set its proper task.
GOETHE

APPARENTLY IT WAS suggested to Osler that his address to Yale students in 1913 should be either moral or religious, but he chose instead to give a simple home-spun message, "a handle to fit your life tools." He recommends developing a way of life based on established habits. He attributes his own successes not to his brains but to the simple habit of living only for the present. He quotes Thomas Carlyle, "Our main business is not to see what lies dimly at a distance, but to do what lies clearly at hand."

With the analogy of a ship closing off watertight compartments to keep afloat, Oster urges learning to control "day-tight" compartments in one's life. By shutting off thoughts of the past or of the future, one may channel all one's energy to the present task. Osler advocates beginning each day without regrets for things done or left undone. Fantasies and dreams of the future should be ignored except on rare occasions. Steady work and concentration on the task at hand, day after day, are his prescription to avoid frantic work, overly long hours, and burnout.

Mental control and a good attitude are necessary to avoid the feelings of inertia that Goethe says "make the morning's lazy leisure usher in a useless day." Osler warns that a poor diet and excesses of tobacco, alcohol, or sex can rob the body of the physical fitness needed for a good outlook. He alludes to Plato's team of horses: unless the driver can master them, the black steed of Passion pulls the white horse of Reason off course.

Osler also urges spiritual concern, prayer, and reading the Bible to make one aware that, although much changes, love, hope, fear, faith, and passion remain unchanged. "The quiet life in day-tight compartments will help you to bear your own and others' burdens with a light heart," guided by the example of physicians of the past.

A WAY OF LIFE

A WAY OF LIFE

FELLOW STUDENTS—EVERY MAN has a philosophy of life in thought, in word, or in deed,[1] worked out in himself unconsciously. In possession of the very best, he may not know of its existence; with the very worst he may pride himself as a paragon. As it grows with the growth it cannot be taught to the young in formal lectures. What have bright eyes, red blood, quick breath, and taut muscles to do with philosophy? Did not the great Stagirite[2] say that young men were unfit students of it?[3]—they will hear as though they heard not, and to no profit.[4] Why then should I trouble you? Because I have a message that may be helpful. It is not philosophical, nor is it strictly moral or religious, one or other of which I was told my address should be, and yet in a way it is all three. It is the oldest and the freshest, the simplest and the most useful, so simple indeed is it that some of you may turn away disappointed as was Naaman the Syrian[5] when told to go wash in Jordan and be clean. You know those composite

An address delivered to Yale students on April 20, 1913. Published by Constable & Co., London, 1913; by Hoeber, New York, 1914; and in Osler's *The Student Life and Other Essays*, London, 1928, 75–99.

1. *in thought, in word, or in deed:* Osler is probably remembering "by thought, word, and deed" from the form of confession found in the Communion service in the *Book of Common Prayer*. However, in the Anglican High Church it has also been customary for a long time for the priest and altar boy(s) to use a form containing the phrase "in thought, word, and deed" before celebrating the Communion, and Osler could conceivably have remembered that from serving for Father Johnson in his boyhood.

2. *the Stagirite:* Aristotle (384–322 B.C.), who was born in Stagira, Greece.

3. Aristotle, *Nicomachean Ethics*, book 1, chap. 3, 1095a:3–10.

4. *they will hear as though they heard not, and to no profit:* This sentence is a reminiscence of a very common Biblical image: Isaiah 6:9 (quoted by Jesus in Matthew 3:14) and 42:20, etc. The words "to no profit" actually occur in 2 Timothy 2:14 but in a different context.

5. *Naaman:* A Syrian captain who was cured of leprosy by Elisha, a Hebrew prophet. Naaman was in-

tools, to be bought for 50 cents, with one handle to fit a score or more of instruments. The workmanship is usually bad, so bad, as a rule, that you will not find an example in any good carpenter's shop; but the boy has one, the chauffeur slips one into his box, and the sailor into his kit, and there is one in the odds-and-ends drawer of the pantry of every well-regulated family. It is simply a handy thing about the house, to help over the many little difficulties of the day. Of this sort of philosophy I wish to make you a present—a handle to fit your life tools. Whether the workmanship is Sheffield or shoddy,[6] this helve will fit anything from a hatchet to a corkscrew.

My message is but a word, *a Way*, an easy expression of the experience of a plain man whose life has never been worried by any philosophy higher than that of the shepherd in *As You Like It*.[7] I wish to point out a path in which the wayfaring man, though a fool, cannot err;[8] not a system to be worked out painfully only to be discarded, not a formal scheme, simply a habit as easy—or as hard!—to adopt as any other habit, good or bad.

I

A few years ago a Xmas card went the rounds, with the legend 'Life is just one "derned" thing after another,' which, in more refined language, is the same as saying 'Life is a habit,' a succession of actions that become more or less automatic. This great truth, which lies at the basis of all actions, muscular or psychic, is the keystone of the teaching of Aristotle, to whom the formation of habits was the basis of moral excellence. 'In a word, habits of any kind are the result of actions of the same kind; and so what we have to do, is to give a certain character to these particular actions.' (*Ethics*.)[9] Lift a seven months old baby to his feet—see him tumble on his nose. Do the same at twelve months—he walks. At two years he runs. The muscles and the nervous system have acquired the habit. One trial after another, one failure after another, has given him power. Put your fin-

---

dignant because Elisha did not come out of his house and lay his hands on him with prayer, but merely sent his servant to tell him to go and wash in the Jordan. Nevertheless, he obeyed the prophet and was cured (2 Kings 5:9–10).

6. Sheffield, a city in Yorkshire, England, is famous for products of superior quality. Osler here uses the alliteration, "*Sh*effield or *sh*oddy." The latter means "of inferior quality."

7. Corin, a shepherd, states his simple philosophy to Touchstone, a clown. William Shakespeare, *As You Like It*, III, ii, 24–32, 76–81.

8. Isaiah 35:8. "And an highway shall be there, and a way, and it shall be called The way of holiness . . . the wayfaring men, though fools, shall not err therein." Osler refers to a path, the way of holiness, as used in the Bible.

9. Aristotle, *Nicomachean Ethics*, book 2, chap. 1, 1103b:21–24.

ger in a baby's mouth, and he sucks away in blissful anticipation of a response to a mammalian habit millions of years old. And we can deliberately train parts of our body to perform complicated actions with unerring accuracy. Watch that musician playing a difficult piece. Batteries, commutators, multipliers, switches, wires innumerable control those nimble fingers, the machinery of which may be set in motion as automatically as in a pianola, the player all the time chatting as if he had nothing to do in controlling the apparatus—habit again, the gradual acquisition of power by long practice and at the expense of many mistakes. The same great law reaches through mental and moral states. 'Character,' which partakes of both, in Plutarch's words, is 'long-standing habit.'[10]

Now the way of life that I preach is a habit to be acquired gradually by long and steady repetition. It is the practice of living for the day only, and for the day's work, *Life in day-tight compartments.*[11] 'Ah,' I hear you say, 'that is an easy matter, simple as Elisha's advice!'[12] Not as I shall urge it, in words which fail to express the depth of my feelings as to its value. I started life in the best of all environments—in a parsonage, one of nine children. A man who has filled Chairs in four universities, has written a successful book,[13] and has been asked to lecture at Yale, is supposed popularly to have brains of a special quality. A few of my intimate friends really know the truth about me, as I know it! Mine, in good faith I say it, are of the most mediocre character. But what about those professorships, &c.? Just habit, a way of life, an outcome of the day's work, the vital importance of which I wish to impress upon you with all the force at my command.

Dr. Johnson[14] remarked upon the trifling circumstances by which men's lives are influenced, 'not by an ascendant planet, a predominating humour, but by the first book which they read, some early conversation which they have heard, or some accident which excited ardour and enthusiasm.'[15] This was my

10. Plutarch, *Moralia: On Moral Virtues* trans. W. C. Helmbold (Cambridge, Mass.: Harvard University Press, 1957), vol. 6, p. 35.

11. Osler coined this term from the watertight compartments in ships.

12. See p. 3.

13. Osler, the youngest son in a family of nine children, was born in a parsonage at Bond Head, Tecumseh, Ontario, Canada. He taught at four universities: McGill, Pennsylvania, Johns Hopkins, and Oxford. Here he refers to his textbook *The Principles and Practice of Medicine,* first published in 1892, which was very popular among medical students of his time. It went through many editions and was translated into German, French, Spanish, and Chinese.

14. Samuel *Johnson* (1709–1784): English critic, author, and lexicographer who compiled the first great English dictionary. He was called the "Great Cham of Literature."

15. It was believed that the ascendant planet at the time of one's birth would have a commanding influence on one's life and fortune. In the old theory of physiology one of the four humors (phlegm, blood, yellow bile, and black bile) was also supposed to determine one's characteristics.

case in two particulars. I was diverted to the Trinity College School, then at Weston, Ontario, by a paragraph in the circular stating that the senior boys would go into the drawing-room in the evenings, and learn to sing and dance — vocal and pedal accomplishments for which I was never designed; but like Saul seeking his asses,[16] I found something more valuable, a man of the White of Selborne type,[17] who knew nature, and who knew how to get boys interested in it. The other happened in the summer of 1871, when I was attending the Montreal General Hospital. Much worried as to the future, partly about the final examination, partly as to what I should do afterwards, I picked up a volume of Carlyle, and on the page I opened there was the familiar sentence — '*Our main business is not to see what lies dimly at a distance, but to do what lies clearly at hand.*'[18] A commonplace sentiment enough, but it hit and stuck and helped, and was the starting-point of a habit that has enabled me to utilize to the full the single talent entrusted to me.

II

The workers in Christ's vineyard were hired by the day;[19] only for this day are we to ask for our daily bread,[20] and we are expressly bidden to take no thought for

Samuel Johnson, "Pope," *Lives of the English Poets*, ed. George Birkbeck Hill (1738; Hildesheim: Georg Olms, 1968), vol. 3, p. 174. Johnson's original passage reads: "Not by an ascendant planet *or* predominating humour, but by the first book which they read, some early conversation which they *heard,* or some accident which excited ardour and emulation" (italics added by editor).

16. Saul, while seeking his father's asses, met Samuel, a prophet, to whom God had revealed that Saul would become the first king of Israel (1 Samuel 9:3–27).

17. Osler is comparing his earliest mentor, Rev. W. A. Johnson, to Gilbert White.

William Arthur *Johnson* (1816–1880): Canadian cleric, schoolmaster, geologist, and naturalist. He was rector of St. Philip's Church, Weston, and founding headmaster of Trinity College School, an independent high school for boys, then at Weston and now at Port Hope. Osler studied there for eighteen months, and his interest in natural science was apparently sparked by Johnson, who owned the first microscope in Toronto and used to take his boys fossil hunting (from Rev. Donald Henderson, Johnson's successor at St. Philip's). He influenced Osler to enter the medical profession. Osler frequently refers to him in his writings; see "Sir Thomas Browne," p. 33.

Gilbert *White* (1720–1793): English naturalist and clergyman. Author of *Natural History and Antiquities of Selborne* (1789), which was one of Osler's favorite books.

18. *Our main business is not to see what lies dimly at a distance, but to do what lies clearly at hand:* Osler's favorite passage; from Thomas Carlyle, "*Signs of the Times,*" *Critical and Miscellaneous Essays* (1829; London: Chapman & Hall, 1899), p. 56. Carlyle's original reads: "Our grand business undoubtedly is," instead of "Our main business is."

19. *The workers in Christ's vineyard were hired by the day:* Matthew 20:1–16.

20. *ask for our daily bread:* Matthew 6:11 and Luke 11:3. The phrase is in the Lord's prayer: "Give us this day our daily bread."

the morrow.[21] To the modern world these commands have an Oriental savour,[22] counsels of perfection[23] akin to certain of the Beatitudes,[24] stimuli to aspiration, not to action. I am prepared on the contrary to urge the literal acceptance of the advice, not in the mood of Ecclesiastes—'Go to now, ye that say to-day or to-morrow we will go into such a city, and continue there a year, and buy and sell and get gain; whereas ye know not what shall be on the morrow;'[25] not in the Epicurean spirit of Omar with his 'jug of wine and Thou,'[26] but in the modernist spirit, as a way of life, a habit, a strong enchantment, at once against the mysticism of the East and the pessimism that too easily besets us. Change that hard saying 'Sufficient unto the day is the evil thereof' into 'the goodness thereof,'[27] since the chief worries of life arise from the foolish habit of looking before and after.[28] As a patient with double vision from some transient unequal action of the muscles of the eye finds magical relief from well-adjusted glasses, so, returning to the clear binocular vision of to-day, the over-anxious student finds peace when he looks neither backward to the past nor forward to the future.

I stood on the bridge of one of the great liners, ploughing the ocean at 25 knots.[29] 'She is alive,' said my companion, 'in every plate; a huge monster with

21. *take no thought for the morrow:* Matthew 6:34. "Take therefore no thought for the morrow: for the morrow shall take thought for the things of itself. Sufficient unto the day *is* the evil thereof."

22. Though sometimes regarded as a distinctive teaching of Christianity, these commands are found in one form or another in many ethical systems. See Omar Khayyám's lines:

> Ah, my Belovèd, fill the Cup that clears
> To-day of past Regret and future Fears:
> To-morrow!—Why, To-morrow I may be
> Myself with Yesterday's Sev'n Thousand Years.

The Rubáiyát of Omar Khayyám, 3rd ed., trans. Edward FitzGerald, (1872), quatrain 20.

23. Matthew 19:21. Jesus tells the rich young man "if thou wilt be perfect, go *and* sell that thou hast, and give to the poor . . . and come *and* follow me." This is one of the precepts of Jesus to be perfect.

24. Matthew 5:3–12 and Luke 6:20–23. Any of the declarations of blessedness pronounced by Jesus in the Sermon on the Mount.

25. *Go to now, ye that say to-day or to-morrow we will go into such a city, and continue there a year, and buy and sell and get gain; whereas ye know not what shall be on the morrow:* James 4:13–14. Osler has miscited this passage as from Ecclesiastes instead of the Epistle of James.

26. *Omar* Khayyám (c.1025–c.1123): Persian poet and astronomer. He symbolizes a person given to indulgences in sensual pleasures, especially drinking and women. *The Rubáiyát of Omar Khayyám,* 3rd ed., trans. Edward FitzGerald, (1872), quatrain 12.

27. Matthew 6:34. See p. 7, n. 21.

28. *looking before and after:* The phrase is a reminiscence of a line of a poem by Percy Bysshe Shelley, "To a Skylark," lines 86–87. The exact quotation is:

> We look before and after
> And pine for what is not:

(cf. William Shakespeare, *Hamlet,* IV, iv, 37).

29. Osler sailed on April 5, 1913, on the *Campania* with William McDougall and F. W. Mott. He wrote

brain and nerves, an immense stomach, a wonderful heart and lungs, and a splendid system of locomotion.' Just at that moment a signal sounded, and all over the ship the watertight compartments were closed. 'Our chief factor of safety,' said the Captain. 'In spite of the *Titanic*,'[30] I said. 'Yes,' he replied, 'in spite of the *Titanic*.' Now each one of you is a much more marvellous organization than the great liner, and bound on a longer voyage. What I urge is that you so learn to control the machinery as to live with 'day-tight compartments' as the most certain way to ensure safety on the voyage. Get on the bridge, and see that at least the great bulkheads are in working order. Touch a button and hear, at every level of your life, the iron doors shutting out the Past—the dead yesterdays. Touch another and shut off, with a metal curtain, the Future—the unborn to-morrows. Then you are safe—safe for to-day! Read the old story in the *Chambered Nautilus*,[31] so beautifully sung by Oliver Wendell Holmes, only change one line to 'Day after day beheld the silent toil.' Shut off the past! Let the dead past bury its dead.[32] So easy to say, so hard to realize! The truth is, the past haunts us like a shadow. To disregard it is not easy. Those blue eyes of your grandmother, that weak chin of your grandfather, have mental and moral counterparts in your make-up. Generations of ancestors, brooding over 'Providence, Foreknowledge, Will and Fate—Fixed fate, free will, foreknowledge, absolute,'[33] may have bred a New England conscience, morbidly sensitive, to heal which some of you had rather sing the 51st Psalm[34] than follow Christ into the slums.[35] Shut out the yesterdays, which have lighted fools the way to dusty death,[36] and have no concern for you personally, that is, consciously. They are there all right, working daily in us, but so are our livers and our stomachs. And the past, in its uncon-

---

this on the steamer for America during the journey (Harvey Cushing, *The Life of Sir Walter Osler*, vol. 2, pp. 349–353).

30. One year before this talk, the *Titanic*, a British passenger steamship, collided with an iceberg and sank on April 14, 1912, and 1,513 lives were lost. The *Titanic* had been believed to be unsinkable because it had several separate watertight compartments; but it struck an iceberg, whose submerged peaks penetrated several compartments and let in enough water to sink the vessel.

31. A poem by Oliver Wendell Holmes in *The Autocrat of the Breakfast Table*, chap. 4, stanza 3, line 1. The exact quotation is: "Year after year beheld the silent toil."

32. Matthew 8:22. The exact quotation is: "But Jesus said unto him, Follow me; and let the dead bury their dead." Osler here replaced "the dead" with "the dead past."

33. John Milton, *Paradise Lost*, book 2, lines 559–560.

34. Psalm 51:1–9, a Psalm of David; a prayer asking for mercy, cleansing, and forgiveness.

35. A "New England conscience" is the kind that characterized the original settlers of New England. They were Calvinist Nonconformists, who emphasized the Reformation doctrine that salvation comes by personally professing a strong faith and avoiding bad habits , with less emphasis on going out and doing good deeds. W. A. Johnson and Osler's other mentors belonged to the school of religion that put equal or greater value on doing good for others.

36. *have lighted fools the way to dusty death:* William Shakespeare, *Macbeth*, V, v, 22–23.

scious action on our lives, should bother us as little as they do. The petty annoyances, the real and fancied slights, the trivial mistakes, the disappointments, the sins, the sorrows, even the joys—bury them deep in the oblivion of each night. Ah! but it is just then that to so many of us the ghosts of the past,

> Night-riding Incubi
> Troubling the fantasy.[37]

come in troops, and pry open the eyelids, each one presenting a sin, a sorrow, a regret. Bad enough in the old and seasoned, in the young these demons of past sins may be a terrible affliction, and in bitterness of heart many a one cries with Eugene Aram, 'Oh God! Could I so close my mind, and clasp it with a clasp.'[38] As a vaccine against all morbid poisons left in the system by the infections of yesterday, I offer 'a way of life.' 'Undress,' as George Herbert says, 'your soul at night,'[39] not by self-examination, but by shedding, as you do your garments, the daily sins whether of omission or of commission, and you will wake a free man, with a new life. To look back, except on rare occasions for stock-taking, is to risk the fate of Lot's wife.[40] Many a man is handicapped in his course by a cursed combination of retro- and intro-spection, the mistakes of yesterday paralysing the efforts of to-day, the worries of the past hugged to his destruction, and the worm Regret allowed to canker[41] the very heart of his life. To die daily,[42] after the manner of St. Paul, ensures the resurrection of a new man, who makes each day the epitome of a life.

III

The load of to-morrow, added to that of yesterday, carried to-day makes the strongest falter. Shut off the future as tightly as the past. No dreams, no visions,

37. Charles Lamb, "Hypochondriacus," lines 30–31. Incubi (plural of incubus) are imaginary demons or evil spirits supposed to descend upon sleeping persons.

38. Eugene *Aram* (1704–1759): A linguist who killed a shoemaker to obtain some insignificant property. The title and hero of a poem by Thomas Hood, "The Dream of Eugene Aram, the Murderer," lines 35–36.

39. George Herbert, "The Church Porch," stanza 76, line 453.

40. Lot's wife was changed into a pillar of salt for looking back during their flight from Sodom (Genesis 19:26).

41. *the worm Regret allowed to canker:* The phrase is a reminiscence of a line of a poem by George Gordon Byron, "On This Day I Complete My Thirty-Sixth Year," stanza 2, lines 5–8. The exact quotation is:

> My days are in the yellow leaf;
> The flowers and fruits of love are gone;
> The worm, the canker, and the grief
> Are mine alone!

42. *die daily:* 1 Corinthians 15:31.

no delicious fantasies, no castles in the air, with which, as the old song so truly says, 'hearts are broken, heads are turned.'[43] To youth, we are told, belongs the future, but the wretched to-morrow that so plagues some of us has no certainty, except through to-day. Who can tell what a day may bring forth? Though its uncertainty is a proverb, a man may carry its secret in the hollow of his hand. Make a pilgrimage to Hades with Ulysses,[44] draw the magic circle, perform the rites, and then ask Tiresias[45] the question. I have had the answer from his own lips. The future is to-day—there is no to-morrow! The day of a man's salvation is *now*[46]—the life of the present, of to-day, lived earnestly, intently, without a forward-looking thought, is the only insurance for the future. Let the limit of your horizon be a twenty-four-hour circle. On the title-page of one of the great

books of science, the *Discours de la Méthode* of Descartes (1637), is a vignette showing a man digging in a garden with his face towards the earth, on which rays of light are streaming from the heavens; beneath is the legend '*Fac et Spera.*'[47] 'Tis a good attitude and a good motto. Look heavenward, if you wish, but never to the horizon—that way danger lies. Truth is not there, happiness is not there, certainty is not there, but the falsehoods, the frauds, the quackeries, the *ignes fatui*[48] which have deceived each generation—all beckon from the horizon, and lure the men not content to look for the truth and happiness that tumble out at their feet. Once while at college climb a mountain-top, and get a general outlook of the land, and make it the occasion perhaps of that careful examination of yourself,[49] that inquisition which Descartes urges every man to hold once in a lifetime—not oftener.

43. *hearts are broken, heads are turned:* Robert Browning, "In a Balcony," line 61, (Constance's line). The exact quotation is:

> What turned the many heads and broke the hearts?
> You are the fate, your minute's in the heaven.

44. *Ulysses:* Latin name for Odysseus (king of Ithaca), one of the heroes of the *Iliad* and the protagonist of the *Odyssey.* After the Trojan War, during his adventures in his ten-year attempt to return home, he made a journey to Hades, the underworld inhabited by departed souls.

45. *Tiresias* (also *Teiresias*): The blind Theban soothsayer who appears in Homer's *Odyssey*, book 11, lines 90–130.

46. *the day of salvation:* 2 Corinthians 6:2.

47. *Fac et Spera:* (Latin) "do (i.e., venture) and hope." René Descartes (1596–1650), French philosopher, mathematician, and scientist, who emphasized reason. Also known for his "principle of certainty: I think, therefore I am" (cogito ergo sum).

48. *ignes fatui:* (Latin) foolish flames; flitting phosphorescent lights seen at night that signify something deluding or misleading; mere illusion.

49. *climb a mountain-top, and get a general outlook of the land, and make it the occasion perhaps of that careful examination of yourself:* Perhaps a reminiscence of Wordsworth, *The Prelude,* book 14, lines 66–69. Wordsworth describes climbing Mount Snowdon in Wales to see the sunrise from the summit, then continues:

Waste of energy, mental distress, nervous worries dog the steps of a man who is anxious about the future. Shut close, then, the great fore and aft bulkheads, and prepare to cultivate the habit of a life of day-tight compartments. Do not be discouraged—like every other habit, the acquisition takes time, and the way is one you must find for yourselves. I can only give general directions and encouragement, in the hope that while the green years are on your heads, you may have the courage to persist.

IV

Now, for the day itself! What first? Be your own daysman! and sigh not with Job for any mysterious intermediary,[50] but prepare to lay your own firm hand upon the helm. Get into touch with the finite, and grasp in full enjoyment that sense of capacity in a machine working smoothly. Join the whole creation of animate things in a deep, heartfelt joy that you are alive, that you see the sun, that you are in this glorious earth which Nature has made so beautiful, and which is yours to conquer and to enjoy. Realize, in the words of Browning, that 'There's a world of capability for joy spread round about us, meant for us, inviting us.'[51] What are the morning sensations?—for they control the day. Some of us are congenitally unhappy during the early hours; but the young man who feels on awakening that life is a burden or a bore has been neglecting his machine, driving it too hard, stoking the engines too much, or not cleaning out the ashes and clinkers. Or he has been too much with the Lady Nicotine, or fooling with Bacchus, or, worst of all, with the younger Aphrodite [52]—all 'messengers of strong prevailment in unhardened youth.'[53] To have a sweet outlook on life you must have a clean body. As I look on the clear-cut, alert, earnest features, and the lithe, active forms of our college men, I sometimes wonder whether or not Socrates and Plato would find the race improved. I am sure they would love to look on such a gathering as

---

It appeared to me the type of a majestic intellect, its acts
And its possessions, what it has and craves,
What in itself it is, and would become.

50. *Be your own daysman! and sigh not with Job for any mysterious intermediary:* Job 9:33. The original reads: "Neither is there any daysman betwixt us, *that* might lay his hand upon us both." The rare and obsolete word "daysman" means "arbitrator" or "mediator." Job here laments that no one can act as an arbitrator between him and God, to ensure that God treats him fairly.
51. Robert Browning, "Cleon," lines 239–241.
52. *Lady Nicotine, Bacchus, and the younger Aphrodite:* They personify tobacco, wine, and sexual passion, respectively. *My Lady Nicotine* (1890) is the title of a collection of humorous essays on smoking by the Scottish essayist and playwright James Barrie.
53. William Shakespeare, *A Midsummer Night's Dream,* I, i, 34–35.

this. Make their ideal yours—the fair mind in the fair body.[54] The one cannot be sweet and clean without the other, and you must realize, with Rabbi Ben Ezra, the great truth that flesh and soul are mutually helpful.[55] The morning outlook—which really makes the day—is largely a question of a clean machine—of physical morality in the wide sense of the term. *C'est l'estomac qui fait les heureux*,[56] as Voltaire[57] says; no dyspeptic[58] can have a sane outlook on life; and a man whose bodily functions are impaired has a lowered moral resistance. To keep the body fit is a help in keeping the mind pure, and the sensations of the first few hours of the day are the best test of its normal state. The clean tongue, the clear head, and the bright eye are birth-rights of each day. Just as the late Professor Marsh[59] would diagnose an unknown animal from a single bone, so can the day be predicted from the first waking hour. The start is everything, as you well know, and to make a good start you must feel fit. In the young, sensations of morning slackness come most often from lack of control of the two primal instincts—biologic habits—the one concerned with the preservation of the individual, the other with the continuance of the species. Yale students should by this time be models of dietetic propriety, but youth does not always reck the rede[60] of the teacher; and I dare say that here, as elsewhere, careless habits of eating are responsible for much mental disability. My own rule of life has been to cut out unsparingly any article of diet that had the bad taste to disagree with me, or to indicate in any way that it had abused the temporary hospitality of the lodging which I had provided. To drink, nowadays, but few students become addicted, but in every large body of men a few are to be found whose incapacity for the day results from the morning clogging of nocturnally-flushed tissues. As moderation is very hard to reach, and as it has been abundantly shown that the best

54. Plato, *Timæus*, 87e.

55. Robert Browning, "Rabbi Ben Ezra," line 72. The exact quotation is:

> Let us cry, 'All good things
> Are ours, nor soul helps flesh more, now, than flesh helps soul!

56. (French) "It is the stomach that makes people happy." This may be from the Greek philosopher Epicurus. See p. 15, n. 75.

57. François Marie Arouet *Voltaire* (1694–1778): French philosopher, historian, and essayist.

58. *dyspeptic:* A person with indigestion (due to local causes or to diseases that are present elsewhere in the body).

59. Othniel Charles *Marsh* (1831–1899): American paleontologist and professor at Yale (1866–1899) who collected fossils on expeditions to the West.

60. *reck the rede:* To say that youth often ignores advice, Osler adapts a line from *Hamlet* (I, iii, 51). The exact quotation is:

> Himself the primrose path of dalliance treads,
> And recks not his own rede.

of mental and physical work may be done without alcohol in any form, the safest rule for the young man is that which I am sure most of you follow—abstinence. A bitter enemy to the bright eye and the clear brain of the early morning is tobacco when smoked to excess, as it is now by a large majority of students. Watch it, test it, and if need be, control it. That befogged, woolly sensation reaching from the forehead to the occiput,[61] that haziness of memory, that cold fish-like eye, that furred tongue, and last week's taste in the mouth—too many of you know them—I know them—they often come from too much tobacco. The other primal instinct is the heavy burden of the flesh which Nature puts on all of us to ensure a continuation of the species. To drive Plato's team[62] taxes the energies of the best of us. One of the horses is a raging, untamed devil, who can only be brought into subjection by hard fighting and severe training. This much you all know as men: once the bit is between his teeth the black steed Passion will take the white horse Reason with you and the chariot rattling over the rocks to perdition.

With a fresh, sweet body you can start aright without those feelings of inertia that so often, as Goethe says, make the morning's lazy leisure usher in a useless day.[63] Control of the mind as a working machine, the adaptation in it of habit, so that its action becomes almost as automatic as walking, is the end of education—and yet how rarely reached! It can be accomplished with deliberation and repose, never with hurry and worry. Realize how much time there is, how long the day is. Realize that you have sixteen waking hours, three or four of which at least should be devoted to making a silent conquest of your mental machinery. Concentration, by which is grown gradually the power to wrestle successfully with any subject, is the secret of successful study. No mind however dull can escape the brightness that comes from steady application. There is an old saying, 'Youth enjoyeth not, for haste'; but worse than this, the failure to cultivate the power of peaceful concentration is the greatest single cause of mental breakdown. Plato pities the young man who started at such a pace that he never reached the goal.[64] One of the saddest of life's tragedies is the wreckage of the career of the young collegian by hurry, hustle, bustle, and tension—the

61. *occiput:* The lower back part of the skull.

62. Plato, *Phaedrus,* 253c–254e.

63. *make the morning's lazy leisure usher in a useless day:* This quote by Goethe has not been identified.

64. Probably Osler refers to Theaetetus, mathematician, friend, and disciple of Plato. He is said to have been fatally wounded during the Corinthian war (390–387 B.C.), which would make the age of his death about twenty. However, the later date, 369, which has also been suggested, makes him a little too old for Socrates' beautiful remark, "that he would most certainly be a great man, if he lived" (Plato, *Theaetetus,* 142c).

human machine driven day and night, as no sensible fellow would use his motor. Listen to the words of a master in Israel, William James:[65]

> Neither the nature nor the amount of our work is accountable for the frequency and severity of our breakdowns, but their cause lies rather in those absurd feelings of hurry and having no time, in that breathlessness and tension, that anxiety of feature and that solicitude of results, that lack of inner harmony and ease, in short, by which the work with us is apt to be accompanied, and from which a European who would do the same work would, nine out of ten times, be free.[66]

Es bildet ein Talent sich in der Stille,[67] but it need not be for all day. A few hours out of the sixteen will suffice, only let them be hours of daily dedication—in routine, in order, and in system, and day by day you will gain in power over the mental mechanism, just as the child does over the spinal marrow in walking, or the musician over the nerve centres. Aristotle somewhere says that the student who wins out in the fight must be slow in his movements, with voice deep, and slow speech,[68] and he will not be worried over trifles which make people speak in shrill tones and use rapid movements. Shut close in hour-tight compartments, with the mind directed intensely upon the subject in hand, you will acquire the capacity to do more and more, you will get into training; and once the mental habit is established, you are safe for life.

Concentration is an art of slow acquisition, but little by little the mind is accustomed to habits of slow eating and careful digestion, by which alone you escape the 'mental dyspepsy'[69] so graphically described by Lowell in the *Fable for Critics.* Do not worry your brains about that bugbear Efficiency, which, sought consciously and with effort, is just one of those elusive qualities very apt to be missed. The man's college output is never to be gauged at sight; all the world's coarse thumb and finger may fail to plumb his most effective work,[70] the casting

---

65. *a master in Israel:* Osler compares William James to Sirach, one of the early scribes, who taught that "wisdom" refers to both practical matters and research in the scriptures and sciences. *The Wisdom of Jesus the Son of Sirach* (Ecclesiasticus 38:24–34; 39:1–11).

William *James* (1842–1910): American psychologist and philosopher. He taught anatomy, physiology, and hygiene, as well as psychology and philosophy, at Harvard University. He is known as one of the founders of pragmatism and also as the brother of the novelist Henry James (1843–1916).

66. William James, "The Gospel of Relaxation," in *Selected Papers on Philosophy* (1917; New York: E. P. Dutton, 1961), p. 31.

67. (German) "A talent forms itself in silence." Goethe, *Torquato Tasso,* I, ii, 66.

68. Aristotle, *Physiognomonica* (Physiognomy), chaps. 2–3, 807a–b.

69. *mental dyspepsy:* Mental indigestion. James Russell Lowell, "A Fable for Critics," line 106.

70. Robert Browning, "Rabbi Ben Ezra," stanza 24, lines 1–2. This poem is warning young people not to be short-sighted in setting guidelines for living and goals for achievement.

of the mental machinery of self-education, the true preparation for a field larger than the college campus. Four or five hours daily—it is not much to ask; but one day must tell another, one week certify another,[71] one month bear witness to another of the same story, and you will acquire a habit by which the one-talent man will earn a high interest, and by which the ten-talent man may at least save his capital.[72]

Steady work of this sort gives a man a sane outlook on the world. No corrective so valuable to the weariness, the fever, and the fret that are so apt to wring the heart of the young. This is the talisman, as George Herbert says,

> The famous stone
> That turneth all to gold,[73]

and with which, to the eternally recurring question, What is Life? you answer, I do not think—I act it; the only philosophy that brings you in contact with its real values and enables you to grasp its hidden meaning. Over the Slough of Despond, past Doubting Castle and Giant Despair, with this talisman you may reach the Delectable Mountains, and those Shepherds of the Mind—Knowledge, Experience, Watchful, and Sincere.[74] Some of you may think this to be a miserable Epicurean doctrine[75]—no better than that so sweetly sung by Horace:

> Happy the man—and Happy he alone,
> He who can call to-day his own,
> He who secure within can say,
> To-morrow, do thy worst—for I have lived to-day.[76]

I do not care what you think, I am simply giving you a philosophy of life that I have found helpful in my work, useful in my play. Walt Whitman, whose

71. *one day must tell another, one week certify another:* This phrase echoes Psalm 19:2 in the *Book of Common Prayer* version: "One day telleth another: one night certifieth another."

72. *a habit by which the one-talent man will earn a high interest, and by which the ten-talent man may at least save his capital:* This phrase is an allusion to Jesus' parable of the talents in Matthew 25:14–30. A talent originally meant a large weight of silver, but from its use in the parable it has come to mean a God-given ability or aptitude. In the parable no servant received ten talents from his master, but one was given five talents and by shrewd investment doubled his money. The servant who received only one talent hid it in the ground; and when the master found this out he reproached him and said he ought at least to have laid it out with the bankers for interest.

73. George Herbert, "The Elixir," stanza 6, lines 21–22. The famous stone refers to the fabled philosophers' stone sought by the alchemists.

74. *the Slough of Despond, past Doubting Castle and Giant Despair:* All of these are names that appear in John Bunyan's *The Pilgrim's Progress,* part 1 (1678; London: George Routledge and Sons, n.d.).

75. *Epicurean doctrine:* The philosophical system of Epicurus (c.342–c.270 B.C.), who taught devotion to a life of pleasure understood as the fruit of temperance.

76. Horace, *Odes,* book 3, no. 29, lines 41–43 (as translated by John Dryden).

physician I was for some years, never spoke to me much of his poems, though occasionally he would make a quotation; but I remember late one summer afternoon as we sat in the window of his little house in Camden there passed a group of workmen whom he greeted in his usual friendly way. And then he said: 'Ah, the glory of the day's work, whether with hand or brain! I have tried

> To exalt the present and the real,
> To teach the average man the glory of his daily work or trade.'[77]

In this way of life each one of you may learn to drive the straight furrow and so come to the true measure of a man.

V

With body and mind in training, what remains?

Do you remember that most touching of all incidents in Christ's ministry, when the anxious ruler Nicodemus[78] came by night, worried lest the things that pertained to his everlasting peace were not a part of his busy and successful life? Christ's message to him is His message to the world—never more needed than at present: 'Ye must be born of the spirit.'[79] You wish to be with the leaders—as Yale men it is your birthright—know the great souls that make up the moral radium of the world.[80] You must be born of their spirit, initiated into their fraternity, whether of the spiritually-minded followers of the Nazarene[81] or of that larger company, elect from every nation, seen by St. John.[82]

Begin the day with Christ and His prayer[83]—you need no other. Creedless, with it you have religion; creed-stuffed, it will leaven any theological dough in which you stick. As the soul is dyed by the thoughts, let no day pass without contact with the best literature of the world. Learn to know your Bible, though not perhaps as your fathers did. In forming character and in shaping conduct, its

---

77. Walt Whitman, "Song of the Exposition," *Leaves of Grass,* canto 7, lines 139–40. Whitman's original passage reads: "the glory of his daily *walk* and trade," instead of "*work or* trade."

78. *Nicodemus:* A pharisee and member of the Sanhedrin; he became a secret follower of Jesus (John 3:1–15).

79. John 3:5.

80. *radium of the world:* "Luminaries of the world." Probably coined by Osler, using the sense of radium as a source of enormous amounts of energy, producing remarkable thermal, electrical, physiological, chemical, and luminous effects without any appreciable change in the original body. The dangers of radium were scarcely appreciated in his time; this phrase carries only beneficial connotations.

81. Jesus Christ.

82. *elect from every nation:* Revelation 5:9 and 7:9–14.

83. The Lord's Prayer, Matthew 6:9–13 and Luke 11:2–4.

touch has still its ancient power. Of the kindred of Ram and sons of Elihu, you should know its beauties and its strength.[84] Fifteen or twenty minutes day by day will give you fellowship with the great minds of the race, and little by little as the years pass you extend your friendship with the immortal dead. They will give you faith in your own day. Listen while they speak to you of the fathers. But each age has its own spirit and ideas, just as it has its own manners and pleasures. You are right to believe that yours is the best university, at its best period. Why should you look back to be shocked at the frowsiness and dullness of the students of the seventies or even of the nineties? And cast no thought forward, lest you reach a period when you and yours will present to your successors the same dowdiness of clothes and times. But while change is the law, certain great ideas flow fresh through the ages, and control us effectually as in the days of Pericles.[85] Mankind, it has been said, is always advancing, man is always the same. The love, hope, fear, and faith that make humanity, and the elemental passions of the human heart, remain unchanged, and the secret of inspiration in any literature is the capacity to touch the chord that vibrates in a sympathy that knows nor time nor place.

The quiet life in day-tight compartments will help you to bear your own and others' burdens with a light heart. Pay no heed to the Batrachians[86] who sit croaking idly by the stream. Life is a straight, plain business, and the way is clear, blazed for you by generations of strong men, into whose labours you enter and whose ideals must be your inspiration. In my mind's eye I can see you twenty years hence—resolute-eyed, broad-headed, smooth-faced men who are in the world to make a success of life; but to whichever of the two great types you belong, whether controlled by emotion or by reason, you will need the leaven of their spirit, the only leaven[87] potent enough to avert that only too common Nemesis to which the Psalmist refers: 'He gave them their heart's desire, but sent leanness withal into their souls.'[88]

84. *Of the kindred of Ram and sons of Elihu, you should know its beauties and its strength:* Elihu is a young man who undertook to argue with Job. "The kindred of Ram" is Elihu's family. Elihu portrayed the beauty and majesty of nature and concluded that its Creator must be far wiser than men, who therefore have no right to question how he governs the universe, as Job had been doing (Job 37).

85. Pericles (c.490–429 B.C.) served as leader of Athens at its highest state intellectually and materially. For further information, see "The Student Life," p. 313, n. 35.

86. Osler probably refers here to *Batrachians* ("The Frogs") performed in 405 B.C. by Aristophanes, who uses frogs croaking noisily by the river Styx to satirize lyric poets. The Yale college yell used at sports events is taken from the refrain of the frogs' chorus in this play. Osler may have added this allusion as especially appropriate for a Yale audience.

87. *leaven:* Osler's favorite word. See "The Leaven of Science," p. 153, n.

88. *He gave them their heart's desire, but sent leanness withal into their souls:* Psalm 106:15. The original

A WAY OF LIFE

I quoted Dr. Johnson's remark about the trivial things that influence.[89] Perhaps this slight word of mine may help some of you so to number your days that you may apply your hearts unto wisdom.[90]

―――
reads: "And he gave them their request; but sent leanness into their soul." Osler changed "their request" to "their heart's desire." He may have been remembering Psalm 21:2, "Thou hast given him heart's desire," or Psalm 20:4, "Grant thee thy heart's desire."

89. *Johnson:* See p. 5–6, n. 15.

90. *apply your hearts into wisdom:* Psalm 90:12.

2

AEQUANIMITAS

Thou must be like a promontory of the sea,
against which, though the waves beat continually,
yet it both itself stands, and about it are those
swelling waves stilled and quieted.
MARCUS AURELIUS, *The Meditations*

I say: Fear not! Life still
Leaves human effort scope.
But, since life teems with ill,
Nurse no extravagant hope;
Because thou must not dream, thou need'st not then despair!
MATTHEW ARNOLD, *Empedocles on Etna*

OSLER GAVE THIS GRADUATION address in 1889 at the University of Pennsylvania Medical School, then the leading center of medical education in the United States. He was about to leave its faculty to create a new medical school at Johns Hopkins University. In this address he urges the graduates to develop *imperturbability* and *equanimity* with regard both to their successes and their failures.

Imperturbability refers to *physical* self-control. It is necessary to ensure clear judgement and to avoid losing a patient's confidence by appearing worried or panicked. Fortunately, this physical trait can be learned, beginning with developing a calm, inscrutable face. Osler stresses that true imperturbability must be based on a wide knowledge of disease and of what needs to be done.

The *mental* equivalent of imperturbability is "cheerful" equanimity (from the Greek Stoics' watchword, "Aequanimitas"). To attain this presence of mind, one must cultivate patience and persistence. A physician must not expect too much from patients, since illness accentuates human frailties and eccentricities. However, the uncertainties of life, the fragmentary nature of truth, and the time demands and the trials of successful practice all make it especially difficult for a physician to maintain equanimity.

Osler admits that his own equanimity has been disturbed by the emotion of his departure from Philadelphia, and he expresses deep gratitude at having been associated with such a distinguished faculty.

AEQUANIMITAS

TO MANY THE FROST of custom has made even these imposing annual ceremonies cold and lifeless. To you, at least of those present, they should have the solemnity of an ordinance—called as you are this day to a high dignity and to so weighty an office and charge. You have chosen your Genius, have passed beneath the Throne of Necessity, and with the voices of the fatal sisters still in your ears, will soon enter the plain of Forgetfulness and drink of the waters of its river.[1] Ere you are driven all manner of ways, like the souls in the tale of Er the Pamphylian,[2] it is my duty to say a few words of encouragement and to bid you, in the name of the Faculty, God-speed on your journey.

I could have the heart to spare you, poor, careworn survivors of a hard struggle, so "lean and pale and leaden-eyed with study;"[3] and my tender mercy

A valedictory address delivered at the University of Pennsylvania, May 1, 1889. *Aequanimitas* is Latin for "even mind, composure." Here it is a reference to the creed of the Stoics, Greek philosophers who elevated reason, repressing passion and feelings.

1. This sentence is based on classical mythology as reshaped by the Greek philosopher Plato (427–347 B.C.). "Genius" is a personal guardian spirit and "Necessity" the goddess whose spindle for making yarn controls the fate of the world. She has three daughters, "the fatal sisters," whose spinning affects people's fates. The souls of the dead go to the plain of "Forgetfulness" to drink from its river "Lethe" and forget their past life before being reborn back into the world. Plato, *Republic*, book 10, 616c–617d, 620d–621a.

2. According to Plato, Er the Pamphylian died in war. Brought back to life on the twelfth day, he told what he had seen in the world of death and how the Fates controlled the lives of people. Plato, *Republic*, book 10, 614–621.

3. Thomas Hood, "The Dream of Eugene Aram, the Murderer," lines 29–30. The exact quotation is:

constrains me to consider but two of the score of elements which may make or mar your lives—which may contribute to your success, or help you in the days of failure.

In the first place, in the physician or surgeon no quality takes rank with imperturbability, and I propose for a few minutes to direct your attention to this essential bodily virtue. Perhaps I may be able to give those of you, in whom it has not developed during the critical scenes of the past month, a hint or two of its importance, possibly a suggestion for its attainment. Imperturbability means coolness and presence of mind under all circumstances, calmness amid storm, clearness of judgment in moments of grave peril, immobility, impassiveness, or, to use an old and expressive word, *phlegm*.[4] It is the quality which is most appreciated by the laity though often misunderstood by them; and the physician who has the misfortune to be without it, who betrays indecision and worry, and who shows that he is flustered and flurried in ordinary emergencies, loses rapidly the confidence of his patients.

In full development, as we see it in some of our older colleagues, it has the nature of a divine gift, a blessing to the possessor, a comfort to all who come in contact with him. You should know it well, for there have been before you for years several striking illustrations, whose example has, I trust, made a deep impression. As imperturbability is largely a bodily endowment, I regret to say that there are those amongst you, who, owing to congenital defects, may never be able to acquire it. Education, however, will do much; and with practice and experience the majority of you may expect to attain to a fair measure. The first essential is to have your nerves well in hand. Even under the most serious circumstances, the physician or surgeon who allows "his outward action to demonstrate the native act and figure of his heart in complement extern,"[5] who shows in his face the slightest alteration, expressive of anxiety or fear, has not his medullary centres[6] under the highest control, and is liable to disaster at any moment. I have spoken of this to you on many occasions, and have urged you to educate your nerve centres so that not the slightest dilator or contractor influence shall pass to the vessels of your face under any professional trial. Far be it from me to urge you,

———

> Much study had made him very lean,
> And pale, and leaden-eye'd.

4. Here Osler used *phlegm* positively in the sense of composure, although a person having a temperament attributed to the predominance of this humor could be considered apathetic, cold, and dull. "Humor" is the old physiological term for one of the four body fluids (along with blood, yellow bile, and black bile) which were thought to determine a person's health and temperament.

5. William Shakespeare, *Othello,* I, i, 63.

6. *medullary centres:* (Obs.) *centrum ovale,* meaning "mass of white matter at the center of each cerebral hemisphere."

ere Time has carved with his hours those fair brows,[7] to quench on all occasions the blushes of ingenuous shame,[8] but in dealing with your patients' emergencies demanding these should certainly not arise, and at other times an inscrutable face may prove a fortune. In a true and perfect form, imperturbability is indissolubly associated with wide experience and an intimate knowledge of the varied aspects of disease. With such advantages he is so equipped that no eventuality can disturb the mental equilibrium of the physician; the possibilities are always manifest, and the course of action clear. From its very nature this precious quality is liable to be misinterpreted, and the general accusation of hardness, so often brought against the profession, has here its foundation. Now a certain measure of insensibility is not only an advantage, but a positive necessity in the exercise of a calm judgment, and in carrying out delicate operations. Keen sensibility is doubtless a virtue of high order, when it does not interfere with steadiness of hand or coolness of nerve; but for the practitioner in his working-day world, a callousness which thinks only of the good to be effected, and goes ahead regardless of smaller considerations, is the preferable quality.

Cultivate, then, gentlemen, such a judicious measure of obtuseness as will enable you to meet the exigencies of practice with firmness and courage, without, at the same time, hardening "the human heart by which we live."[9]

In the second place, there is a mental equivalent to this bodily endowment, which is as important in our pilgrimage as imperturbability. Let me recall to your minds an incident related of that best of men and wisest of rulers, Antoninus Pius,[10] who, as he lay dying, in his home at Lorium in Etruria, summed up the philosophy of life in the watchword, *Aequanimitas*.[11] As for him, about to pass *flammantia moenia mundi*[12] (the flaming ramparts of the world), so for you,

---

7. *ere Time has carved with his hours those fair brows:* William Shakespeare, "Sonnet 19," line 9. The exact quotation is:

> Oh, carve not with thy hours my love's fair brow,
>
> Nor draw no lines there with thine antique pen.

8. *quench on all occasions the blushes of ingenuous shame:* Thomas Gray, "Elegy Written in a Country Churchyard," line 70. The exact quotation is:

> The struggling pangs of conscious truth to hide,
>
> To quench the blushes of ingenuous shame.

9. William Wordsworth, "Ode: Intimations of Immortality from Recollections of Early Childhood," stanza 11, line 201.

10. *Antoninus Pius* (86–161 A.D.): Esteemed Roman emperor who had a peaceful reign. His character is described by his nephew and adoptive son Marcus Aurelius in *The Meditations,* book 1, sect. 16; book 6, sect. 30.

11. *aequanimitas:* See p. 000, n. 000. The anecdote about Antoninus Pius comes from his "Life" in the *Scriptores Historiae Augustae,* chap. 12, sect. 6, trans. David Magie (London: William Heneimann; New York: E. P. Dutton, 1921), p. 131.

12. *flammantia moenia mundi:* (Latin) every mortal had to pass "the flaming walls of the world," a sphere

fresh from Clotho's spindle,[13] a calm equanimity is the desirable attitude. How difficult to attain, yet how necessary, in success as in failure! Natural temperament has much to do with its development, but a clear knowledge of our relation to our fellow-creatures and to the work of life is also indispensable. One of the first essentials in securing a good-natured equanimity is not to expect too much of the people amongst whom you dwell. "Knowledge comes, but wisdom lingers,"[14] and in matters medical the ordinary citizen of to-day has not one whit more sense than the old Romans, whom Lucian[15] scourged for a credulity which made them fall easy victims to the quacks of the time, such as the notorious Alexander,[16] whose exploits make one wish that his advent had been delayed some eighteen centuries. Deal gently then with this deliciously credulous old human nature in which we work, and restrain your indignation, when you find your pet parson has triturates of the 1000th potentiality[17] in his waistcoat pocket, or you discover accidentally a case of Warner's Safe Cure[18] in the bedroom of your best patient. It must needs be that offences of this kind come; expect them, and do not be vexed.

Curious, odd compounds are these fellow-creatures, at whose mercy you will be; full of fads and eccentricities, of whims and fancies; but the more closely we study their little foibles of one sort and another in the inner life which we see, the more surely is the conviction borne in upon us of the likeness of their weaknesses to our own. The similarity would be intolerable, if a happy egotism did not often render us forgetful of it. Hence the need of an infinite patience and of an ever-tender charity toward these fellow-creatures; have they not to exercise the same toward us?

A distressing feature in the life which you are about to enter, a feature which will press hardly upon the finer spirits among you and ruffle their equanimity, is

---

of fire thought to encircle the earth, to get into the regions of heaven. The reference is to Lucretius, *De Rerum Natura*, book 1, line 73.

13. *Clotho:* One of Necessity's three daughters (the three fates); Clotho controls the present. See p. 21.

14. Alfred Tennyson, "Locksley Hall," lines 141, 143.

15. *Lucian* (c.125-c.200 A.D.): Greek sophist and satirist of human follies and superstition.

16. *Alexander* of Abonoteichus (c.2nd cent. A.D.): Mystic denounced by Lucian for his quackery and mystical rites and for claiming divine aid from the Greek god of medicine, Asclepius. He was the idol of the people of the day. Lucian, "Alexander the False Prophet," in *Lucian*, trans. A. M. Harmon (Cambridge, Mass: Harvard University Press, 1959), vol. 4, pp. 175–253.

17. A quack medicine.

18. At the time of an epidemic of kidney and liver failure in the United States in the 1880s, H. H. Warner of Rochester, N.Y., manufactured "Warner's Safe Kidney and Liver Cure," which became popular among people of the day. Osler here refers to quack medicines. Stewart Hall Holbrook, *The Golden Age of Quackery* (New York: Macmillan, 1959), p. 90.

the uncertainty which pertains not alone to our science and art, but to the very hopes and fears which make us men. In seeking absolute truth we aim at the unattainable, and must be content with finding broken portions. You remember in the Egyptian story, how Typhon with his conspirators dealt with good Osiris;[19] how they took the virgin Truth, hewed her lovely form into a thousand pieces, and scattered them to the four winds; and, as Milton says, "from that time ever since, the sad friends of truth, such as durst appear, imitating the careful search that Isis made for the mangled body of Osiris, went up and down gathering up limb by limb still as they could find them. We have not yet found them all,"[20] but each one of us may pick up a fragment, perhaps two, and in moments when mortality weighs less heavily upon the spirit, we can, as in a vision, see the form divine, just as a great Naturalist, an Owen or a Leidy,[21] can reconstruct an ideal creature from a fossil fragment.

It has been said that in prosperity our equanimity is chiefly exercised in enabling us to bear with composure the misfortunes of our neighbours. Now, while nothing disturbs our mental placidity more sadly than straightened[22] means, and the lack of those things after which the Gentiles seek,[23] I would warn you against the trials of the day soon to come to some of you—the day of large and successful practice. Engrossed late and soon in professional cares, getting and spending, you may so lay waste your powers that you may find, too late, with hearts given away, that there is no place in your habit-stricken souls for those gentler influences which make life worth living.

It is sad to think that, for some of you, there is in store disappointment, perhaps failure. You cannot hope, of course, to escape from the cares and anxieties incident to professional life. Stand up bravely, even against the worst. Your very hopes may have passed on out of sight, as did all that was near and dear

19. *Typhon, Osiris* and *Isis:* In Egyptian mythology Osiris, a good king of Egypt, was murdered by his brother Set (identified with the Greek Typhon, a monster with one hundred serpent heads), who cut his body into pieces. The scattered pieces were collected and buried by Isis, Osiris' sister and wife.

20. John Milton "*Areopagitica,*" in *Complete Prose Works of John Milton,* ed. Ernest Sirluck (New Haven, Conn.: Yale University Press, 1959), vol. 2 p. 549.

21. Richard *Owen* (1804–1892): English naturalist. Author of *Lectures on the Comparative Anatomy and Physiology of Invertebrates* (1843).

Joseph *Leidy* (1823–1891): Professor of anatomy at the University of Pennsylvania Medical School, known also as a fine naturalist. For further information, see "The Leaven of Science," p. 155, n. 10 and pp. 160–162, where Osler expresses admiration for him not only as a naturalist but also as a man.

22. *straightened* (properly *straitened*): Having inadequate means of living; living in poverty.

23. Matthew 6:31–33. The exact quotation is: "Therefore take no thought, saying, What shall we eat? or, What shall we drink? or, Wherewithal shall we be clothed? (For after all these things do the Gentiles seek) for your heavenly Father knoweth that ye have need of all these things. But seek ye first the kingdom of God, and his righteousness; and all these things shall be added unto you."

to the Patriarch at the Jabbok[24] ford, and, like him, you may be left to struggle in the night alone. Well for you, if you wrestle on, for in persistency lies victory, and with the morning may come the wished-for blessing. But not always; there is a struggle with defeat which some of you will have to bear, and it will be well for you in that day to have cultivated a cheerful equanimity. Remember, too, that sometimes "from our desolation only does the better life begin."[25] Even with disaster ahead and ruin imminent, it is better to face them with a smile, and with the head erect, than to crouch at their approach. And, if the fight is for principle and justice, even when failure seems certain, where many have failed before, cling to your ideal, and, like Childe Roland[26] before the dark tower, set the slug-horn to your lips, blow the challenge, and calmly await the conflict.

It has been said that "in patience ye shall win your souls,"[27] and what is this patience but an equanimity which enables you to rise superior to the trials of life? Sowing as you shall do beside all waters,[28] I can but wish that you may reap the promised blessing of quietness and of assurance forever, until

> Within this life,
> Though lifted o'er its strife,[29]

you may, in the growing winters, glean a little of that wisdom which is pure, peaceable, gentle, full of mercy and good fruits, without partiality and without hypocrisy.

The past is always with us, never to be escaped; it alone is enduring; but, amidst the changes and chances[30] which succeed one another so rapidly in this life, we are apt to live too much for the present and too much in the future. On such an occasion as the present, when the *Alma Mater*[31] is in festal array, when we joy in her growing prosperity, it is good to hark back to the olden days and gratefully to recall the men whose labours in the past have made the present possible.

---

24. *Jabbok:* Jacob wrestled with the angel on the banks of the river Jabbok, a tributary of the Jordan, in Gilead, and received a new name, "Israel" (Genesis 32:22–26).

25. William Shakespeare *Antony and Cleopatra*, V, ii, 1–2. Cleopatra says to Charmian and Iras:
> My desolation does begin to make
> A better life.

26. Robert Browning, "Childe Roland to the Dark Tower Came," stanza 34, lines 199–204.

27. Luke 21:19. Osler's quotation comes from the Revised Version (1885).

28. Isaiah 32:20. The exact quotation is: "Blessed are ye that sow beside all waters"

29. Robert Browning, "Rabbi Ben Ezra," stanza 17, lines 97–98.

30. An allusion to the first collect at the end of the Communion service in the *Book of Common Prayer*. The exact quotation is: "Among all the changes and chances of this mortal life."

31. *Alma Mater:* (Latin) literally, "nourishing mother"; here refers to the University of Pennsylvania.

The great possession of any University is its great names. It is not the "pride, pomp and circumstance"[32] of an institution which bring honour, not its wealth, nor the number of its schools, not the students who throng its halls, but the *men* who have trodden in its service the thorny road through toil, even through hate, to the serene abode of Fame, climbing "like stars to their appointed height."[33] These bring glory, and it should thrill the heart of every alumnus of this school, of every teacher in its faculty, as it does mine this day, reverently and thankfully to recall such names amongst its founders as Morgan, Shippen,[34] and Rush,[35] and such men amongst their successors as Wistar, Physick, Barton, and Wood.[36]

Gentlemen of the Faculty — *Noblesse oblige.*[37]

And the sad reality of the past teaches us to-day in the freshness of sorrow at the loss of friends and colleagues, "hid in death's dateless night."[38] We miss

32. William Shakespeare, *Othello,* III, iii, 354. The exact quotation is:

> Farewell the neighing steed and the shrill trump,
>
> The spirit-stirring drum, the ear-piercing fife,
>
> The royal banner and all quality,
>
> Pride, pomp, and circumstance of glorious war!

33. Percy Bysshe Shelley, "Adonais," stanza 44, line 390. The exact quotation is:

> The splendours of the firmament of time
>
> May be eclipsed, but are extinguished not;
>
> Like stars to their appointed height they climb.

34. John *Morgan* (1735–1789) and William *Shippen* (1736–1808): They both studied in Edinburgh with John and William Hunter. Morgan then founded the University of Pennsylvania Medical School, and Shippen taught anatomy and surgery there using Hunter's new practice — the dissection of human bodies. For further information, see "The Leaven of Science," p. 157, n. 23, pp. 155–156, n. 16, and pp. 156–157.

35. Benjamin *Rush* (1745–1813): Physician, patriot, and humanitarian; student of Shippen and Morgan at the University of Pennsylvania Medical School and later professor of chemistry there.

36. *Wistar, Physick, Barton, and Wood:* Early professors at the University of Pennsylvania Medical School or at its associated hospitals.

Caspar *Wistar* (1761–1818): Professor of anatomy and midwifery. For further information, see "The Leaven of Science," pp. 157–159.

Phylip Syng *Physick* (1768–1837): Professor of surgery who made many improvements in surgical procedures and instruments. For further information, see "The Leaven of Science," pp. 156–157.

John Rhea *Barton* (1794–1871): At Pennsylvania Hospital he did pioneer surgery on hip joints and immobilizing fractured jaws.

George Bacon *Wood* (1797–1879): Professor of pharmacy as well as theory and practice of medicine, he wrote *The Dispensatory of the United States* (1833) with Franklin Bache.

37. *Noblesse oblige:* (French) nobility brings with it the obligation to behave nobly. Duc de Lévis, "Sur la noblesse," in *Réflexions.* Osler refers to the faculty members as having the moral obligation to display honorable deeds.

38. William Shakespeare, "Sonnet 30," line 6. The exact quotation is:

> Then can I drown an eye, unused to flow,
>
> For precious friends hid in death's dateless night.

from our midst one of your best known instructors, by whose lessons you have profited, and whose example has stimulated many. An earnest teacher, a faithful worker, a loyal son of this University, a good and kindly friend, Edward Bruen [39] has left behind him, amid regrets at a career untimely closed, the memory of a well-spent life.

We mourn to-day, also, with our sister college,[40] the grievous loss which she has sustained in the death of one of her most distinguished teachers, a man who bore with honour an honoured name, and who added lustre to the profession of this city. Such men as Samuel W. Gross [41] can ill be spared. Let us be thankful for the example of a courage which could fight and win; and let us emulate the zeal, energy, and industry which characterized his career.

Personally I mourn the loss of a preceptor, dear to me as a father, the man from whom more than any other I received inspiration, and to whose example and precept I owe the position which enables me to address you to-day. There are those present who will feel it no exaggeration when I say that to have known Palmer Howard [42] was, in the deepest and truest sense of the phrase, a liberal education—

> Whatever way my days decline,
> I felt and feel, tho' left alone,
> His being working in mine own,
> The footsteps of his life in mine.[43]

While preaching to you a doctrine of equanimity, I am, myself, a castaway. Recking not my own rede,[44] I illustrate the inconsistency which so readily besets us. One might have thought that in the premier school of America, in this Civitas Hippocratica,[45] with associations so dear to a lover of his profession, with

39. Edward Tunis *Bruen* (1851–1889): Colleague of Osler at the University of Pennsylvania Medical School.

40. Jefferson Medical College in Philadelphia.

41. Samuel Weissell *Gross* (1837–1889): Professor of surgery at Jefferson Medical College. He developed a radical operation for cancer and was one of the first to use antiseptic surgery; he was Osler's friend and colleague on the "News" Board. In fact, it was his idea to offer a professorship at the University of Pennsylvania to Osler. (See "L'Envoi," p. 351.) In 1892 his widow Grace Revere married Osler.

42. Robert Palmer *Howard* (1823–1889): Professor of medicine and dean of the faculty at McGill University. He was Osler's undergraduate teacher and was revered by him as a father figure and mentor. In a later address, "The Student Life," Osler portrays him as a wonderful man (pp. 327–328).

43. Alfred Tennyson, "In Memoriam A.H.H.," part 85, stanza 11.

44. *Recking not my own rede:* "Not following my own advice." William Shakespeare, *Hamlet,* I, iii, 51. Osler is admitting that although he is advising imperturbability he is emotionally moved by the occasion.

45. *Civitas Hippocratica* (Latin): "Hippocratic society." Osler compares Philadelphia, in 1889 the leading

colleagues so distinguished, and with students so considerate, one might have thought, I say, that the Hercules Pillars[46] of a man's ambition had here been reached. But it has not been so ordained, and to-day I sever my connexion with this University. More than once, gentlemen, in a life rich in the priceless blessings of friends, I have been placed in positions in which no words could express the feelings of my heart, and so it is with me now. The keenest sentiments of gratitude well up from my innermost being at the thought of the kindliness and goodness which have followed me at every step during the past five years. A stranger—I cannot say an alien—among you, I have been made to feel at home—more you could not have done. Could I say more? Whatever the future may have in store of success or of trials, nothing can blot the memory of the happy days I have spent in this city, and nothing can quench the pride I shall always feel at having been associated, even for a time, with a Faculty so notable in the past, so distinguished in the present, as that from which I now part.

Gentlemen,—Farewell, and take with you into the struggle the watchword of the good old Roman—*Aequanimitas.*

American center of medical training, to Cos, one of the Greek Dodecanese Islands, where Hippocrates, the most famous physician of antiquity, taught and practiced medicine.

46. *Hercules Pillars:* The promontories flanking the east entrance to the Strait of Gibraltar, regarded by the ancients as the western limits of the mortal world. They were named after the Greek hero Hercules (son of Zeus), who sailed to the Hesperides.

3

SIR THOMAS BROWNE

THIS AND OTHER BIOGRAPHICAL essays were part of Osler's mission to resurrect the literary heroes of medicine. When Osler was a pupil at Trinity College School, he was introduced by a favorite teacher to Sir Thomas Browne's work *Religio Medici*. Osler recommends that medical students read Browne's writings for his advice on aiming for perfection, self-mastery, devotion to duty, and on having a deep interest in things human.

Browne was born in 1605, almost three hundred years before this talk. After Oxford, he studied in Europe where he obtained a doctor's degree at Leiden in the Netherlands in 1633. This experience gave him an unusual breadth of cultural understanding and mastery of languages.

Browne returned to England in 1634 because of poor health. Before he was thirty, he wrote the book *Religio Medici*, which put him in contact with many of the leading philosophers, more so than with the great physicians, of that time. Like Milton, he wrote that nature should have been populated "without feminine," decrying nature's method for propagation. Ironically, in 1641 he married, and later had ten children.

In his forty-five years of medical practice he was a keen observer rather than an experimentalist. He had a strong interest in history, archaeology, literature, and philosophy. Browne was made an honorary Fellow of the Royal College of Physicians and was knighted. He died unexpectedly from colic on his seventy-seventh birthday.

The *Religio Medici* attempted to combine "daring skepticism with humble faith in the Christian religion," from the standpoint of a loyal but unprejudiced son of the Church of England. Some of Browne's ideas, such as hope for the ultimate salvation of the race and efficacy of prayers for the dead, were then viewed in many quarters as heretical. Sir Kenelm Digby read Browne's book while in prison and allegedly the same night wrote a book-length criticism that was subsequently published with the *Religio Medici*.

The *Religio Medici* was written without thought of publication and initially was circulated just to friends. However, in 1642 an unauthorized copy with many errors was printed. Browne then released an authorized edition which became popular, was translated into several languages, and was reprinted several times.

SIR THOMAS BROWNE

The value of this essay escapes me

A
S A BOY IT WAS my good fortune to come under the influence of a
parish priest of the Gilbert White[1] type, who followed the seasons
of Nature no less ardently than those of the Church, and whose
excursions into science had brought him into contact with physic
and physicians. Father Johnson,[2] as his friends loved to call him, founder and
Warden of the Trinity College School, near Toronto, illustrated that angelical
conjunction[3] (to use Cotton Mather's words) of medicine and divinity more
common in the sixteenth and seventeenth centuries than in the nineteenth. An
earnest student of Sir Thomas Browne, particularly of the *Religio Medici*, he
often read to us extracts in illustration of the beauty of the English language,
or he would entertain us with some of the author's quaint conceits, such as the
man without a navel (Adam),[4] or that woman was the rib and crooked piece

An address delivered at the Physical Society of Guy's Hospital in London, October 12, 1905. Published
in the *British Medical Journal*, 1905, ii, 993–998; as the "Religio Medici" in *The Library*, London, 1906,
vii, 1; reprinted by the Chiswick Press in 1906 as "Sir Thomas Browne" in *An Alabama Student*. Unless
otherwise stated, notes about Browne's passages are from *The Works of Sir Thomas Browne* (1928), ed.
Geoffrey Keynes (Chicago: The University of Chicago Press, 1964), and are abbreviated as "Keynes."

1. Gilbert *White* (1720–1793): English naturalist and clergyman. See "A Way of Life," p. 6, n. 17.
2. William Arthur *Johnson* (1816–1880): For biographical information, see "A Way of Life," p. 6, n. 17.
According to Cushing, "The appellation 'Father' Johnson, as his friends loved to address him, was one
which in those days a Protestant might have regarded as a term of reproach—a reproach in which Johnson, however, would have gloried" (Cushing, vol. 1, p. 29, note). As an Anglo-Catholic or "Tractarian,"
Johnson would have encouraged it.
3. Cotton Mather, *Essays to Do Good* (1710; London: J. Dennett, 1808), pp. 84f.
4. *Pseudodoxia Epidemica* (1646), book 5, chap. 5, Keynes, vol. 2, pp. 346–347; and *Religio Medici* (1643),
part 2, sect. 10, Keynes, vol. 1, p. 86.

of man.[5] The copy which I hold in my hand (J. T. Fields's edition of 1862), my companion ever since my schooldays, is the most precious book in my library. I mention these circumstances in extenuation of an enthusiasm which has enabled me to make this almost complete collection of the editions of his works I show you this evening, knowing full well the compassionate feeling with which the bibliomaniac is regarded by his saner colleagues.

I. The Man

The little Thomas was happy in his entrance upon the stage, October 19, 1605. Among multiplied acknowledgements, he could lift up one hand to Heaven (as he says) that he was born of honest parents, 'that modesty, humility, patience, and veracity lay in the same egg, and came into the world'[6] with him. Of his father, a London merchant, but little is known. There is at Devonshire House a family picture which shows him to have been a man of fine presence, looking not unworthy of the future philosopher, a child of three or four years, seated on his mother's knee. She married a second time, Sir Thomas Dutton,[7] a man of wealth and position, who gave his stepson every advantage of education and travel. We lack accurate information of the early years—of the schooldays at Winchester, of his life at Broadgate Hall, now Pembroke College, Oxford, and of the influences which induced him to study medicine. Possibly he got his inspiration from the Regius Professor of Medicine, the elder Clayton,[8] the Master of Broadgate Hall and afterwards of Pembroke College. That he was a distinguished undergraduate is shown in his selection at the end of the first year in residence to deliver an oration at the opening of Pembroke College. Possibly between the years 1626, when he took the B.A., and 1629, when he commenced M.A., he may have been engaged in the study of medicine; but Mr. Charles Williams,[9] of Norwich, who is perhaps more familiar than any one living with the history of our author, does not think it likely that he began until he went abroad. In these years he could

5. *Religio Medici*, part 2, sect. 9, Keynes, vol. 1, p. 83; and *Pseudodoxia Epidemica*, book 6, chap. 1, Keynes, vol. 2, p. 399.

6. *that modesty, humility, patience, and veracity lay in the same egg, and came into the world:* The quote is unknown.

7. Thomas *Dutton* (c.1575–1634): A quarrelsome man who killed his colonel, Sir Hatton Cheke, in a duel before he married Browne's mother.

8. Thomas *Clayton* (1575–1647): First Master of Pembroke College. He was also a musician and linguist. As Regius professor of medicine at Oxford, he is said to have cared for the souls as well as the bodies of his patients.

9. Charles *Williams* (1829–1907): Author of *The Measurements of the Skull of Sir T. Browne* (London: Jarrold & Sons, 1895) and *Souvenir of Sir Thomas Browne* (Norwich: Jarrold & Sons, 1905).

at least have 'entered upon the physic line'[10] and could have proceeded to the M.B. He was too early to participate in the revival of science in Oxford,[11] but even after that had occurred Sydenham[12] flung the cruel reproach at his Alma Mater[13] that he would as soon send a man to her to learn shoemaking as practical physic. It was possible, of course, to pick up a little knowledge of medicine from the local practitioners and from the Physic Garden,[14] together with the lectures of the Regius Professor,[15] who, as far as we know, had not at any rate the awkward failing of his more distinguished son,[16] who could not look upon blood without fainting, and in consequence had to hand over his anatomy lectures to a deputy.

Clayton's studies and work would naturally be of a somewhat mixed character, and at that period even many of those whose chief business was theology were interested in natural philosophy, of which medicine formed an important part. Burton[17] refers to an address delivered about this time by Clayton dealing with the mutual relations of mind and body. The *Anatomy of Melancholy*, which appeared in 1621, must have proved a stimulating bonne-bouche[18] for the

10. *Physic:* Refers to medicine practiced by physicians. See "Physic and Physicians as Depicted in Plato," p. 127, n.

11. The *revival of science* took place in the mid-seventeenth century at Oxford with anatomist William Petty (1623–1687), John Wilkins (1614–1672), Jonathan Goddard (1617–1675), John Wallis (1616–1703), and Seth Ward (1617–1689), some of whom, together with Robert Boyle (1627–1691), founded in 1660 the Royal Society, the oldest scientific society in Great Britain.

12. Thomas *Sydenham* (1624–1689): English physician, often called "the English Hippocrates." His insistence on clinical observation rather than theory was the basis for his criticism of Oxford. He was also a friend of John Locke and Robert Boyle.

13. Literally, a kind or nurturing mother, but usually referring to a college or university attended. Here the term refers specifically to Oxford University. Sydenham was connected with Magdalen College and later with All Souls' (at Oxford). This passage is quoted in the *Diary of the Rev. John Ward,* ed. Charles Severn (London: H. Colburn, 1839), p. 100. John Ward, an English cleric, served as vicar of Stratford-upon-Avon from 1648 to 1679.

14. The botanic garden at Oxford, set up at the beginning of the seventeenth century, was the oldest in Britain, intended to grow plants for study for medicine and other scientific use.

15. Thomas Clayton: p. 34, n. 8.

16. Thomas *Clayton* (1612–1693): The younger Clayton was also warden of Merton College, Oxford (1661–1693). He was an old acquaintance and correspondent of Browne's. On June 20, 1679, Browne wrote to his son Edward in London: "I receaved a Letter yesterday from my old acquaintance Sr Thomas Clayton, now warden of Merton colledge in Oxford. You were beholden to him in Oxford; and still are, for his good report of you" (Keynes, vol. 4, p. 118).

17. Robert *Burton* (1577–1640): English cleric. Author of *The Anatomy of Melancholy* (1621), a medical treatise on the causes, symptoms, and cure of melancholy (caused by love, hypochondriasis, superstition, and madness). This was one of Osler's favorite sources.

18. *bonne-bouche:* Literally, "an appetizer, a tasty morsel"; here a book that awakened the appetite for knowledge.

Oxford men of the day, and I like to think of the eagerness with which so ardent a student as Browne of Pembroke would have pounced on the second and enlarged edition which appeared in 1624. He may, indeed, have been a friend of Burton, or he may have formed one of a group of undergraduates to watch Democritus Junior [19] leaning over the bridge and laughing at the bargees as they swore at each other. It is stated, I know not on what authority, that Browne practised in Oxford for a time.

After a visit to Ireland with his stepfather he took the grand tour—France, Italy, and Holland—spending two years in study. Of his Continental trip our knowledge is very meagre. He went to Montpellier, still famous, but failing, where he probably listened to the teaching of Rivière,[20] whose *Praxis* was for years the leading textbook in Europe—thence to Padua, where he must have heard the celebrated Sanctorius [21] of the Medicina Statica—then on to Leyden, just rising into prominence, where it is said he took his doctor's degree in 1633. Of this, however, there is no certainty. A few years ago I looked through the register of that famous University,[22] but failed to find his name. At the end of two years' travel he may have had cobwebs in his pocket, and the Leyden degree was expensive, as that quaint old contemporary of Browne, the Rev. John Ward,[23] of Stratford-on-Avon, tells us (*Diary*): 'Mr. Burnet [24] had a letter out of the Low Countries [25] of the charge of a doctor's degree, which is at Leyden about £16, besides feasting the professors; at Angers in France, not above £9, and feasting not

19. The pseudonym adopted by Burton in the 1621 (first) edition of *The Anatomy of Melancholy*. Bishop Kennett in *Register and Chronicle* (1728) tells how as a student Burton would become despondent and seek to lift his spirits by going to the bridge and listening to the bargemen swear.

20. Lazare *Rivière* (1589–1655): French physician. Author of the medical textbook *Praxis Medica Cum Theoria* (1640).

21. *Sanctorius* (usually called Satorio Santorio) (1561–1636): Italian physician and professor of theoretical medicine at the University of Padua, and author of *De Statica Medicina* (1614). He laid the foundation for the modern study of metabolism, and was the first to develop a scaled thermometer and attempt to measure body temperature in health and illness. He left Padua and returned to Venice in 1625. If Browne did see him, it seems unlikely that it was in Padua.

22. *Leyden* (now Leiden): University founded by William of Orange in 1575, in Leiden, South Holland Province. This is the same city where the Elzevir family of printers were located. The original note at the end of this chapter reads: "Since Osler vainly searched the Leyden register, Browne's M.D. has been recognized under the disguise, 'Braun, Thomas, Anglus Londinensis, 3 Dec. 1633.'"

23. John *Ward:* See p. 35, n. 13. The quote is unknown.

24. Probably Thomas *Burnet* (1635–1715), who studied medicine at Montpellier. His son, also Thomas Burnet, obtained his M.D. from Leiden in 1691 and later became Charles II's physician. He wrote of a *Thesaurus of Medicinæ Practicæ* (1673).

25. *the Low Countries:* The region comprising the three present states of the Netherlands, Belgium, and Luxemburg.

necessary neither.'[26] No doubt the young Englishman got of the best that there was in the teaching of the day, and from the *Religio* one learns that he developed from it an extraordinary breadth of culture, and a charity not always granted to travellers. He pierced beneath the shell of nationalism into the heart of the people among whom he lived, feeling at home everywhere and in every clime; hence the charity, rare in a Protestant, expressed so beautifully in the lines: 'I can dispense with my hat at the sight of a cross, but scarce with the thought of my Saviour.'[27]

He must have made good use of his exceptional opportunities; as he was able to boast, in a humble way it is true, that he understood six languages.

Returning to England in 1634 he settled at Shibden Dale, close to Halifax,[28] not, as Mr. Charles Williams has pointed out, to practise his profession, but to recruit his health, somewhat impaired by shipwreck and disease. Here, in Upper Shibden Hall, he wrote the *Religio Medici*, the book by which to-day his memory is kept green among us. In his travels he had doubtless made many observations on men, and in his reading had culled many useful memoranda. He makes it quite clear—and is anxious to do so—that the book was written while he was very young. He says: 'My life is a miracle of thirty years.'[29] 'I have not seen one revolution of Saturn.'[30] 'My pulse hath not beat thirty years.'[31] Indeed, he seems to be of Plato's opinion that the pace of life slackens after this date,[32] and there is a note of sadness in his comment, that while the radical humour[33] may contain sufficient oil for seventy,[34] 'in some it gives no light past thirty,'[35] and he adds that those dying at this age should not complain of immaturity.[36] In the quiet Yorkshire valley, with 'leisurable hours for his private exercise and satis-

26. The phrase means "not necessary either." The double negative is used here for emphasis.

27. *Religio Medici*, part 1, sect. 3, Keynes, vol. 1, p. 13. Although he was willing to respect the customs in Catholic lands, travel there did not change his Protestant faith.

28. *Halifax:* A city in northern England, in Yorkshire. *Shibden Hall* is the name of the house where Browne lived.

29. *Religio Medici*, part 2, sect. 11, Keynes, vol. 1, p. 87.

30. *Religio Medici*, part 1, sect. 41, Keynes, vol. 1, p. 52. Saturn was thought to take thirty years to make its orbit around the sun.

31. Ibid.

32. Plato, *Laws*, book 6, 785b; see also *Republic*, book 5, 460e. Plato defines the prime of life as a period of about thirty years in a man's life.

33. *radical humour:* In mediæval philosophy, the humor or moisture naturally inherent in all plants and animals, where its presence is a necessary condition of their vitality (*OED*).

34. *Religio Medici*, part 1, sect. 43, Keynes, vol. 1, p. 53.

35. Ibid.

36. Ibid.

faction,'[37] the manuscript was completed, 'with,' as he says, 'such disadvantages that (I protest) from the first setting pen to paper I had not the assistance of any good book.'[38] 'Communicated to one it became common to many,'[39] and at last in 1642, seven years after its completion, reached the press in a depraved form.

In 1637, at the solicitation of friends,[40] Browne moved to Norwich,[41] with which city, so far as we know, he had had no previous connexion. At that date the East Anglian capital had not become famous in the annals of medicine. True, she had given Caius[42] to the profession, but he had only practised there for a short time and does not seem to have had any special influence on her destinies. Sir Thomas Browne may be said to be the first of the long list of worthies who have in the past two and a half centuries made Norwich famous among the provincial towns of the kingdom. Here for forty-five years he lived the quiet, uneventful life of a student-practitioner,[43] absorbed, like a sensible man, in his family, his friends, his studies, and his patients. It is a life of singular happiness to contemplate. In 1641 he married Dorothy Mileham, 'a lady of such a symmetrical proportion to her worthy husband—that they seemed to come together by a kind of natural magnetism.'[44] In the *Religio* he had said some hard things of the gentle goddess and had expressed himself very strongly against Nature's method for the propagation of the race. He believed, with Milton, that the world should have been populated 'without feminine,'[45] and in almost identical words they wish that some way less trivial and vulgar had been found to generate mankind.[46]

37. *Religio Medici*, "To the Reader," Keynes, vol. 1, p. 9.

38. Ibid., p. 10.

39. Ibid., p. 9.

40. One of the "friends" was Dr. Lushington, his tutor, then rector of Barnham Westgate in the neighborhood. Samuel Johnson, "The Life of Sir Thomas Browne," in *Sir Thomas Browne: The Major Works* (1756; London: Cox & Wyman, 1977), p. 489.

41. *Norwich:* A city in England, in Norfolk. Norwich and Bristol were the largest towns after London in Browne's time.

42. John *Caius* (Kayes) (1510–1573): English scholar and physician born in Norwich. He was anatomical lecturer for the London company of surgeons and later physician to Edward VI, Mary I, and Elizabeth I. Author of *A History of the University of Cambridge* (1568), he was the first of the eminent men who practiced medicine in Norwich.

43. Thomas Browne held a similar attitude to Osler's and gives an example of it in a letter dated 1646, which was probably written to Dr. Henry Power (1623–1668).

44. Samuel Johnson, "The Life of Sir Thomas Browne," p. 489. This phrase is in John Whitefoot's "Some Minutes for the Life of Sir Thomas Browne," prefixed to Browne's *Posthumous Works* (1712).

45. In John Milton's *Paradise Lost* (book 10, lines 889–893), Adam wishes that God had filled the earth only with men. The exact quotation is: "O why did God . . . not fill the World at once With men as Angels without Feminine."

46. *Religio Medici*, part 2, sect. 9, Keynes, vol. 1, p. 83.

Dame Dorothy proved a good wife, a fruitful branch, bearing ten children. We have a pleasant picture of her in her letters to her boys and to her daughter-in-law, in a spelling suggestive of Pitman's[47] phonetics. She seems to have had in full measure the simple piety and the tender affection mentioned on her monument in St. Peter's Church. The domestic correspondence (Wilkin's edition of the *Works*) gives interesting glimpses of the family life, the lights and shadows of a cultured English home. The two boys were all that their father could have wished. Edward,[48] the elder, had a distinguished career, following his father's footsteps in the profession and reaching the dignity of the Presidency of the Royal College of Physicians. Inheriting his father's tastes, as the letters between them prove, his wide interests in natural history and archaeology are shown in his well-known book of *Travels*,[49] and I am fortunate in possessing a copy of the *Hydriotaphia* with his autograph.

Edward's son, the 'Tommy'[50] of the letters, the delight of his grandfather, also became a physician, and practised with his father. He died in 1710 in rather unfortunate circumstances, and with him the male line of Sir Thomas ended. Of the younger son[51] we have, in the letters, a charming picture—a brave sailor-lad with many of his father's tastes, who served with great distinction in the Dutch wars,[52] in which he met (it is supposed) a sailor's death. The eldest daughter married Henry Fairfax,[53] and through their daughter, who married the Earl of Buchan, there are to-day among the Buchans and Erskines the only existing representatives of Sir Thomas.

The waves and storms of the Civil War[54] scarcely reached the quiet Norwich home. Browne was a staunch Royalist, and his name occurs among the citi-

47. Isaac *Pitman* (1813–1897): English inventor of an original system of shorthand, based on phonetics.

48. Edward *Browne* (1642–1708): Thomas Browne's eldest son, who practiced medicine in London and was made physician to Charles II. He became president of the College of Physicians, London, and a Fellow of the Royal Society.

49. Edward Browne wrote *An Account of Several Travels Through a Great Part of Germany: In Four Journeys* (1677) and *A Brief Account of Some Travels in Hungaria, Servia, Bulgaria, Macedonia, Thessaly, Austria, Styria, Carinthia, Carinola, and Friuli* (1673).

50. Thomas *Browne* (1673–1710): Edward Browne's eldest child, who became a physician and a Fellow of the Royal Society. His death "in rather unfortunate circumstances" probably refers to the fact that he fell off his horse and died, possibly drunk.

51. Thomas *Browne* (1647–c.1667): Thomas Browne's second son, who was a lieutenant on the warship *Mary Rose*. His father corresponded with him until his death during the war of 1663–1667.

52. The naval wars between England and Holland, 1652–1653 and 1663–1667.

53. *Henry Fairfax* married Thomas Browne's daughter Anne, and Anne's daughter Frances (thus Browne's granddaughter) married David Erskine, earl of Buchan.

54. The war in Great Britain between the English Parliamentarians and Scottish Covenanters on the one side and the Royalists on the other, 1642–1652.

zens who in 1643 refused to contribute to a fund for the recapture of the town of Newcastle. It is astonishing how few references occur in his writings to the national troubles, which must have tried his heart sorely. In the preface to the *Religio* he gives vent to his feelings, lamenting not only the universal tyranny of the Press, but the defamation of the name of his Majesty, the degradation of Parliament, and the writings of both 'depravedly, anticipatively, counterfeitedly, imprinted.'[55] In one of the letters he speaks of the execution of Charles I as 'horrid murther,'[56] and in another he calls Cromwell a usurper.[57] In civil wars physicians of all men suffer least, as the services of able men are needed by both parties, and time and again it has happened that an even-balanced soul, such as our author, has passed quietly through terrible trials, doing the day's work with closed lips. Corresponding with the most active decades of his life, in which his three important works were issued, one might have expected to find in them reference to the Civil War, or, at least, echoes of the great change wrought by the Commonwealth, but, like Fox,[58] in whose writings the same silence has been noticed, whatever may have been his feelings, he preserved a discreet silence. His own rule of life, no doubt, is expressed in the advice to his son: 'Times look troublesome, but you have an honest and peaceable profession which may employ you, and discretion to guide your words and actions.'[59]

Busy with his professional work, interested in natural history, in archaeology, and in literature, with a wide circle of scientific friends and correspondents, the glimpses of Browne's life, which we have from the letters, are singularly attractive. He adopted an admirable plan in the education of his children, sending them abroad, and urging them to form early habits of independence. His younger boy, Thomas, he sent at the age of fourteen to France, alone, and he remarks in one of his letters to him: 'He that hath learnt not in France travelleth in vain.'[60] Everywhere in the correspondence with his children there is evidence of good, practical sense. He tells one of the boys to 'cast off *pudor rusticus,* and to have a handsome garb of his body.'[61] Even the daughters were taken to France. In

---

55. *Religio Medici*, "To the Reader," Keynes, vol. 1, p. 9.

56. In a letter to his son Thomas in France, dated January 4, 1661[/2], Keynes, vol. 4, p. 16.

57. In a letter to his son Thomas in France, dated January 31, 1660[/1], Keynes, vol. 4, p. 5.

58. George *Fox* (1624–1691): English religious leader who founded the Society of Friends (Quakers). Author of *Journal* (1694).

59. In a letter to his son Edward in London, dated December 15, 1679, Keynes, vol. 4, p. 144.

60. In a letter to his son Thomas in France, dated November 1, 1661, Keynes, vol. 4, p. 14. Browne actually wrote "learneth" where Osler has "hath learnt."

61. The phrase means to "rid yourself of the shyness of the rustic and acquire instead the accomplishments of cultured life." This advice was something that Browne wrote several times to his son Thomas. It is found in one letter dated December 22, 1660, another dated January 31, 1660[/1], and a third dated November 1, 1661, Keynes, vol. 4, p. 4, 5, and 14.

his souvenir of Sir Thomas Browne, Mr. Charles Williams[62] has given an illustration of his house, a fine old building which was unfortunately torn down some years ago, though the handsome mantelpiece has been preserved.

An interesting contemporary account has been left by Evelyn,[63] who paid a visit to Sir Thomas in 1673. He says:

> The whole house being a paradise and a cabinet of rarities, and that of the best collections, especially medails, books, plants, and natural things. Amongst other curiosities, Sir Thomas had a collection of the eggs of all the foule and birds he could procure, that country, especially the promintory of Norfolck, being frequented, as he said, by several kinds which seldom or never go further into the land, as cranes, storkes, eagles, and a variety of other foule.[64]

After Dr. Edward Browne[65] was established in London, the letters show the keen interest Sir Thomas took in the scientific work of the day. Writing of his son's lecture on anatomy at the Chirurgical Hall,[66] he warns him that he would have more spectators than auditors, and after that first day, as the lecture was in Latin, 'very many will not be earnest to come here-after.'[67] He evidently takes the greatest interest in his son's progress, and constantly gives him suggestions with reference to new points that are coming up in the literature. Here and there are references to important medical cases, and comments upon modes of treatment. It is interesting to note the prevalence of agues, even of the severe haemorrhagic types, and his use of Peruvian bark.[68] In one of the letters a remarkable case of pneumothorax is described: 'A young woman who had a julking and fluctuation in her chest so that it might be heard by standers-by.'[69] Evidently he had a large and extensive practice in the Eastern Counties, and there are nu-

62. Charles *Williams:* See p. 34, n. 9.

63. John *Evelyn* (1620–1706): English Royalist and government official, known as a traveler and connoisseur of art and architecture. He was also one of the founders of the Royal Society. He chronicled contemporary events in his *Diary* (1640–1706).

64. John Evelyn, *The Diary,* entry for October 17, 1671, ed. E. S. de Beer (1640–1706; Oxford: Clarendon Press, 1955), vol. 3, pp. 594–595.

65. Thomas Browne's eldest son. See p. 39, n. 48.

66. The *Chirurgical Hall* (or Surgeons' Hall) stood in the Old Bailey in London until 1809.

67. In a letter to his son Edward in London, dated February 14 [1678/9], Keynes, vol. 4, p. 92.

68. *Peruvian bark:* Specifically in medicine (also Jesuits'). The bark of various species of the cinchona tree, from which quinine is procured, formerly ground into powder and taken as a febrifuge (*OED*).

69. In a letter to his son Edward in London, dated January 5 [1679/80], Keynes, vol. 4, p. 146.

julking: (Obs.) splashing; striking. This is a dialect word that means "giving out a sloshing sound, like a cask of liquor that is not quite full when it is shaken" (*The English Dialect Dictionary,* ed. Joseph Wright [London: Oxford University Press, 1898]).

merous references to the local physicians. There is a poem extolling his skill in the despaired-of case of Mrs. E. S., three or four of the lines of which are worth quoting:

> He came, saw, cur'd![70] Could Caesar's self do more;
> Galen,[71] Hippocrates,[72] London's four-score
> Of ffamous Colledge[73] . . . had these heard him read
> His lecture on this Skeliton,[74] half dead;
> And seen his modest eye search every part,
> Judging, not seeing.[75]

The correspondence with his son is kept up to the time of his death. Only part of the letters appear in Wilkin's *Life,* and there are many extant worthy of publication.

In 1671 he was knighted by Charles II. In 1664 he was made an honorary Fellow of the Royal College of Physicians, with which, through his son, he had close affiliations. His name does not appear in the roll of the Royal Society, with the spirit and objects of which he must yet have had the warmest sympathy. He was in correspondence with many of the leading men of the day—Evelyn, Grew, Elias Ashmole, Dugdale, Paston, Aubrey, and others.[76] The letters deal with a remarkable variety of subjects—natural history, botany, chemistry, magic and archaeology, &c. The *Pseudodoxia Epidemica* (1646)[77] extended his reputation

70. *came, saw, cur'd*: An echo of the famous line of Caesar "veni, vidi, vici" ("I came, I saw, I conquered"), meaning that Caesar himself could not have done greater deeds. The original phrase is in Lucius Annaeus Seneca's *Suasoriae* (Discourses), book 2, sect. 22.

71. Claudius *Galen* (c.130–c.200): Greek physician. See "Teaching and Thinking," pp. 181–182, n. 27.

72. *Hippocrates* (c.460–c.375 B.C.): Greek physician. See "The Master-Word in Medicine," p. 274, n. 108.

73. Probably the Royal College of Physicians.

74. *skeliton* (emaciated person): Refers to a woman named Mrs. E. S., whom he was having difficulties treating.

75. Author of the poem is not known.

76. John *Evelyn*: See p. 41, n. 64.

Obadiah *Grew* (1607–1689): English nonconformist religious writer who wrote *A Sinner's Justification* (1670).

Elias *Ashmole* (1617–1692): English antiquarian whose collection of curiosities formed the nucleus of the Ashmolean Museum in Oxford.

William *Dugdale* (1605–1686): English antiquarian and royalist who wrote a lengthy work on English monasticism. He consulted Browne for his work *The History of Imbanking and Drayning* (1662).

Robert *Paston*, 1st earl of Yarmouth (1631–1683): Fellow of the Royal Society who fought in the Civil War. It was through him that Browne's correspondence with Evelyn began.

John *Aubrey* (1626–1697): English antiquarian. Author of *Miscellanies* (1696) and *Minutes of Lives* (1669–1696), portrayals of Bacon, Milton, Raleigh, Hobbes, and others.

77. *The Epidemic of Presumed (but False) Truths* (1646) by Browne, which is described by Osler on pp.

among all classes and helped to bring him into close relationship with the virtuosi of the period. There is in the Bodleian[78] a delightful letter from Mr. Henry Bates,[79] a wit of the court, a few extracts from which will give you an idea of the extravagant admiration excited by his writings:

> Sir,—Amongst those great and due acknowledgements this horizon owes you for imparting your sublime solid phansie to them in that incomparable piece of invention and judgement, R. M.[80] gives mee leave, sir, here at last to tender my share, which I wish I could make proportionable to the value I deservedly sett upon it, for truly, sir, ever since I had the happiness to know your religion I have religiously honoured you; hug'd your Minerva[81] in my bosome, and voted it my *vade mecum*.[82] . . . I am of that opinion still, that next the *Legenda Dei*,[83] it is the master piece of Christendome; and though I have met sometimes with some *omnes sic ego vero non sic*[84] men, prejudicating pates, who bogled at shadowes in 't, and carpt at atoms, and have so strappadoed[85] me into impatience with their senseless censures, yet this still satisfied my zeal toward it, when I found *non intelligunt*[86] was the nurse of theire *vituperant*,[87] and they onely stumbled for want of a lanthorne.[88,89]

51–52. But the book is usually known in English as *Vulgar Errors,* where "vulgar" means "common" and a strict translation of the Latin title would be "Epidemic False Teachings."

78. The library of Oxford University, reestablished by Sir Thomas Bodley (1545–1613). For further information, see "The Old Humanities and the New Science," p. 78, n. 100.

79. Henry *Bates:* Assumed not to be well known, because Osler identifies him only as "a wit of the court."

80. *R. M.: Religio Medici.*

81. *Minerva:* Olympian goddess of wisdom.

82. *vade mecum:* (Latin) "go with me." In English it refers to a book one carries with oneself at all times.

83. *Legenda Dei:* (Latin) the phrase means "God's things to be read" or "what is read of God." Bates is ranking the *Religio Medici* next to the Bible.

84. *omnes sic ego vero non sic:* (Latin) "everyone thus, but I not thus." Or, more loosely, the sentence means "everyone else behaves in this way, but I do not behave this way."

85. *strappado:* (Obs.) a form of punishment to obtain confession. The strappado was inflicted by securing the victim in ropes (usually by the wrists), hauling him up, and then letting him fall until the rope went taut.

86. *non intelligunt:* (Latin) "they do not understand."

87. *vituperant:* (Latin) "they censure."

88. *lanthorne:* (Obs.) lantern.

89. Osler's original note reads: "Wilkin, vol. i, p. 353." Browne corresponded with many of the leading men of the day, and this is an extract from Henry Bates' letter, which is in the Bodleian. In it he says that he was impatient with complaints and criticisms; but when he discovered that some of the denunciations were not intelligent but merely based on ignorance ("and they onely stumbled for want of a lanthorne"), he felt pleased.

While interested actively in medicine, Browne does not seem to have been on intimate terms with his great contemporaries—Harvey, Sydenham, or Glisson[90]—though he mentions them, and always with respect. He was a prudent, prosperous man, generous to his children and to his friends. He subscribed liberally to his old school at Winchester, to the rebuilding of the Library of Trinity College, Cambridge, and to the repairs at Christ Church, Oxford. A life placid, uneventful, and easy, without stress or strain, happy in his friends, his family, and his work, he expressed in it that harmony of the inner and of the outer man which it is the aim of all true philosophy to attain, and which he inculcated so nobly and in such noble words in the *Religio Medici* and in the *Christian Morals.*

A description of him given by his friend, the Rev. John Whitefoot,[91] is worth quoting:

> He was never seen to be transported with mirth or dejected with sadness; always cheerful but rarely merry, at any sensible rate; seldom heard to break a jest, and when he did he would be apt to blush at the levity of it. His gravity was natural, without affectation.[92]

The end came unexpectedly in his seventy-seventh year, after a sharp attack of colic, on his birthday, October 19, 1682—a curious possibility of which he speaks in the *Letter to a Friend:*

> But in persons who outlive many years, and when there are no less than 365 days to determine their lives every year—that the first day should make the last, that the tail of the snake should return into its mouth precisely at that time, and they should wind up upon the day of their nativity[93]—is, indeed, a remarkable coincidence, which, though astrology hath taken witty pains to solve, yet hath it been very wary in making predictions of it.[94]

90. William *Harvey* (1578–1657): English physician and anatomist who discovered the circulation of the blood. For further information, see "Teacher and Student," p. 116, n. 22.

Sydenham: See p. 35, n. 12.

Francis *Glisson* (1597–1677): English physician and anatomy lecturer, known for his study on rickets.

91. John *Whitefoot* (1610–1699): Rector of Heigham and Hellesdon and an old and intimate friend of Browne's. He wrote *Some Minutes for the Life of Sir Thomas Browne.* Dr. Johnson quotes extensively from this memoir.

92. Quoted from Whitefoot in Samuel Johnson's "The Life of Sir Thomas Browne," p. 503.

93. Browne has in mind a picture of a snake with its tail in its mouth, which was taken by the Greeks to symbolize eternity or a complete cycle of time. It is originally found in Egyptian hieroglyphics. Browne himself died on his birthday, October 19, 1682.

94. *A Letter to Friend,* Keynes, vol. 1, p. 105.

There are three good portraits of Sir Thomas; one in the College of Physicians, London, which is the best known and has been often reproduced, and from which is taken the frontispiece in Greenhill's edition of the *Religio Medici*; a second is in the Bodleian,[95] and this also has frequently been reproduced; the third is in the vestry of St. Peter's Mancroft, Norwich. Through the kindness of Mr. Charles Williams, it is here reproduced. In many ways it is the most pleasing of the three, and Browne looks in it a younger man, closer to the days of the *Religio*. There is a fourth picture, the frontispiece to the fifth edition of the *Pseudodoxia*, but it is so unlike the others that I doubt very much if it could have been Sir Thomas. If it was, he must have suffered from the artist, as did Milton, whose picture in the frontispiece to the *Poems*,[96] 1645, is a base caricature; but Browne has not had the satisfaction of Milton's joke and happy revenge.

II. The Book

As a book the *Religio Medici* has had an interesting history. Written at 'leisurable hours and for his private exercise and satisfaction,'[97] it circulated in manuscript among friends, 'and was by transcription successively corrupted, until it arrived in a most depraved copy at the press.'[98] Two surreptitious editions were issued by Andrew Crooke[99] in 1642, both in small octavo, with an engraved frontispiece by Marshall[100] representing a man falling from a rock (the earth) into the sea of eternity, but caught by a hand issuing from the clouds, under which is the legend, *A Coelo Salus*.[101] Johnson suggests that the author may not have been ignorant of Crooke's design, but was very willing to let a tentative edition be issued— 'a stratagem by which an author panting for fame, and yet afraid of seeming to challenge it, may at once gratify his vanity and preserve the appearance of modesty.'[102]

There are at least six manuscripts of the *Religio* in existence, all presenting minor differences, which bear out the author's contention that by transcrip-

---

95. *Bodleian* Library in Oxford.

96. The 1645 edition of Milton's poems had as a frontispiece an ugly portrait by William Marshall (fl. 1630–1650). Milton, in revenge, arranged for the artist to engrave some Greek verses ridiculing the picture as caricature.

97. Both quotations from *Religio Medici*, "To the Reader," Keynes, vol. 1, p. 9.

98. Ibid.

99. Andrew *Crooke* (d. 1674): One of the leading publishers of his day in England.

100. William *Marshall* (fl. 1630–1650): Prolific early English engraver. His portraits include those of Milton, Donne, and Shakespeare.

101. *A Coelo Salus*: (Latin) "from heaven, salvation."

102. Samuel Johnson, "The Life of Sir Thomas Browne," pp. 485–486.

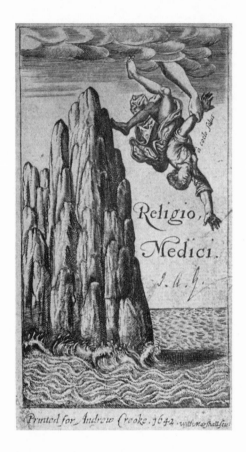

tion they had become depraved. One in the Wilkin collection, in the Castle Museum,[103] Norwich, is in the author's handwriting. Had Browne been party to an innocent fraud, he would scarcely have allowed Crooke to issue within a year a second imperfect edition—not simply a second impression, as the two differ in the size and number of the pages, and present also minor differences in the text. The authorized edition appeared in the following year by the same publisher and with the same frontispiece, with the following words at the foot of the plate: 'A true and full copy of that which was most imperfectly and surreptitiously printed before under the name of *Religio Medici*'.[104] It was issued anonymously, with a preface, signed 'A. B.'; 'To such as have or shall peruse the observations upon a former corrupt copy of this Booke.'[105] A curious incident here links together two men, types of the intellectual movement of their generation—both students, both mystics—the one a quiet observer of nature, an

103. The original note at the end of this chapter reads: "the Castle Museum MS. is no longer believed to be autograph."

104. *Religio Medici* (1643, 2nd ed.), the engraved title page.

105. Ibid.

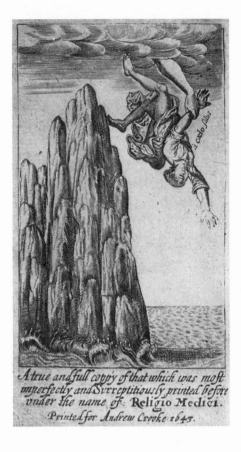

A true and full coppy of that which was most imperfectly and Svrreptitiously printed before vnder the name of Religio Medici.
Printed for Andrew Crooke 1643.

antiquary, and a physician; the other a restless spirit, a bold buccaneer, a politician, a philosopher, and an amateur physician. Sir Kenelm Digby,[106] committed to Winchester House[107] by the Parliamentarians, had heard favourably from the Earl of Dorset[108] of the *Religio Medici.* Though late in the day, 'the magnetic motion,' as he says 'was impatience to have the booke in his hands,' so he sent at once to St. Paul's churchyard for it. He was in bed when it came.

> This good natur'd creature I could easily perswade to be my bedfellow and
> to wake me as long as I had any edge to entertain myselfe with the delights
> I sucked in from so noble a conversation. And truly I closed not my eyes
> till I had enricht myselfe with (or at least exactly surveyed) all the treasures
> that are lapt up in the folds of those new sheets.[109]

106. Kenelm *Digby* (1603–1665): English author, naval commander, and diplomat. A very versatile man, he was also the author of *Observations upon Religio Medici* (1643).

107. Digby was imprisoned on suspicion of a too active royalism.

108. Probably Richard *Sackville,* 5th earl of Dorset (1622–1677): Author of an elegy in memory of Ben Jonson.

109. Kenelm Digby, *Observations upon Religio Medici* (London: Printed by R. C. for Daniel Frere, 1643).

Sir Kenelm holds the record for reading in bed; not only did he read the *Religio* through, but he wrote *Observations* upon it the same night in the form of a letter to his friend, which extends to three-fourths of the size of the *Religio* itself. As Johnson remarks, he 'returned his judgement of it not in the form of a letter but of a book.'[110] He dates it at the end 'the 22nd (I think I may say the 23rd, for I am sure it is morning and I think it is day) of December, 1642.'[111] Johnson says that its principal claim to admiration is that it was written within twenty-four hours, of which part was spent in procuring Browne's book and part in reading it.[112] Sir Kenelm was a remarkable man, but in connexion with his statements it may be well to remember the reputation he had among his contemporaries, Stubbs[113] calling him 'the Pliny[114] of our age for lying.' However this may be, his criticisms of the work are exceedingly interesting and often just. This little booklet of Sir Kenelm has floated down the stream of literature, reappearing at intervals attached to editions of the *Religio*, while his weightier tomes are deep in the ooze at the bottom.

The *Religio Medici* became popular with remarkable rapidity. As Johnson remarks, 'It excited attention by the novelty of paradoxes, the dignity of sentiment, the quick succession of images, the multitude of abstrusive allusions, subtility of disquisition, and the strength of language.'[115] A Cambridge student, Merryweather,[116] travelling in Europe, translated it into Latin, and it was published in 1644 by Hackius[117] at Leyden in a very neat volume. A second impression appeared in the same year, and also a Paris edition, a reprint of the Leyden. The continental scholars were a good deal puzzled, and not altogether certain of the orthodoxy of the work. Merryweather, in a very interesting letter (1649)

110. Samuel Johnson, "The Life of Sir Thomas Browne," p. 275.

111. Digby, *Observations upon Religio Medici*. Digby claims that he wrote *Observations* in a single sitting on December 22, 1642.

112. Samuel Johnson, "The Life of Sir Thomas Browne."

113. Probably Henry *Stubbs* (also Stubbe) (1632–1676): English physician and classicist, of Christ Church, Oxford, who wrote against monarchy, ministers, and universities. These words apparently come from Henry Stubbs' *A Specimen of Some Animadversions upon . . . Plus Ultra . . . by Mr Joseph Glanvil* (1670). Osler, however, probably found the quote in the article on Digby in the *Dictionary of National Biography (DNB)*.

114. *Pliny:* Pliny the Elder (Gaius Plinius Secundus, c.23–c.79): He was notorious for the errors and credulity in his thirty-seven-volume work, *Naturalis Historia* (Natural History). Here Stubbs is questioning Digby's reliability.

115. Samuel Johnson, "The Life of Sir Thomas Browne."

116. John *Merryweather* (c.1644–c.1881): Cambridge scholar whose Latin translation of *Religio Medici* greatly contributed to its fame among continental scholars.

117. Petrus *Hackius* (date unknown): The pseudonym of a Leiden publisher; he also published the Dutch version of the Bible.

says that he had some difficulty in getting a printer at Leyden. Salmasius,[118] to whom Haye,[119] a book merchant, took it for approbation, said 'that there was in it many things well said, but that it contained also many exorbitant conceptions in religion and would probably find much frowning entertainment, especially amongst the ministers.'[120] Two other printers also refused it. The most interesting continental criticism is by that distinguished member of the profession, Gui Patin,[121] professor in the Paris Faculty of Medicine. In a letter to Charles Spon[122] of Lyons, dated Paris, October 21, 1644, he mentions having received a little book called the *Religio Medici*, written by an Englishman, 'a very mystical book containing strange and ravishing thoughts.'[123] In a letter, dated 1645, he says, 'the book is in high credit here; the author has wit, and there are abundance of fine things in the book. He is a humorist[124] whose thoughts are very agreeable, but who, in my opinion, is to seek for a master in religion may in the end find none.' Patin thought the author in a parlous state, and as he was still alive he might grow worse as well as better. Evidently, however, the work became a favourite one with him, as in letters of 1650-3-7 he refers to it again in different editions. It is remarkable that he nowhere mentions the author by name, but subsequently, when Edward Browne[125] was a student in Paris, Patin sends kindly greetings to his father.

Much discussion occurred on the Continent as to the orthodoxy of the *Religio*. It is no slight compliment to the author that he should have been by one claimed as a Catholic, by another denounced as an Atheist, while a member of the Society of Friends[126] saw in him a likely convert. The book was placed on the 'Index.'[127] In England, with the exception of Digby's *Observations*,[128] there

118. Claude de *Saumaise* (*Salmasius* is the Latin version of his French name) (1588–1653): Professor at Leiden whose defense of King Charles I was attacked by Milton in *A Defence of the People of England* (1651).

119. *Haye, a book merchant:* Unknown.

120. In a letter from Merryweather to Browne, dated October 1, 1649.

121. Gui *Patin* (1601–1672): French physician and professor of surgery at the Paris Faculty of Medicine. He was opposed to novelties in medicine and the use of chemicals, but supported bloodletting. His letters to other physicians tell about topics of science and also social customs in his time. Osler enjoyed reading his letters, saying "I am perfectly enchanted with the old rascal" (Cushing, vol. 2, p. 48)

122. Charles *Spon* (1609–1684): French physician who wrote prognostics of Hippocrates in verse.

123. Gui Patin's letter to Charles Spon of Lyons, Paris, dated October 21, 1644.

124. *humorist:* Person of a whimsical disposition. The sense derives from the old medical theory of the four humors, whose proportions were thought to determine an individual's temperament.

125. Edward *Browne:* Thomas Browne's eldest son. See p. 39, n. 48.

126. The formal designation of the Quakers, a sect founded by George Fox in about 1650.

127. *Index Librum Prohibitorum* (Index of Prohibited Books): A list of books that Roman Catholics are forbidden to read without special permission, or unless the books have been expurgated or corrected.

128. See p. 47, n. 109.

were no adverse criticisms of any note. Alexander Ross,[129] that interesting old Southampton schoolmaster, who seems always to have been ready for an intellectual tilt, wrote a criticism entitled *Medicus Medicatus, or the Physician's Religion cured by a Lenitive or Gentle Potion.*

In England there were two reprints in 1645, and it appeared again in the years 1656, 1659, 1669, 1672, and in 1682, the year of Browne's death. A comparison of the early editions shows that all have the same frontispiece and are, with slight variations, reprints of that of 1643. The work also began to be reprinted with the *Pseudodoxia Epidemica* (third edition, 1659). The Latin editions followed each other rapidly. As I mentioned, it first appeared at Leyden in 1644, and was reprinted the same year there and in Paris; then in 1650 in Leyden again, in 1652 in Strassburg, and in the same place in 1665 and 1667. The most important of these editions was that of Strassburg, 1652, with elaborate notes by Moltkius,[130] of which Gui Patin speaks as 'miserable examples of pedantry,' and indeed stigmatizes the commentator as a fool. The Dutch translation appeared in 1655 and a French in 1668, so that altogether during the author's lifetime there were at least twenty editions of the work.

In the seventeenth century there were in all twenty-two editions. In the eighteenth century there were four English editions, one Latin, and one German. Then a long interval of seventy-seven years elapsed, until in 1831 Thomas Chapman,[131] a young Exeter College man, brought out a neat little edition, my own copy of which is made precious by many marginal notes by S. T. Coleridge, who was one of the earliest and most critical among the students of Sir Thomas. In the same year the first American edition was published, edited by the Rev. Alexander Young,[132] of Boston. In 1838 appeared an excellent edition by J. A. St. John,[133] 'traveller, linguist, author, and editor,' and in 1844 Longmans' edition by John Peace,[134] the librarian of the City Library, Bristol. This edition was republished

129. Alexander *Ross* (1590–1654): Scottish writer and schoolmaster. In *Medicus Medicatus* (1645) he criticized Browne for his application of "rhetorical phrase" to religious subjects, for his tendency toward judicial astrology, and generally on the score of heresy.

130. *Moltkius:* The preface of the annotated 1652 Latin edition of *Religio Medici* is signed with the initials "L.N.M.E.M.," which the British Library Catalogue expands as "Levinus Nicolas *Moltkius* (or Moltkenius) Eques Misniensis." The name has not beeen identified.

131. Thomas *Chapman* (1812–1834): He edited *Religio Medici* (Oxford: J. Vincent, 1831).

132. Alexander *Young* (1801–1854): American antiquarian and Unitarian minister. Critical printer of source material such as *Chronicles of the Pilgrim Fathers* (1841).

133. James Augustus *St. John* (1801–1875): English author who wrote about the life of Sir Walter Raleigh and about his own travel to Egypt and other countries, mostly on foot. He edited *Religio Medici* (London: J. Rickerby, 1838).

134. John *Peace* (1785–1861): The librarian of the City Library, Bristol. He edited *Religio Medici* and its sequel *Christian Morals* (London: Longman, Brown, and Longmans, 1844).

in America by the house of Lea & Blanchard,[135] Philadelphia, the only occasion, I believe, on which the *Religio* has been issued by a firm of medical publishers. In 1845 appeared Pickering's beautiful edition, edited, with many original notes, by the Rev. Henry Gardiner,[136] in many ways the most choice of nineteenth-century issues. In 1862 James Ticknor Fields,[137] the well-known Boston scholar and publisher, brought out a very handsome edition, of which, for the first time in the history of the book, an *édition de luxe* was printed on larger paper. In 1869 appeared Sampson Low & Co.'s edition by Willis Bund;[138] and in 1878 Rivingtons' edition edited by W. P. Smith.[139] Then in 1881 there came what must always remain the standard edition, edited by Dr. Greenhill[140] for the Golden Treasury Series, and reprinted repeatedly by Macmillan & Co. To his task Dr. Greenhill brought not only a genuine love of Sir Thomas Browne, but the accuracy of an earnest, painstaking scholar. Since the year 1881 a dozen or more editions have appeared, of which I may mention the excellent one by Dr. Lloyd Roberts,[141] of Manchester. I may finish this dry summary by noting the contrast between the little parchment-covered surreptitious edition of 1642 and the sumptuous folio of the Vale Press. In all, including those which have appeared with the collected works, there have been about fifty-five editions. Browne states that the work had also been translated into High Dutch[142] and into Italian, but I can find no record of these editions, nor of a German translation, 1680, mentioned by Watt.[143]

Space will allow only a brief reference to Browne's other writings. *Pseudodoxia Epidemica: or, Enquiries into very many received Tenents and commonly presumed Truths,* appeared in 1646 in a small folio. In extent this is by far the

135. *Lea & Blanchard:* Osler's original note reads: "They did not issue an edition in 1848, as is stated by Greenhill on the authority of J. T. Fields."

136. Henry *Gardiner* (1815–1864): He edited *Religio Medici* (London: William Pickering, 1845).

137. James Ticknor *Fields:* Osler seems to have confused the editor and his publishing company.

   James Thomas *Fields* (1817–1881): His publishing firm of Ticknor and Fields in Boston printed *Religio Medici,* which he edited, in 1862.

138. John William *Willis Bund* (1843–1928): Barrister, writer, and agriculturist. He edited *Religio Medici* (London: Sampson Low, 1869).

139. Walter Percy *Smith* (1848–1922): Master at Winchester College. His Rivingtons' edition was first published in 1874 and reissued by Longmans in 1893.

140. Edward Headlam *Greenhill* (1814–1888): Physician who practiced in London and wrote on, among other things, Addison's disease and chronic bronchitis. He edited *Religio Medici* (London: Macmillan, 1881).

141. David Lloyd *Roberts* (1835–1920): Consulting obstetric physician of the Manchester Royal Infirmary. He edited *Religio Medici* (London: David Scott, 1892).

142. *High Dutch* refers to the German language.

143. Robert *Watt* (1774–1819): Scottish bibliographer. He compiled *Catalogue of Medical Books for the Use of Students Attending Lectures on the Principles & Practice of Medicine* (1812).

most pretentious of Browne's works. It forms an extraordinary collection of old wives' fables and popular beliefs in every department of human knowledge, dealt with from the standpoint of the science of that day. In a way it is a strong protest against general credulity and inexactness of statement, and a plea for greater accuracy in the observation of facts and in the recording of them. Walter Pater [144] has drawn attention to the striking resemblance between Browne's chapter on the sources of Error and Bacon's doctrine of the Idola [145] — shams which men fall down and worship. He discusses cleverly the use of doubts; but, as Pater remarks, 'Browne was himself a rather lively example of entertainments of the Idols of the Cave [146] — Idola Specus — and, like Boyle, Digby, and others,[147] he could not quite free himself from the shackles of alchemy and a hankering for the philosopher's stone.'[148] The work was very popular, and extended the reputation of the author very widely. Indeed, in 1646 Browne was not known at large as the author of the *Religio,* as his name had not appeared on the title-page of any edition issued at that date. The *Pseudodoxia* was frequently reprinted, a sixth edition being published in 1672, and it appeared in French both in France and in Holland.

Equalling in popularity among certain people the *Religio,* certainly next to it in importance, is the remarkable essay known as *Hydriotaphia — Urne-Buriall: or A Discourse of the Sepulchrall Urnes lately found in Norfolk* (1658). Printed with it is *The Garden of Cyrus,*[149] a learned discourse on gardens of all forms in all ages. Naturally, when an unusual number of funeral urns were found at Walsingham,[150] they were brought to the notice of Browne, the leading antiquary of the county. Instead of writing a learned disquisition upon their date—

52

SIR THOMAS

BROWNE

144. Walter Horatio *Pater* (1839–1894): English critic, essayist, novelist, and humanist. Author of *Marius the Epicurean* (1885), *Studies in the History of the Renaissance* (1873), and *Plato and Platonism* (1893).

145. Literally, "idols." Francis Bacon discusses the idola in his *Novum Organum* (1620), book 1, aphorisms 39–62.

146. "The Idols of the Cave" are those originating from the individual and his own environment.

147. Robert *Boyle* (1627–1691): English natural philosopher and chemist. *Digby:* See p. 47, n. 109.

148. *the philosopher's stone:* An imaginary stone that was believed to have the power of turning everything to gold. Concerning this stone sought by the alchemists in the middle ages, Browne writes that "it is not impossible to be procured" (*Pseudodoxia Epidemica,* book 3, chap. 12, Keynes, vol. 2, p. 197).

Osler here is paraphrasing Pater rather than quoting him. Walter Horatio Pater, "Sir Thomas Browne," *Appreciations* (1886; London: Macmillan, 1910), pp. 148–149.

149. *Cyrus* (c.424–401 B.C.): Persian prince famous for his garden; he is said to have been the first person to plant a quincunx (an arrangement of five trees or other objects in an X-shape, with four at the corners and one in the middle), but Browne in *The Garden of Cyrus* claims that it belongs to more remote antiquity.

150. *Walsingham:* A town in Norfolk County, England, where the Virgin is thought to have appeared in 1061, an event still commemorated in an annual pilgrimage to her shrine.

he thought them Roman, they were in reality Saxon—with accurate measurements and a catalogue of the bones, he touches upon the whole incident very lightly, but, using it as a text, breaks out into a noble and inspiring prose poem, a meditation upon mortality and the last sad rites of all nations in all times, with learned comments on modes of sepulchre, illustrated with much antiquarian and historical lore. Running through the work is an appropriate note of melancholy at the sad fate which awaits the great majority of us, upon whom 'the iniquity of oblivion must blindly scatter her poppy.'[151] 'The greater part must be content to be as though they had not been, to be found in the register of God, not in the record of man.'[152]

Nowhere in his writings does the prose flow with a more majestic roll. Take, for example, this one thought:

If the nearness of our last necessity brought a nearer conformity unto it, there were a happiness in hoary hairs and no calamity in half senses. But the long habit of living indisposeth us for dying, when avarice makes us the sport of death, when even David grew politically cruel,[153] and Solomon could hardly be said to be the wisest of men.[154] But many are too early old and before the days of age. Adversity stretcheth our days, misery makes Alcemena's nights,[155] and time hath no wings unto it.[156]

Closely connected in sentiment with the *Urn-Burial* is the thin folio pamphlet—the rarest of all Browne's works, printed posthumously in 1690—*A Letter to a Friend upon Occasion of the Death of his Intimate Friend*. It is a splendid dissertation on death and modes of dying, and is a unique study of the slow progress to the grave of a consumptive. It is written in his most picturesque and characteristic vein, with such a charm of diction that some critics have given it the place of honour among his works. Pater, in most enthusiastic terms,

151. Browne actually wrote: "But the iniquity of oblivion blindely scattereth her poppy." *Hydriotaphia, Urn-Burial* (1658), chap. 5, Keynes, vol. 1, p. 167. For further information, see "The Master-Word in Medicine," p. 261, n. 41.

152. Ibid.

153. *David:* King of all Israel. The following passage shows the cruelty of David: "And he smote Moab, and measured them with a line, casting them down to the ground; even with two lines measured he to put to death, and with one full line to keep alive. And so the Moabites became David's servants and brought gifts" (2 Samuel 8:2).

154. *Solomon,* the son of David, is famous for his wisdom. Possibly Browne is referring to Solomon's building of shrines to foreign gods (1 Kings 11: 6–10).

155. *Alcemena* (also *Alcmene*): Zeus tripled the length of the night when he slept with Alcmene, the mother of Hercules. *Hydriotaphia,* chap. 5, Keynes, vol. 1, p. 165.

156. Ibid.

speaks of it with the *Urn-Burial* as 'the best justification of Browne's literary reputation.'[157]

The tender sympathy with the poor relics of humanity which Browne expresses so beautifully in these two meditations has not been meted to his own. 'Who knows the fate of his bones or how often he is to be buried?'[158] he asks. In 1840, while workmen were repairing the chancel of St. Peter Mancroft, the coffin of Sir Thomas was accidentally opened, and one of the workmen took the skull, which afterwards came into the possession of Dr. Edward Lubbock,[159] who deposited it in the Museum of the Norfolk and Norwich Infirmary. When I first saw it there in 1872 there was on it a printed slip with these lines from the *Hydriotaphia:* 'To be knaved out of our graves, to have our skulls made drinking-bowls, and our bones turned into pipes, to delight and sport our enemies, are tragical abominations escaped in burning burials.'[160] The skull has been carefully described by Mr. Charles Williams,[161] to whom I am indebted for the loan of photographs.[162]

In addition to the *Letter to a Friend*, there are three posthumous works, *Certain Miscellany Tracts* (1684), edited by Archbishop Tenison,[163] and *Posthumous Works* (1712),[164] containing chiefly papers of antiquarian interest. In the same year, 1712, appeared the *Christian Morals*, edited by Archdeacon Jeffrey of Norwich,[165] from a manuscript found among Browne's papers. Probably a work of his later life, it forms a series of ethical fragments in a rich and stately prose which, in places, presents a striking parallelism to passages in the Hebrew

157. Walter Horatio *Pater*, "Sir Thomas Browne," *Appreciations* (1886) (London: Macmillan, 1910), p. 152.

158. *Hydriotaphia*, dedication letter "To My Worthy and Honoured Friend Thomas Le Gros of Crostwick Esquire," Keynes, vol. 1, p. 131.

159. Edward *Lubbock* (1805–1847): The Lubbocks were a very old family in Norfolk, and this Edward Lubbock was probably related to the Lubbocks who are Barons Avebury; but he is not mentioned in the account of their family in Burke's *Peerage*. Bernard Burke (1814–1892), *Burke's Genealogical and Heraldic History of Peerage, Baronetage and Knightage*, 105th ed., ed. Peter Townend (London: Burke's Peerage, Ltd., 1970).

160. *Hydriotaphia*, chap. 3, Keynes, vol. 1, p. 155.

161. Charles *Williams:* See p. 34, n. 9.

162. The original note reads: "The skull was reburied in 1922.–ED."

163. Thomas *Tenison* (1636–1715): Archbishop of Canterbury. Author of works against Roman Catholicism, and philanthropist, political writer, and prominent figure in the effort to urge moderation toward Protestant dissenters from the Church of England. *Certain Miscellany Tracts*, ed. Thomas Tenison (London: printed for Charles Mearn, 1683[*sic*]).

164. Edited probably by Edmund Curll. Geoffrey Keynes, *Bibliography of Sir Thomas Browne*, 2d ed. (Oxford: Clarendon Press, 1968), p. 109.

165. John *Jeffery* (also *Jeffrey*) (1647–1720): Archdeacon of Norwich, who published devotional works.

poetry. The work is usually printed with the *Religio,* to which in reality it forms a supplement.

Of the collected editions of Browne's works, the first, a fine folio, appeared in 1686. In 1836, Simon Wilkin,[166] himself a Norwich man, edited the works with the devotion of an ardent lover of his old townsman, and with the critical accuracy of a scholar. All students of Sir Thomas remain under a lasting debt to Mr. Wilkin, and it is pleasant to know, that through the kindness of his daughter-in-law, Mrs. Wilkin, of Sidmouth, a Sir Thomas Browne Library has been founded in connexion with the Castle Museum, Norwich, in which Mr. Simon Wilkin's collections have been placed.

III. Appreciation

Critics from Johnson[167] to Walter Pater[168] have put on record their estimate of Browne and of his place in literature. Among these for keenness of appreciation Pater takes the first rank. Lamb and Coleridge[169] dearly loved the old Norwich physician, in whom they found a kindred spirit. In America the New England writers, Ticknor, Fields, Holmes, and Lowell,[170] were ardent students of

166. Simon *Wilkin* (1790–1862): Editor of *Sir Thomas Browne's Works* (London: William Pickering, 1835–1836), he was a scholar of ancient and modern languages. When he lost his fortune, he became a printer in Norwich, and began the Norfolk and Norwich Literary Institution.

167. Samuel *Johnson* (1709–1784): See "A Way of Life," p. 5, n. 14.

168. Walter *Pater:* See p. 52, nn. 144 and 148.

169. Charles *Lamb* (1775–1834): English essayist and critic. Author of *Tales from Shakespeare* (1807) and *Essays of Elia* (1823).

Samuel Taylor *Coleridge* (1772–1834): English poet, critic, and philosopher. Among his most notable works are *Poems on Various Subjects* (1796) and *Lyrical Ballads* (1798).

Lamb and Coleridge were lifelong friends; Lamb was one of the young admirers of Coleridge when he attended Christ's Hospital School in London. Coleridge once wrote in a letter, "Sir Thomas Browne is among my first Favorites. Rich in various Knowledge, exuberant in conceptions and conceits, contemplative, imaginative, often truly great and magnificent in his style and diction." *Collected Letters of Samuel Taylor Coleridge,* ed. Leslie Griggs (Oxford: Clarendon Press, 1956), pp. 566–567. There are numerous Brownean allusions in Lamb's writings, too.

170. George *Ticknor* (1791–1871): American educator and historian, professor of French, Spanish, and belles-lettres at Harvard (1819–1835), and a founder of the Boston Public Library.

James Thomas *Fields* See p. 51, n. 137.

Oliver Wendell *Holmes* (1809–1894): American man of letters and physician. He taught anatomy and physiology at Dartmouth and at Harvard Medical School. Osler included Holmes's *Breakfast-Table* series in the list of ten books which he recommended to medical students. (See "Bed-side Library for Medical Students," p. 371.)

James Russell *Lowell* (1819–1891): American poet, essayist, and diplomat. Author of *A Year's Life* (1841), *A Fable for Critics* (1848), and *The Biglow Papers* (1848, 1867).

his works. Lowell in particular is fond of apt quotations from him, and in one place speaks of him as 'our most imaginative mind since Shakespeare.'[171] But no one has put so briefly and so clearly the strong characters of our author as the French critic, Taine:[172]

> Let us conceive a kindred spirit to Shakespeare's, a scholar and an observer instead of an actor and a poet, who in place of creating is occupied in comprehending, but who, like Shakespeare, applies himself to living things, penetrates their internal structure, puts himself in communication with their actual laws, imprints in himself fervently and scrupulously the smallest details of their figure; who at the same time extends his penetrating surmises beyond the region observation, discerns behind visible phenomena a world obscure yet sublime, and trembles with a kind of veneration before the vast, indistinct, but populous abyss on whose surface our little universe hangs quivering. Such a one is Sir Thomas Browne, a naturalist, a philosopher, a scholar, a physician, and a moralist, almost the last of the generation which produced Jeremy Taylor[173] and Shakespeare. No thinker bears stronger witness to the wandering and inventive curiosity of the age. No writer has better displayed the brilliant and sombre imagination of the North. No one has spoken with a more elegant emotion of death, the vast night of forgetfulness, of the all-devouring pit of human vanity which tries to create an immortality out of ephemeral glory or sculptured stones. No one has revealed in more glowing and original expressions the poetic sap which flows through all the minds of the age.[174]

The growing popularity of Browne's writings testifies to the assured position he holds, if not in the hearts of the many, at least in the hearts of that saving remnant which in each generation hands on the best traditions of our literature. We, who are members of his profession, may take a special pride in him. Among physicians, or teachers of physic, there is, perhaps, but one name in the very first rank. Rabelais[175] stands apart with the kings and queens of literature.

171. James Russell Lowell, *Among My Books* (Boston: Fields, Osgood, 1870), pp. 152–153.

172. Hippolyte Adolphe *Taine* (1828–1893): French philosopher and critic. Among his most notable works are *La Fontaine et ses fables* (1861), *Les Philosophes français du XIXe siècle* (1857), and *Histoire de la littérature anglaise* (1865).

173. Jeremy *Taylor* (1613–1667): English cleric and author of *The Golden Grove* (1655), *Liberty of Prophesying* (1646), and *The Rule and Exercises of Holy Living* (1650).

174. H. A. Taine, *History of English Literature*, trans. Henry van Laun (New York: The Colonial Press, 1900), vol. 1, pp. 252–253.

175. François *Rabelais* (c.1494–1553): French physician, better known as a humorist and satirist. He studied medicine at Montpellier and practiced in Lyons. He edited various medical treatises and wrote the novels *Pantagruel* (1533) and *Gargantua* (1535).

Among the princes of the blood there are differences of opinion as to rank, but Sir Thomas Browne, Holmes, and John Brown[176] of Edinburgh, form a group together high in the circle. Of the three, two were general practitioners; Oliver Wendell Holmes only in the early part of his life, and for forty years a teacher of anatomy; but all three have far closer ties with us than Goldsmith, Smollett, or Keats,[177] whose medical affiliations were titular rather than practical.

Burton, Browne, and Fuller[178] have much in common—a rare quaintness, a love of odd conceits, and the faculty of apt illustrations drawn from out-of-the-way sources. Like Montaigne's[179]—Burton's even more—Browne's bookishness is of a delightful kind, and yet, as he maintains, his best matter is not picked from the leaves of any author, but bred among the 'weeds and tares'[180] of his own brain. In his style there is a lack of what the moderns call technique, but how pleasant it is to follow his thoughts, rippling like a burn, not the stilted formality of the technical artist in words, the cadencies of whose precise and mechanical expressions pall on the ear.

As has been remarked, the *Religio Medici* is a *tour de force*,[181] an attempt to combine daring scepticism with humble faith in the Christian religion. Sir Thomas confesses himself to be 'naturally inclined to that which misguided zeal

176. *Holmes:* See p. 55, n. 170.

John *Brown* (1735–1788): Scottish physician and author of *Elementa Medicinæ* (1780). His Brunonian system of medicine held that many paradoxical symptoms were really evidence of debility that called for supportive treatment.

177. Oliver *Goldsmith* (1728–1774): Irish poet, playwright, and novelist, who wrote *The Vicar of Wakefield* (1766). He ran an unsuccessful medical practice in London, and was known as having been an apothecary's assistant and a poor physician (with a questionable foreign diploma).

Tobias George *Smollett* (1721–1771): Scottish novelist who gave up medicine to write novels, such as *The Expedition of Humphry Clinker* (1771).

John *Keats* (1795–1821): English poet. In 1810 Keats' guardian took him out of the school where he was studying literature to have him apprenticed with a surgeon in Edmonton for five years. He then took up medical studies at Guy's Hospital, London. In 1816 he passed his examinations but never practiced medicine.

178. *Burton:* See p. 35, n. 17.

Thomas *Fuller* (1608–1661): English cleric who preached sermons advocating the maintenance of peace between the king and parliament. Author of *History of the Holy Warre* (i.e., the Crusades, 1639), *The Holy State and Profane State* (1642), and *Worthies of England* (1662).

179. Michel Eyquem de *Montaigne* (1533–1592): French essayist. Author of *Essais* (the first two books were written between 1571–1580 and the third from 1585–1588), a work that exercised considerable influence on French and English literature. Osler lists Montaigne third in his "Bed-side Library for Medical Students."

180. *bred among the 'weeds and tares':* The quote from Walter Horatio Pater: See p. 000, n. 000. The word *tares* means a particular type of weeds found in grain fields, which are often injurious. *Religio Medici*, part 1, sect. 36, Keynes, vol. 1, p. 47.

181. *tour de force:* (French) a feat of unusual strength, skill, or ingenuity.

terms superstition.'[182] He 'cannot hear the Ave Maria bell without an elevation.'[183] He has no prejudices in religion, but subscribes himself a loyal son of the Church of England. In clear language he says, 'In brief, where the Scripture is silent the Church is my text; where that speaks it is but my comment. When there is a joint silence of both, I borrow not the rules of my religion from Rome or Geneva, but from the dictates of my own reason.'[184] He is hard on the controversialist in religion—'every man is not a proper champion for truth, nor fit to take up the gauntlet in the cause of verity,'[185] &c. While he disclaims any 'taint or tincture' of heresy,[186] he confesses to a number of heretical hopes, such as the ultimate salvation of the race, and the efficacy of prayers for the dead. He freely criticizes certain seeming absurdities in the Bible narrative. His travels have made him cosmopolitan and free from all national prejudices.

> I feel not in myself those common antipathies that I can discover in others, those national repugnancies do not touch me, nor do I behold with prejudice the French, Italian, Spaniard, or Dutch; but where I find their actions in balance with my countrymen's, I honour, love, and embrace them in the same degree. I was born in the eighth climate,[187] but seem for to be framed and constellated unto all. I am no plant that will not prosper out of a garden; all places, all airs, make unto me one country; I am in England, everywhere, and under any meridian.[188]

Only the 'fool multitude'[189] that chooses by show he holds up to derision as 'that numerous piece of monstrosity, which, taken asunder, seem men, and the reasonable creatures of God; but confused together, make but one great beast, and a monstrosity more prodigious than Hydra.'[190,191] He has a quick sympathy with the sorrows of others, and, though a physician, his prayer is with the hus-

---

182. *Religio Medici*, part 1, sect. 3, Keynes, vol. 1, p. 13.

183. Ibid. The *Ave Maria bell* tolls at six and twelve every day. When people hear the bell, they are supposed to pray to God.

184. *Religio Medici*, part 1, sect. 5, Keynes, vol. 1, p. 14.

185. *Religio Medici*, part 1, sect. 6, Keynes, vol. 1, p. 15.

186. Ibid. The exact quotation is: "By this means I leave no gap for Heresies, Schisms, or Errors, of which, at present, I hope I shall not inquire Truth to say, I have no taint or tincture."

187. Ibid. *The eighth climate* is England. "Climate" here refers to a zone between two parallels of latitude. Browne means that he comes from England, which lies in relatively high latitudes. The whole passage is quoted in "Chauvinism in Medicine," p. 227.

188. *Religio Medici*, part 2, sect. 1, Keynes, vol. 1, p. 70.

189. Shakespeare, *The Merchant of Venice*, II, ix, 26.

190. *Hydra:* The nine-headed serpent slain by Hercules. For further information, see "Chauvinism in Medicine," p. 234, n. 21.

191. *Religio Medici*, part 2, sect. 1, Keynes, vol. 1, p. 71.

bandman and for healthful seasons. No one has put more beautifully the feeling which each one of us has had at times about patients:

> Let me be sick myself, if sometimes the malady of my patient be not a disease unto me; I desire rather to cure his infirmities than my own necessities; where I do him no good, methinks it is scarce honest gain; though I confess 'tis but the worthy salary of our well-intended endeavours.[192]

He has seen many countries, and has studied their customs and politics. He is well versed in astronomy and botany. He has run through all systems of philosophy but has found no rest in any. As death gives every fool gratis the knowledge which is won in this life with sweat and vexation, he counts it absurd to take pride in his achievements, though he understands six languages besides the patois [193] of several provinces.[194]

As a scientific man Browne does not take rank with many of his contemporaries. He had a keen power of observation, and in the *Pseudodoxia* and in his letters there is abundant evidence that he was an able naturalist. He was the first to observe and describe the peculiar substance known as adipocere,[195] and there are in places shrewd flashes, such as the suggestion that the virus of rabies may be mitigated by transmission from one animal to another. But we miss in him the clear, dry light of science as revealed in the marvellous works of his contemporary, Harvey.[196] Busy as a practical physician, he was an observer, not an experimenter to any extent, though he urges: 'Join sense unto reason and experiment unto speculation, and so give life unto embryon truths and verities yet in their chaos.'[197] He had the highest veneration for Harvey, whose work he recognized as epoch making—'his piece, *De Circul. Sang.*,[198] which discovery I prefer to that of Columbus.'[199] He recognized that in the faculty of observation

192. *Religio Medici*, part 2, sect. 9, Keynes, vol. 1, p. 85.

193. *patois:* Dialects.

194. *Religio Medici*, part 2, sect. 8, Keynes, vol. 1, p. 82. Browne knew "six modern languages (French, Italian, Spanish, Portuguese, Dutch and Danish), not to mention Hebrew and especially Latin and Greek." C. A. Patrides, " 'Above Atlas His Shoulders': An Introduction to Sir Thomas Browne," in *Sir Thomas Browne: The Major Works* (London: Cox & Wyman, 1977), p. 33. Browne once wrote "On Languages, and Particularly the Saxon Tongue," printed in *Sir Thomas Browne's Works*, ed. S. Wilkin (London: William Pickering, 1835), vol. 4, pp. 195–212.

195. *adipocere:* A brown, waxlike substance formed in animal tissues that have been buried in a moist place.

196. *Harvey:* See p. 44, n. 90.

197. *Join sense unto reason and experiment unto speculation, and so give life unto embryon truths and verities yet in their chaos:* The quote has not been identified.

198. *The Circulation of the Blood.*

199. In a letter to Dr. Henry Power (1623–1668), dated to 1646 (Keynes, vol. 4, p. 255).

the old Greeks were our masters, and that we must return to their methods if progress were to be made. He had a much clearer idea than had Sydenham[200] of the value of anatomy, and tells his young friend, Power of Halifax,[201] to make *Autopsia*[202] *his fidus Achates.*[203]

That he should have believed in witches, and that he should have given evidence in 1664 which helped to condemn two poor women, is always spoken of as a blot on his character; but a man must be judged by his times and his surroundings.[204] While regretting his credulity, we must remember how hard it was in the sixteenth and seventeenth centuries not to believe in witches—how hard, indeed, it should be to-day for any one who believes implicitly the Old Testament!—and men of the stamp of Reginald Scot and Johannes Wierus,[205] who looked at the question from our point of view, were really anomalies, and their strong presentation of the rational side of the problem had very little influence on their contemporaries.

For the student of medicine the writings of Sir Thomas Browne have a very positive value. The charm of high thoughts clad in beautiful language may win some readers to a love of good literature; but beyond this is a still greater advantage. Like the 'Thoughts of Marcus Aurelius'[206] and the *Enchiridion* of Epictetus,[207] the *Religio* is full of counsels of perfection which appeal to the mind of

200. *Sydenham:* See p. 35, n. 12.

201. Henry *Power* (1623–1668): One of Browne's earliest correspondents who later became a noted physician at Halifax and a naturalist. Author of *Experimental Philosophy, in Three Books: Containing New Experiments Microscopical, Mercurial, Magnetical* (London: printed by T. Roycroft, for J. Martin and J. Allestry, 1664), the first work on microscopy published in England.

202. *Autopsia:* Autopsy.

203. *fidus Achates:* A devoted, trustworthy friend. *Achates* was the faithful comrade of Aeneas, the Trojan protagonist in Virgil's *Aeneid.* The phrase is from the letter to Dr. Henry Power dated to 1646 (Keynes, vol. 4, p. 225). The exact quotation is: "Lay your foundation in anatomy, wherein autopsia must be your fidus Achates" (*Aeneid,* book 1, line 188).

204. The original note at the end of this chapter reads: "The witches are now known to have been condemned in spite of, not with the help of, Browne's evidence."

205. Reginald Scot (c.1538–1599): English writer who argued against belief in witches. Author of *The Discovery of Witchcraft* (1584).

Johannes *Wierus* (also Johann *Weyer* or *Wyer*) (1515–1588): Dutch physician, sometimes called the founder of medical psychiatry. Author of *De praestigiis daemonum* (1563), in which "he maintained that witches were merely poor people who had lost control of their emotions and whose minds had become distorted" (Arturo Castiglioni, *A History of Medicine,* trans. E. B. Krumbhaar [New York: A. A. Knopf, 1941], pp. 498–499).

206. Osler refers to *The Meditations* by Marcus Aurelius.

207. Literally, a handbook written by Flavius Arrian, the historian of Alexander the Great, about the doctrines of his teacher, the eminent Stoic philosopher Epictetus's (c.60–140 A.D.). Epictetus' advice was that to lead a peaceful life one should endure and abstain and do good works (*Encyclopaedia Britannica*).

youth, still plastic and unhardened by contact with the world. Carefully studied, from such books come subtle influences which give stability to character and help to give a man a sane outlook on the complex problems of life. Sealed early of this tribe of authors, a student takes with him, as *compagnons de voyage,* life-long friends whose thoughts become his thoughts and whose ways become his ways. Mastery of self, conscientious devotion to duty, deep human interest in human beings—these best of all lessons you must learn now or never: and these are some of the lessons which may be gleaned from the life and from the writings of Sir Thomas Browne.

61

SIR THOMAS
BROWNE

4

THE OLD HUMANITIES
AND THE NEW SCIENCE

IN 1919, THE LAST YEAR of his life, Osler became president of the prestigious Classical Association of Oxford, where he delivered this address. The focus of his talk is that teachers of the humanities have largely ignored science and its advances. He argues that both science and the humanities would benefit from more interaction.

By analogy with the leavening that raises bread dough, Osler poses these questions: How can scientists be given the leaven of the humanities to prevent overspecialization and narrowness? How can the humanities be leavened with science? Osler urges that liberal education should contain more of both.

He recounts the rapid advances of science in his lifetime as "light triumphed over darkness." This period involved increasing humanistic concern and growing intellectual excitement, especially about the theory of evolution. Then World War I raised questions about whether science could rule without causing ruin.

Osler points out that Germany had not been saved in the war by its strong religion or its high levels of science, medicine, and the humanities. He attributes Germany's downfall to fantasies of wealth and power, which neither religion nor science managed to hold in check.

Given the changed social conditions seen by 1919, what was the role for scholars of the classical humanities? Osler compares them to the protected, well-cared-for larvae in a nest of ants. The nectar or hormones (that is, the humanities) that they secrete provides energy to the community. The humanities can bring people into contact with the master minds, especially the ancient Greeks, who formed the root of our civilization and its religions, philosophies, literature, our ideals of democratic freedom, the fine arts, and the fundamentals of science.

Osler chides Oxford for letting the humanities curriculum become stagnant. He particularly decries the lack of emphasis on the impact that science, especially evolution, has had on modern thought. Religion can be blamed for the divorce between science and the humanities. He also blames religion for the attitude that all important knowledge is known and only needs to be transmitted. Osler laments that students from areas other than literature and history are ignored at Oxford, and he urges the establishment of an Honour School for the study of the evolution of modern scientific thought. He argues that scientific and classical students both should go to primary sources and be taught the connection between the past and the present. He hopes that the two areas of study can be more compatible in the future.

Finally, Osler refers to the stories of the free cities of Greece to demonstrate how a love of a better way of life can exist in a democracy. He says that perceived conflicts between religious and democratic ideals can be resolved. He suggests that the solution to the longings of humanity lies in the combination of philanthropy with technical knowledge, and he concludes by adding that it also lies in joy in working as prescribed by Hippocrates.

THE OLD HUMANITIES & THE NEW SCIENCE

I

ARLY IN THE SIXTEENTH CENTURY a literary joke sent inextinguishable laughter[1] through the learned circles of Europe. The *Epistolae Obscurorum* Virorum[2] is great literature, to which I refer for two reasons— its standard is an exact gauge of my scholarship, and had *Magister Nostrandus Ortuinus Gratius*[3] of Cologne, to whom most of the letters are addressed, been asked to join that wicked Erfurt Circle,[4] he could not have been more surprised than I was to receive a gracious invitation to preside over this gathering of British scholars. I felt to have been sailing under false colours to have ever, by pen or tongue, suggested the possession of even the traditional small Latin and less Greek.[5] Relieved by the assurance that in alternate years

The presidential address delivered before the Classical Association at Oxford, May 16, 1919. Printed in the *British Medical Journal*, ii, 1919. Reprinted in London, 1919; Boston, 1920, with an introduction by Harvey Cushing.

1. *inextinguishable laughter:* Homer, *Iliad*, book 1, lines 599–600. The gods are at a banquet and have begun to quarrel over how the Trojan War is going; and Hephaestus reminds them how Zeus once before got angry and threw him out of heaven and so lamed him. Then Hephaestus hobbles around refilling all the others' cups, and he looks so funny that the other gods cannot stop laughing at him and all make peace.

2. A satirical humanist work published in 1515–1517, consisting of an anonymous collection of letters in medieval Latin purporting to be written by various bachelors and masters in theology, in which they incidentally expose themselves to ridicule. The letters were attributed principally to Ulrich von Hutten (1488–1523), humanist and supporter of Luther. The English title of the work is *Epistles of Obscure Men*.

3. *Ortuinus Gratius* (c.1480–1542): A famous opponent of the new learning and the alleged addressee of the *Epistolae Obscurorum Virorum*.

4. The circle of Humanists who composed the *Epistolae*.

5. *small Latin and less Greek:* Ben Jonson, "To the Memory of My Beloved, the Author Mr. William Shakespeare: And What He Hath Left Us," line 31.

the qualification of your President was an interest in education and literature, I gladly accepted, not, however, without such anticipatory qualms as afflict an amateur at the thought of addressing a body of experts. Not an educated man in the Oxford sense, yet faint memories of the classics linger—the result of ten years of such study as lads of my generation pursued, memories best expressed in Tom Hood's lines:

> The weary tasks I used to con!
> The hopeless leaves I wept upon!
> Most fruitless leaves to me![6]

In a life of teaching and practice, a mere picker-up of learning's crumbs[7] is made to realize the value of the humanities in science not less than in general culture.

To have a Professor of Medicine in this Chair gives to the Oxford meeting an appropriate Renaissance—shall we say medieval?—flavour, and one may be pardoned the regret that the meeting is not being held in May 1519, to have had the pleasure of listening to an address from a real Oxford scholar-physician,[8] an early teacher of Greek in this University, and the founder of the Royal College of Physicians, whose *Rudimenta Grammatices*[9] and *De Emendata Structura Latini Sermonis*[10] upheld for a generation, on the Continent at least, the reputation of English scholarship. These noble walls, themselves an audience—indeed, most appreciative of audiences—have storied memories of Linacre's voice, and the basis of the keen judgement of Erasmus[11] may have been formed by intercourse with him in this very school. In those happy days, to know Hippocrates[12]

6. Thomas Hood, "Ode on a Distant Prospect of Clapham Academy," lines 16–18.

7. *picker-up of learning's crumbs:* Robert Browning, "An Epistle," line 1. Browning in turn was thinking of Matthew 15:27 and Mark 7:28, where the Syro-Phoenician woman begging for Jesus' help compares herself to a dog eating the crumbs that fall from its master's table.

8. Thomas *Linacre* (c.1460–1524): English physician and classical scholar. At Oxford he prepared translations of Galen's work from the original Greek. He served as the attending physician for Henry VIII, and was the founder and first president of the Royal College of Physicians of London. He is one of three famous older physicians whom Osler greatly admired. For further information, see "The Master-Word in Medicine," p. 265, n. 63.

9. *Rudimenta Grammatices* (The Rudiments of Grammar) (c.1523).

10. *De Emendata Structura Latini Sermonis* (On the Corrected Structure of Latin Speech) (1524).

11. Desiderius *Erasmus* (c.1467–1536): Dutch humanist, theologian, and satirist who was regarded as a leader of learning in northern Europe during the Renaissance. He criticized the clergy for their lack of study and teaching. He aimed at reform, but within the Roman Catholic Church. He is known as the author of *Encomium Moriæ* (Praise of Folly).

12. *Hippocrates* (c.460–c.375 B.C.): Greek physician. For further information, see "The Master-Word in Medicine," p. 274, n. 108.

Claudius *Galen* (c.130–c.200): Greek physician. For further information, see "Teaching and Thinking," pp. 181–182, n. 27.

and Galen was to know disease and to be qualified to practise; and my profession looks back in grateful admiration to such great medical humanists as Linacre and Caius and Rabelais.[13] Nor can I claim to speak for pure science, some salt of which remains from early association, and from a lifelong attempt to correlate with art a science which makes medicine, I was going to say the only—but it is more civil to say the most—progressive of the learned professions.

To have lived right through an epoch matched only by two in the story of the race,[14] to have shared in its long struggle, to have witnessed its final victory (and in my own case, to be left, I trust, with wit enough to realize its significance)—to have done this has been a wonderful privilege. To have outgrown age-old theories of man and of nature, to have seen West separated from East[15] in the tangled skein of human thought, to have lived in a world re-making— these are among the thrills and triumphs of the Victorian of my generation. To a childhood and youth came echoes of the controversy that Aristarchus[16] began, Copernicus continued, and Darwin ended, that put the microcosm into line with the macrocosm, and for the golden age of Eden substituted the *tellus dura*[17] of Lucretius.[18] Think of the Cimmerian darkness[19] out of which our generation has, at any rate, blazed a path! Picture the mental state of a community which could produce *Omphalos*[20]—*an attempt to untie the geological knot!*[21] I heard warm

13. John *Caius* (1510–1573): See "Sir Thomas Browne," p. 38, n. 42.

François *Rabelais* (c.1494–1553): See "Sir Thomas Browne," p. 56, n. 175.

14. *two in the story of the race:* The classical period and the Renaissance.

15. Osler is implying that the rise of scientific thought has sundered the Western from the Eastern world. Perhaps compare for this attitude Rudyard Kipling's "The Ballad of East and West," which begins, "Oh, East is East, and West is West, and never the twain shall meet."

16. *Aristarchus* of Samos (late 3rd cent. B.C.): Greek astronomer. He was the first to maintain that the earth rotates on its own axis and revolves around the sun.

17. *tellus dura:* (Latin) "hard earth," from Lucretius' *De Rerum Natura* 5, line 926. Osler is referring to the difference between the paradise of the biblical Eden and the hard world of Lucretius' early human beings.

18. Titus *Lucretius* Carus (c.96–55 B.C.): See p. 86, n. 155.

19. *the Cimmerian darkness:* Intense utter darkness, where the Cimmerians, a mythical people in the Homeric poems, were believed to dwell, in the far west where the sun never shone. Homer, *Odyssey,* book 11, lines 13–19. Osler, however, was more likely thinking of John Milton's "L'Allegro," line 10: "In dark Cimmerian desert ever dwell."

20. *Omphalos:* (Greek) navel. The word alludes to the question of whether Adam had had one, because he was not born from a woman's womb like all later men, but was created directly by God as a fullgrown adult. This question was debated quite seriously by older Christian thinkers such as Sir Thomas Browne.

21. Osler's original note reads: "By the well-known naturalist, Philip Henry Gosse."

Philip Henry *Gosse* (1810–1888) was a pioneer collector and a student of marine specimens and fossils, as well as a minister of the Plymouth Brethren, a puritanical and fundamentalist sect. His book *Omphalos* (1857) was an attempt to reconcile his studies with his beliefs. Gosse accepted the argument that, as the prototype of humanity, Adam must have looked like all other men, despite his unique origin. He then

clerical discussions on its main thesis, that the fossils were put into the earth's strata to test man's faith in the Mosaic account of the creation, and our Professor of Natural Theology[22] lectured seriously upon it! The intellectual unrest of those days wrapped many in that 'divyne cloude of unknowynge',[23] by which happy phrase Brother Herp[24] designates medieval mysticism; and not a bad thing for a young man to live through, as sufficient infection usually remains to enable him to understand, if not to sympathize with, mental states alien or even hostile.

An Age of Force followed the final subjugation of Nature. The dynamo replaced the steam-engine, radiant energy revealed the hidden secrets of matter, to the conquest of the earth was added the control of the air and the mastery of the deep. Nor was it only an age of Force. Never before had man done so much for his brother, the victory over the powers of Nature meant also glorious victories of peace; pestilences were checked, the cry of the poor became articulate, and to help the life of the submerged half became the sacred duty of the other. How full we were of the pride of life![25] In 1910 at Edinburgh I ended an address on 'Man's Redemption of Man' with the well-known lines of Shelley beginning 'Happiness and Science dawn though late upon the earth.'[26] And now! having survived the greatest war in history,[27] and a great victory, with the wreckage of medieval autonomy to clear up, our fears are lest we may fail to control the fretful forces of Caliban,[28] and our hopes are to rebuild Jerusalem in this green and pleasant land.[29]

---

tried to apply this argument to the world, arguing that God brought it into existence when the Bible said he did (the date was generally calculated as 4004 B.C.) but with as it were a built-in past, looking and functioning as if it had already existed for millions of years. His book was derided from all sides. Osler's account of Gosse's reasoning seems to be based on hostile reviews at the time.

22. *our Professor of Natural Theology:* James Bovell (1817–1880), who was the professor of natural theology, physiology, and chemistry at Trinity College in Osler's time. He taught physiology based on his *Outlines of Natural Theology* (1859). Osler greatly admires him, but here he disparages his opinions rather than his person. For biographical information on Bovell, see "The Master-Word in Medicine," p. 258, n. 17.

23. "The Divine Cloud of Unknowing" is a fourteenth-century Middle English religious mystical treatise on what separates man from a full understanding of God. The author of this work maintained that "unknowing" was a stage one had to pass through to attain knowledge of God.

24. Henricus *Harphius* (also De *Herp* or *Erp*) (c.1400–1478): Author of *Directorium aureum contemplationum,* which includes "the divyne cloude of unknowynge."

25. *the pride of life:* 1 John 2:16.

26. Percy Bysshe Shelley, "The Daemon of the World," line 461.

27. World War I (1914–1918).

28. *Caliban:* A character Shakespeare's *The Tempest* who is a subhuman, half-savage creature, son of the witch Sycorax, who is the slave of Prospero. He enters into an unsuccessful conspiracy to kill his master.

29. *rebuild Jerusalem* (Ezekiel 36:28): A symbol for the ideal capital for the people and the kingdom of God. William Blake, "Milton," line 16. The original quotation is:

Never before in its long evolution has the race realized its full capacity. Our fathers have told us, and we ourselves have known, of glorious sacrifices; but the past four years have exhausted in every direction the possibilities of human effort. And, as usual, among the nations the chief burden has fallen on that weary Titan, the Motherland,

> Bearing on shoulders immense,
> Atlantean, the load,
> Wellnigh not to be borne,
> Of the too vast orb of her fate.[30]

Not alone did she furnish the sinews of war, but she developed a spirit that made defeat impossible.

No wonder war has advocates, to plead the heroic clash of ideals, the purging of a nation's dross in the fire of suffering and sacrifice, and the welding in one great purpose of a scattered people. Even Montaigne, sanest of men, called it 'the greatest and most magnificent of human actions,'[31] and the glamours of its pride, pomp, and circumstance[32] still captivate. But there are other sides which we should face without shrinking. Why dwell on the horrors such as we doctors and nurses have had to see? Enough to say that war blasts the soul, and in this great conflict the finer sense of humanity has been shocked to paralysis by the helplessness of our civilization and the futility of our religion to stem a wave of primitive barbarism. Black as are the written and unwritten pages of history, the concentrated and prolonged martyrdom surpasses anything man has yet had to endure. What a shock to the proud and mealy-mouthed[33] Victorian who had begun to trust that Love was creation's final law,[34] forgetting that Egypt and Babylon are our contemporaries and of yesterday in comparison with the hundreds of thousands of years since the cave-dwellers left their records on

---

Till we have built Jerusalem

In England's green and pleasant land.

30. Matthew Arnold, "Heine's Grave," lines 93–96. Atlas, condemned by Zeus, had to carry the globe on his shoulders because he took part in the rebellion of the Titans.

31. Michel Eyquem de *Montaigne* (1533–1592): See "Sir Thomas Browne," p. 57, n. 179.

32. William Shakespeare, *Othello,* III, iii, 354.

33. *mealy-mouthed:* Afraid to speak one's mind or use plain terms.

34. *Love was creation's final law:* The passage is reminiscent of the lines of a poem by Alfred Tennyson, "In Memoriam A.H.H.," part 126, stanzas 2–30. The exact quotation is:

"Love is and was my King and Lord,

And will be, tho' as yet I keep

Within his court on earth, and sleep

Encompass'd by his faithful guard.

This sentiment was common among Victorian writers.

walls and bones. In the mystic shadow of the Golden Bough,[35] and swayed by the emotions of our savage ancestors, we stand aghast at the revelation of the depth and ferocity of primal passions which reveal the unchangeableness of human nature.

When the wild beast of Plato's dream[36] becomes a waking reality, and a herd-emotion of hate sweeps a nation off its feet, the desolation that follows is wider than that in France and Belgium, wider even than the desolation of grief, and something worse—the hardened heart, the lie in the soul[37]—so graphically described in Book II of the *Republic*—that forces us to do accursed things, and even to defend them! I refer to it because, as professors, we have been accused of sinning against the light.[38] Of course we have. Over us, too, the wave swept, but I protest against the selection of us for special blame. The other day, in an address on 'The Comradeship of Letters' at Turin, President Wilson is reported to have said: 'It is one of the great griefs of this war that the universities of the Central Empires used the thoughts of science to destroy mankind; it is the duty of the universities of these states to redeem science from this disgrace, and to show that the pulse of humanity beats in the classroom, and that there are sought out not the secrets of death but the secrets of life.'[39] A pious and worthy wish! but once in war a nation mobilizes every energy, and to say that science has been prostituted in discovering means of butchery is to misunderstand the situation. Slaughter, wholesale and unrestricted, is what is sought, and to accomplish this the discoveries of the sainted Faraday[40] and of the gentle Dalton[41] are utilized to the full, and to their several nations scientific men render this service freely,

35. A branch of mistletoe, which in mythology served as a pass to the underworld. James George Frazer, an English anthropologist, wrote *The Golden Bough* (1890–1915), a comparative study of the folklore, mythology, and religion of mankind. His work deals with the history of supernatural beliefs and symbolic rituals.

36. Plato, *Republic,* book 9, 571c. "The wild beast" represents uncontrolled human appetites and passions.

37. *the hardened heart, the lie in the soul:* Plato, *Republic,* book 2, 382.

38. The *light* means the truth. It is also commonly used in reference to the word of God and in reference to Jesus Christ as the light of the world, as in John 3:19. The exact quotation is: "And this is the condemnation, that light is come into the world, and men loved darkness rather than light, because their deeds were evil."

Sinning against the light is a common and longstanding idiom, in which the light may be taken as either that of divine revelation or inspiration or that of the natural understanding.

39. Woodrow *Wilson* (1856–1924): Twenty-eighth President of the United States (1913–1921). The quote is from his address on "The Comradeship of Letters" at Turin.

40. Michael *Faraday* (1791–1867): English chemist and physicist who contributed to the study of electricity and magnetism. A deeply religious man, he was a member of the Sandemanian sect.

41. John *Dalton* (1766–1844): English physicist and chemist, noted for his formulation of the atomic theory. He was also considered a natural philosopher.

if not gladly. That the mental attitude engendered by science is apt to lead to a gross materialism is a vulgar error! Scientific men, in mufti[42] or in uniform, are not more brutal than their fellows, and the utilization of their discoveries in warfare should not be a greater reproach to them than is our joyous acceptance of their success.

What a change of heart after the appalling experience of the first gassing in 1915! Nothing more piteously horrible than the sufferings of the victims has ever been seen in warfare.[43] Surely we could not sink to such barbarity! Is thy servant a dog?[44] But martial expediency soon compelled the Allies to enlist the resources of chemistry; the instruction of our enemies was soon bettered, and before the armistice there were developments in technique and destructive force that would have delighted Nisroch,[45] who first invented aerial 'machinations to plague the sons of men.'[46] A group of medical men representing the chief universities and medical bodies of the United Kingdom was innocent enough to suggest that such an unclean weapon—the use of lethal gases, 'condemning its victims to death by long-drawn-out torture,' and with infinite possibilities for its further development—should be for ever abolished. 'Steeped in folly by theories and prepossessions,' failure to read the 'lessons of war which should have sufficed to convince a beetle'—such were among the newspaper comments; and in other ways we were given to understand that our interference in such matters was most untimely. All the same, it is gratifying to see that the suggestion has been adopted at the Peace Congress.

With what a howl of righteous indignation the slaughter of our innocent women and children by the bombing of open towns was received. It was a dirty

42. *in mufti:* In plain clothes, not in uniform; the word is of Anglo-Indian origin.

43. As Osler mentioned, poison gas was first used in warfare by the Germans in 1915. Osler's original note reads: "I am sorry to have seen Sargent's picture, 'Gassed,' in this year's Academy. It haunts the mind like a nightmare."

John Singer *Sargent* (1856–1925) is mainly known for his portraits as well as for his sunlit landscapes. The painting Osler refers to is a twenty-foot-long oil on canvas depicting "gassed and blindfolded soldiers" being led to a dressing station after an attack of poison gas (1918–1919).

44. A modification of the Bible, 2 Kings 8:13. The exact quotation is: "And Hazael said, But what, *is* thy servant a dog, that he should do this great thing?" Elisha has been ordered by God to anoint Hazael and reveal to him that he will become king of Syria; but the prophet weeps, foreseeing the atrocities that Hazael will commit against the Israelites. Hazael protests that he is not so base as to do such things; yet when the time comes, he does.

45. *Nisroch:* The Assyrian god in whose temple King Sennacherib (705–681 B.C.) was worshipping when he was slain (2 Kings 19:37). Perhaps Osler believed the Assyrians were the first people to employ catapults and similar machines in warfare, and fancifully attributed the idea to the promptings of their national god.

46. John Milton, *Paradise Lost*, book 6, lines 504–505.

and bloody business, worthy of the Oxydracians,[47] who by means of Levin-bolts[48] and Thunders[49] more horrible, more frightful, more diabolical, maiming, breaking, tearing, and slaying more folk, confounded men's senses and threw down more walls than would a hundred thunderbolts (Rabelais, Bk. IV, ch. 1xi).

Against reprisals there was at first a strong feeling. Early in 1916 I wrote to *The Times:*

> The cry for reprisals illustrates the exquisitely hellish state of mind into which war plunges even sensible men. Not a pacifist, but a 'last ditcher,'[50] yet I refuse to believe that as a nation, how bitter soever the provocation, we shall stain our hands in the blood of the innocent. In this matter let us be free from bloodguiltiness, and let not the undying reproach of humanity rest on us as on the Germans.

Two years changed me into an ordinary barbarian. A detailed tally of civilians killed by our airmen has not, I believe, been published, but the total figures quoted are not far behind the German. Could a poll have been taken a week before the armistice as to the moral justification of the bombing of Berlin—for which we were ready—how we should have howled at the proposer of any doubt. And many Jonahs[51] were displeased that a city greater than Nineveh,[52] with more than the three score and ten thousand who knew not the right hand from the left, had been spared.[53] We may deplore the necessity and lament, as did a certain great personage:[54]

yet public reason just—
Honour and empire with revenge enlarged

47. The people in *Pantagruel* (1533) by François Rabelais, (book 4, chap. 61), who use the unprecedent-edly effective instruments of destruction and war invented by the character Gaster to destroy their enemies.

48. *Levin-bolts:* Lightning bolts.

49. *Thunders:* One of the means of destruction devised by Gaster in Rabelais's account.

50. *last ditcher:* Someone willing to fight to the last extremity, to defend to the death the last bit of trench that the enemy has not taken. The *OED* attributes the phrase "to die in the last ditch" to Gilbert Burnet, Bishop of Salisbury (1643–1715), in his *History of His Own Times,* vol. 1, p. 457; but it was probably a soldiers' idiom already in use in his time.

51. *Jonah:* Hebrew prophet who was angry with God because he relented and spared Nineveh when the people repented, thereby discrediting the prediction that he had ordered Jonah to make (Jonah 4).

52. *Nineveh:* Capital of ancient Assyria.

53. *a city greater than Nineveh, with more than the three score and ten thousand who knew not the right hand from the left, had been spared:* Osler paraphrased Jonah: 4:11. The original reads: "And should not I spare Nineveh, that great city, wherein are more than sixscore thousand persons that cannot discern between their right hand and their left hand; *and* also much cattle?"

54. *a certain great personage:* Satan.

>   . . . compels me now
> To do what else, though damned, I should abhor.[55]

All the same, we considered ourselves 'Christians of the best edition, all picked and culled,'[56] and the churches remained open, prayers rose to Jehovah, many of whose priests—even His bishops!—were in khaki,[57] and quit themselves like men[58]—yes, and scores died the death of heroes! Into such hells of inconsistency does war plunge the best of us!

Learning—new or old—seems a vain thing to save a nation, but possibly as a set-off science, as represented by cellulose and sulphuric acid, may yet prove the best bulwark of civilization. In his *History of the Origin of Medicine* (1778, p. 30) Lettsom[59] maintains that the invention of firearms has done more to prevent the destruction of the human species than any other discovery. He says: 'Invention and discernment of mind have made it possible to reverse the ancient maxim that strength has always prevailed over wisdom.'[60] Science alone may prevent a repetition of the story of Egypt, of Babylonia, of Greece, and of Rome. The suggestion seems brazen effrontery when we have not even given the world the equivalent of the Pax Romana.[61] Ah! what a picture of self-satisfied happiness in Plutarch![62] One envies that placid life in the midst of the only great peace the world has known, spanning a period of more than two hundred years. And he could say, 'No tumults, no civil sedition, no tyrannies, no pestilences nor calamities depopulating Greece, no epidemic disease needing powerful and choice drugs and medicines,'[63] though as a Delphic priest[64] there is a pathetic la-

55. John Milton, *Paradise Lost*, book 4, lines 389–392.

56. François Rabelais, *Gargantua et Pantagruel*, book 4, chap. 50, trans. Peter Anthony Motteux (Chicago: Encyclopaedia Britannica, 1952), p. 292.

57. *in khaki:* In uniform, therefore enlisted in the forces.

58. *quit themselves like men:* The phrase is a reminiscence of 1 Samuel 4:9. The original reads: "Be strong, and quit yourselves like men . . . and fight." (Also, 1 Corinthians 16:13).

59. John Coakley *Lettsom* (1744–1815): English physician who supported Jenner on vaccination, pioneered a study on drug addiction, and made the first description of neuritis.

60. *History of the Origin of Medicine: An Oration:* Speech delivered at the anniversary meeting of the Medical Society of London, January 19, 1778.

61. The *Pax Romana:* (Latin) the peace that prevailed between the peoples making up the Roman Empire. Osler's point is that the Romans succeeded in imposing peace throughout the Western civilized world, and the modern civilization in his time had failed to do the same. Seneca, *De Clementia* (On Clemency), book 1, chap. 4, sect. 2.

62. *Plutarch* (c.46–c.125): Greek biographer, known for his works *Moralia* and *Parallel Lives*. Osler lists Montaigne third and Plutarch fourth in his "Bed-Side Library for Medical Students."

63. Plutarch, *Moralia: On Moral Virtues*, 186e, trans. William W. Goodwin (Boston: Little Brown, 1874), vol. 3, p. 100.

64. *a Delphic priest:* Osler refers to Plutarch, who was an honorary member of the college of priests at Delphi.

ment that the Pythian priestess[65] has now only commonplace questions to deal with.[66] Surely those cultivated men of his circle must have felt that their house could never be removed. Has Science reached such control over Nature that she will enable our civilization to escape the law of the Ephesian,[67] written on all known records—*panta rei?*[68] Perhaps so, now that material civilization is worldwide, cataclysmic forces, powerful enough in centres of origin, may weaken as they pass out in circles. Let this be our hope in the present crisis. At any rate, in the free democracies in which Demos[69] with safety says *L'État c'est moi,*[70] it has yet to be determined whether Science, as the embodiment of a mechanical force, can rule without invoking ruin. Two things are clear: there must be a very different civilization or there will be no civilization at all; and the other is that neither the old religion combined with the old learning, nor both with the new science, suffice to save a nation bent on self-destruction. The suicide of Germany, the outstanding fact of the war, followed an outburst of national megalomania.[71] For she had religion—it may shock some of you to hear! I mean the people, not the writers or the thinkers, but the people for whom Luther[72] lived and Huss[73] died. Of the two devotional ceremonies which stand supreme in my memory one was a service in the Dom, Berlin, in which 'not the great nor well bespoke, but the mere uncounted folk'[74] sang Luther's great hymn,[75] *Ein' feste Burg ist unser Gott.*[76] With the Humanities Germany never broke, and the proportion of students in her schools and universities who studied Greek and Latin has been

65. *Pythian priestess:* Priestess of Delphi in ancient Greece who delivered the oracles of Apollo.

66. Osler's original note reads: "Why the Pythian priestess, &c. (Plutarch's *Morals,* vol. iii, p. 100, Goodwin's edition.)"

67. *the Ephesian:* Refers to Heraclitus (c.540–c.470 B.C.), who was a citizen of Ephesus. The *law of the Ephesian* is the aphorism that follows, *panta rei.* For further information, see "The Student Life," p. 321, n. 79.

68. *panta rei* (properly spelled *rhei*): (Greek) "all things are in a state of flux." Attributed by Aristotle to Heraclitus.

69. *Demos:* The word means the common people in ancient Greece, but Osler is not restricting his reference to the ancient Greeks.

70. A phrase spoken by Louis XIV (1638–1715), King of France, which means "I am the state."

71. *megalomania:* A psychosis characterized by delusions of greatness.

72. Martin *Luther* (1483–1546): German leader of the Protestant Reformation.

73. John *Huss* (c.1369–1415): Bohemian religious reformer and martyr who was burned as a heretic.

74. *not the great nor well bespoke, but the mere uncounted folk:* The quote has not been identified.

75. *Luther's great hymn:* This hymn is based on Psalm 46. The two well-known English versions are Thomas Carlyle's, beginning "A safe stronghold our God is still," and that of Frederic Henry Hedge, beginning "A mighty fortress is our God." Music to this hymn was arranged by Johann Sebastian Bach (1685–1750).

76. Osler's original note reads: "And the other, how different! The crowded Blue Mosque of Cairo, and the crowded streets with the thousands of kneeling Moslems awaiting the cry of the Muezzin from the tower."

higher than in any other country. You know better than I the innumerable classical studies of her scholars. In classical learning relating to science and medicine she simply had the field, for one scholar in other countries she had a dozen, and the monopoly of journals relating to the history of these subjects. And she had science, and led the world in the application of the products of the laboratory to the uses of everyday life—in commerce, in the Arts, and in war. Withal, like Jeshurun,[77] she waxed fat;[78] and did ever such pride go before such destruction![79] What a tragedy that the successors of Virchow and Traube and Helmholtz and Billroth [80] should have made her a byword among the nations! 'Lilies that fester smell far worse than weeds.'[81]

II

So much preliminary to the business before us, to meet changed conditions as practical men, with the reinforcement born of hope or with the strong resolution of despair.

For what does this Classical Association stand? What are these classical interests that you represent? Take a familiar simile. By a very simple trick, you remember, did Empedocles [82] give Menippus in the moon-halt [83]—the first stage

77. *Jeshurun:* Another name for Israel.

78. *she waxed fat:* The song of Moses (Deuteronomy 32:15). The exact quotation is: "But Jeshurun waxed fat, and kicked . . . then he forsook God *which* made him, and lightly esteemed the Rock of his salvation."

79. *pride go before such destruction:* Proverbs 16:18. Osler's point is that pride led the Germans to disaster just as it had the ancient Israelites.

80. Rudolf L. K.*Virchow* (1821–1902): German father of pathology and professor of pathological anatomy in Würzburg and Berlin. He carried out research on blood (leukemia, etc.), phlebitis, tuberculosis, etc. He was very influential in the field of public health, making sanitary reforms in Berlin (the establishment of sewers). He was also a political leader who was elected to parliament and opposed Bismarck.

Ludwig *Traube* (1818–1876): German clinician and pathologist, known for his Traube's curves, membrane, space, etc. He promoted use of percussion and auscultation and of thermometry in physical diagnosis. He was working in the Royal Charité when Osler studied in Berlin.

Herman Ludwig Ferdinand von *Helmholtz* (1821–1894): German physicist, anatomist, and physiologist known for numerous contributions, including work in areas of physics closely related to physiology, especially acoustics and optics. Helmholtz frequently wrote about the conditions for scientific research in Germany, especially his "On Academic Freedom in German Universities" in *Popular Lectures on Scientific Subjects,* 2nd series, trans. E. Atkinson, (New York: D. Appleton, 1881). He was teaching in the Royal Charité when Osler was in Berlin in 1873.

Christian A. T. *Billroth* (1824–1894): Austrian surgeon, known for his Billroth's disease, mixture, operation, strands, suture, etc. Osler visited him in Vienna in 1874.

81. William Shakespeare, "Sonnet 94," line 14.

82. *Empedocles* (c.495–c.435 B.C.): Greek philosopher and poet. See "Physic and Physicians as Depicted in Plato," p. 127, n. 3.

83. Empedocles shows Menippus, a cynic philosopher, the whole world from the moon. Lucian, "Icaro-

of his memorable trip—such long and clear vision that he saw the tribes of men like a nest of ants, a seething mass going to and fro at their different tasks.[84] Of the function of the classical members in this myrmecic[85] community there can be no question. Neither warriors, nor slaves, nor neuters, you live in a well-protected social environment, heretofore free from enemies, and have been well taken care of. I hate to speak of you as larvae, but as such you perform a duty of the greatest importance in this trophidium[86] stage of your existence. Let me explain. From earliest days much attention has been paid by naturalists to the incredible affection—'incredible στοργή,'[87] Swammerdam[88] calls it—which ants display in feeding, licking, and attending the larvae. Disturb a nest, and the chief care is to take them to a place of safety. This attention is what our symphilic community—to use a biological term—bestows on you. So intensely altruistic, apparently, is this behaviour, that for the very word στοργή, which expresses the tenderest of all feelings, there is a difficulty in finding an equivalent; indeed, Gilbert White[89] used it almost as an English word. The truth is really very different. It has been shown that the nursing function—or instinct—is really trophallactic.[90] In the case of the ant the nurse places the larva on its back, and the broad ventral surface serves as a trough for the food, often predigested. The skill and devotion with which this is done are among the wonders in the life of the insect to which moralists have never tired of urging a visit. But listen to the sequel! The larva is provided with a pair of rich honey-bags in the shape of salivary glands, big exudatoria from which is discharged an ambrosia greedily lapped up by the nurse, who with this considers herself well paid for her care. In the same manner, when the assiduous V.A.D.[91] wasp distributes food to the larvae, the heads of which

---

menippus," sects. 13–14, in *Lucian*, trans. A. M. Harmon (London: Heinemann, 1913), vol. 2, pp. 289–323.

84. Ibid., p. 301, where Menippus compares the people he sees to a nest of ants.

85. *myrmecic:* Ant-like.

86. *trophidium:* The Greek element "troph," used to form compound words, means "nourishment." The "trophidium stage" is presumably the nurturing stage; Osler may have intended it to mean "cocoon," in which a larva lies encased while it feeds and grows.

87. στοργή: (Greek) (Storgê) the kind of love or affection instinctively felt for one's kindred, as between parents and children.

88. Jan *Swammerdam* (1637–1680): Dutch anatomist and entomologist who was a pioneer in microscopic studies and gave the first description of red blood corpuscles. He also studied the morphology and metamorphosis of insects. He wrote *History of Insects* (1685), and his descriptions and drawings were published by Hermann Boerhaave as *Biblia Naturae* (1737–1738) after his death.

89. Gilbert *White* (1720–1793): See "A Way of Life," p. 6, n. 17.

90. *trophallactic:* Characteristic of the mutual exchange of food material or other secretions between adult insects and larvae.

91. V.A.D. (Voluntary Aid Detachment) was a voluntary aid organization of women who nursed wounded

eagerly protrude from their cells, she must be paid by a draught of nectar from their exudatoria, while if it is not forthcoming the wasp seizes the head of the larva in her mandibles and jams it back into its cell and compels it to pay up. The lazy males will play the same game and even steal the much sought liquid without any compensatory gift of nourishment.[92]

What does the community at large, so careful of your comforts, expect from you? Surely the honey-dew and the milk of paradise[93] secreted from your classical exudatoria, which we lap up greedily in recensions, monographs, commentaries, histories, translations, and brochures. Among academic larvae you have for centuries absorbed the almost undivided interest of the nest, and not without reason, for the very life of the workers depends on the hormones you secrete. Though small in number, your group has an enormous kinetic value, like our endocrine organs. For man's body, too, is a humming hive of working cells, each with its specific function, all under central control of the brain and heart, and all dependent on materials called hormones (secreted by small, even insignificant-looking structures) which lubricate the wheels of life. For example, remove the thyroid gland just below the Adam's apple, and you deprive man of the lubricants which enable his thought-engines to work—it is as if you cut off the oil-supply of a motor—and gradually the stored acquisitions of his mind cease to be available, and within a year he sinks into dementia. The normal processes of the skin cease, the hair falls, the features bloat, and the paragon of animals is transformed into a shapeless caricature of humanity. These essential lubricators, of which a number are now known, are called hormones—you will recognize from its derivation how appropriate is the term.[94]

Now, the men of your guild secrete materials which do for society at large what the thyroid gland does for the individual. The Humanities are the hormones. Our friend Mr. P. S. Allen[95] read before this Association a most suggestive paper on the historical evolution of the word Humanism. I like to think of the pleasant-flavoured word as embracing all the knowledge of the ancient

---

soldiers during the First World War. Osler's idea is that the v.a.d. nurses handed out supplies in the same manner as the female wasp hands out food.

92. Osler's original note reads: "Professor Wheeler in *Proceedings of Amer. Phil. Soc.*, vol. lvii, No. 4, 1918." Benjamin Ide *Wheeler* (1854–1927): Professor of classical and comparative philology at Cornell University. He became president of the University of California in 1899.

93. *the honey-dew and the milk of paradise:* The phrase echoes "Kubla Khan," lines 53–54, by Samuel Taylor Coleridge. The exact lines read:

> For he on honey-dew hath fed,
> And drunk the milk of Paradise.

94. The Greek word *hormôn* means "setting in motion, exciting, and stimulating."

95. Percy Stafford *Allen* (1869–1933): Erasmian scholar and president of Corpus Christi College, Oxford.

classical world—what man knew of Nature as well as what he knew of himself. Let us see what this University means by the *Literae Humaniores*.[96] The 'Greats' papers [97] for the past decade make interesting study. With singular uniformity there is diversity enough to bear high tribute to the ingenuity of the examiners. But comparing the subjects in 1918 with those in the first printed papers of the School in 1831, one is surprised to find them the same—practically no change in the eighty-seven years! Compare them, again, with the subjects given in John Napleton's [98] *Considerations*, 1773—no change! and with the help of Rashdall [99] we may trace the story of the studies in Arts, only to find that as far back as 1267, with different names sometimes, they have been through all the centuries essentially the same—Greek and Latin authors, logic, rhetoric, grammar, and the philosophies, natural, moral, and metaphysical—practically the seven liberal Arts for which, as you may see by the name over the doors, Bodley's building provided accommodation.[100] Why this invariableness in an ever-turning world? One of the marvels, so commonplace that it has ceased to be marvellous, is the deep rooting of our civilization in the soil of Greece and Rome—much of our dogmatic religion, practically all the philosophies, the models of our literature, the ideals of our democratic freedom, the fine and the technical arts, the fundamentals of science, and the basis of our law. The Humanities bring the student into contact with the master minds who gave us these things—with the dead who never die, with those immortal lives 'not of now or of yesterday but which always were.'[101] As true to-day as in the fifth century B.C. the name of Hellas [102] stands no longer for the name of a race, but as the name of knowledge; or, as more tersely put by Maine, 'Except the blind forces of Nature, nothing

96. *Literae Humaniores:* Oxford name for classical literature (Greek and Latin) considered as a subject for study; "humane letters."

97. *Greats' papers:* Colloquialism at Oxford for the final examination for the degree of B.A.; now applied especially to the examination for Honours in Literae Humaniores (*OED*).

98. John *Napleton* (c.1738–1817): English theologian and educational reformer, canon of Hereford, and author of various sermons and pamphlets on student life at Oxford, including "Considerations on the public exercises for the first and second degrees in the University of Oxford" (1773).

99. Hastings *Rashdall* (1858–1924): English theologian, philosopher, and historian of universities. Author of *The Universities of Europe in the Middle Ages* (1895).

100. *Bodley's building:* Bodleian Library, the central library of Oxford University, which was reestablished by Sir Thomas Bodley (1545–1613). Over the various doors opening from the quadrangle are inscriptions SCHOLA LOGICAE, SCHOLA METAPHYSICAE, and so on, as Osler says, comprising the traditional branches of learning. Osler refers to these on p. 000 below as "mocking inscriptions" because these doors do not in fact lead to rooms where these subjects are studied.

101. *not of now or of yesterday but which always were:* Job 8:8–9.

102. *Hellas:* The word meant "all the homeland of the Greeks" in the classical period. *Ellas* in modern Greek means the modern Greek state.

moves in this world that is not Greek in origin.'[103] Man's anabasis[104] from the old priest-ridden civilizations of the East began when 'the light of reason lighted up all things,'[105] with which saying Anaxagoras expressed our modern outlook on life.

The Humanities have been a subject of criticism in two directions. Their overwhelming prominence, it is claimed, prevents the development of learning in other and more useful directions; and the method of teaching is said to be antiquated and out of touch with the present needs. They control the academic life of Oxford. An analysis of the Register for 1919 shows that of the 257 men comprising the Heads and Fellows[106] of the twenty-three colleges (including St. Edmund Hall), only fifty-one are scientific, including the mathematicians.

It is not very polite perhaps to suggest that as transmitters and interpreters they should not bulk quite so large in a modern university. 'Twas all very well

> in days when wits were fresh and clear
> And life ran gaily as the sparkling Thames[107]

in those happy days when it was felt that all knowledge had been garnered by those divine men of old time, that there was nothing left but to enjoy the good things harvested by such universal providers as Isidore, Rabanus Maurus, and Vincent of Beauvais,[108] and those stronger dishes served by such artists as Albertus Magnus and St. Thomas Aquinas[109]—delicious blends of such skill that

---

103. Henry James Sumner *Maine* (1822–1888): English jurist, professor of civil law at Cambridge, professor of jurisprudence at Oxford, and author of *Village-Communities in the East and West* (New York: Henry Holt, 1876), p. 238.

104. *anabasis:* Journey upward.

105. *Anaxagoras* (c.500–428 B.C.): Greek philosopher whose pupils included Pericles, Euripides, and Socrates. No such saying is ascribed to Anaxagoras in Kirk's standard work on the pre-Socratic philosophers. Theodor Gomperz (in *Greek Thinkers*, trans. Laurie Magnus [London: John Murray, 1901], vol. 1, pp. 215–216), summarizes Anaxagoras' teaching about *Nous* or Reason and says he regarded it as a Prime Mover, similar to the one postulated by Aristotle. Osler may be vaguely remembering that passage.

106. *fellows:* Scholars and teachers who are associated with the Heads in governing the colleges of Oxford and Cambridge

107. Matthew Arnold, "The Scholar Gypsy," lines 201–202.

108. *Isidore* of Seville (c.570–636): Spanish churchman and scholar who wrote an encyclopedia called *Etymologiae*, which kept alive ancient lore and texts throughout the Middle Ages. He also wrote *De Natura Rerum*, which dealt with medieval astronomy.

Rabanus *Maurus* (776–856): German theologian at the time of the Carolingian revival of learning. He wrote on etymology, the Bible, and education.

Vincent of *Beauvais* (c.1190–1264): Medieval Latin scholar who compiled the encyclopedia of medieval knowledge, *Speculum Majus.*

109. Albertus *Magnus* (1206–1280): A Dominican who taught in Paris and Cologne. He was learned in works of Aristotle and Jewish and Arabic scientists, and he was Aquinas' teacher.

only the palate of an Apicius[110] could separate Greek, Patristic, and Arabian savours.

It is not the dominance, but the unequal dominance that is a cause of just complaint. As to methods of teaching—by their fruits ye shall know them.[111] The product of 'Greats'[112] needs no description in this place. Many deny the art to find the mind's construction in the face, but surely not the possibility of diagnosing at a glance a 'first in Greats'! Only in him is seen that altogether superior expression, that self-consciousness of having reached life's goal, of having, in that pickled sentence of Dean Gaisford's[113] Christmas sermon, done something 'that not only elevates above the common herd, but leads not unfrequently to positions of considerable emolument.'[114] 'Many are the wand-bearers, few are the mystics,'[115] and a system should not be judged by the exceptions. As a discipline of the mind for the few, the system should not be touched, and we should be ready to sacrifice a holocaust of undergraduates every year to produce in each generation a scholar of the type of, say, Ingram Bywater.[116] 'Tis Nature's method—does it not cost some thousands of eggs and fry to produce one salmon?

But the average man, not of scholar timber, may bring one railing accusation against his school and college. Apart from mental discipline, the value of the ancient languages is to give a key to their literatures. Yet we make boys and young men spend ten or more years on the study of Greek and Latin, at the end of which time the beauties of the languages are still hidden because of the pernicious method in which they are taught. It passes my understanding how the more excellent way of Montaigne, of Milton, and of Locke should have been neglected until recently. Make the language an instrument to play with and to play with thoroughly, and recognize that except for the few in 'Mods.'[117] and

St. Thomas *Aquinas* (c.1225–1274): Italian philosopher and theologian of the Roman Catholic Church. Author of *Summa Theologiae* (1265–1273), which, while professing to treat theology, was designed to form a complete and systematic summary of the knowledge of the time.

110. Marcus Gabius (also Gavius) *Apicius* (1st cent. A.D.): Roman gourmet during the reign of Tiberius.

111. *by their fruits ye shall know them:* Matthew 7:20.

112. *Greats:* See p. 78, n. 97.

113. Thomas *Gaisford* (1779–1855): Regius professor of Greek at Oxford and dean of Christ Church Cathedral.

114. William Tuckwell, *Reminiscences of Oxford* (London: Cassell, 1907), p. 129. The exact quotation is: "Which not only elevates above the vulgar herd, but leads not infrequently," etc. Osler may have got this anecdote from oral tradition in Oxford rather than from Tuckwell.

115. Plato, *Phaedrus,* 69c–d.

116. Ingram *Bywater* (1840–1914): English classical scholar and Regius professor of Greek at Oxford. He edited Aristotle's *Poetics* and contributed to the compilation of the *Oxford English Dictionary.*

117. *Mods:* Colloquialism for "moderations," the First Public Examination for the degree of B.A., conducted by the Moderators (*OED*).

'Greats'[118] it is superfluous to know how the instrument is constructed, or to dissect the neuro-muscular mechanism by which it is played. It is satisfactory to read that the Greek Curriculum Committee thinks 'it is possible in a comparatively short time to acquire a really valuable knowledge of Greek, and to learn with accuracy and fair fluency some of the most important works in Greek literature.' I am sure of it, if the teacher will go to school to Montaigne[119] and feed fat against[120] that old scoundrel Protagoras[121] a well-earned grudge for inventing grammar—*pace* Mr. Livingstone,[122] every chapter in whose two books appeals to me, except those on grammar, against which I have a medullary prejudice. I speak, of course, as a fool among the wise, and I am not pleading for the 'Greats' men, but for the average man, whom to infect with the spirit of the Humanities is the greatest single gift in education. To you of the elect this is pure *camouflage*—the amateur talking to the experts; but there is another side upon which I feel something may be said by one whose best friends have been the old Humanists, and whose breviary is Plutarch, or rather Plutarch gallicized by Montaigne.[123] Paraphrasing Mark Twain's comment upon Christian Science,[124] the so-called Humanists have not enough Science, and Science sadly lacks the Humanities. This unhappy divorce, which should never have taken place, has been officially recognized in the two reports edited by Sir Frederic Kenyon,[125]

118. *Greats:* See p. 78, n. 97.

119. Michel Eyquem *Montaigne:* See "Sir Thomas Browne," p. 57, n. 179.

120. The phrase *feed fat against . . . grudge* is taken from Shylock who says, "I will feed fat the ancient grudge I bear him." William Shakespeare, *The Merchant of Venice*, I, iii, 48.

121. *Protagoras* (c.483–c.414 B.C.): Greek philosopher and sophist. Dealing with science in school, Osler expressed himself in another address as follows: "How I have cursed the memory of Protagoras since finding that he introduced grammar into the curriculum, and forged the fetters which chained generations of schoolboys in the cold formalism of words." *The School-World* (a journal of higher education published by Macmillan in London), vol. 18, 1916, pp. 41–44 (Cushing, vol. 1, p. 34). For further information on Protagoras, see "Physic and Physicians as Depicted in Plato," p. 000, n. 000.

122. Richard Winn *Livingstone* (1880–1960): English classical scholar who was a professor of classics at Oxford. Author of *The Greek Genius and Its Meaning to Us* (1912) and *A Defence of Classical Education* (1916).

123. These two were Osler's favorite authors. He recommended Montaigne and Plutarch following the Old and New Testaments and Shakespeare in a list of ten books which he put down as a "Bed-side Library for Medical Students," p. 371.

   Plutarch See p. 73, n. 62.

   Michel Eyquem de *Montaigne:* See "Sir Thomas Browne," p. 57, n. 179.

124. Mark Twain, *Christian Science* (New York: Harper & Brothers, 1899). We cannot find anything like this in Twain's *Christian Science*. Osler may be paraphrasing the whole force of Twain's criticism, rather than one passage.

125. Osler's original note reads: "*Education, Scientific and Humane*, 1917, and *Education, Secondary and University*, 1919."

which have stirred the pool, and cannot but be helpful. To have got constructive, anabolic action from representatives of interests so diverse is most encouraging. While all agree that neither in the Public Schools nor in the older Universities are the conditions at present in keeping with the urgent scientific needs of the nation, the specific is not to be sought in endowments alone, but in the leaven which may work a much needed change [126] in both branches of knowledge.

III

The School of Literae Humaniores excites wonder in the extent and variety of the knowledge demanded, and there is everywhere evidence of the value placed upon the ancient models; but this wonder pales before the gasping astonishment at what is not there. Now and again a hint, a reference, a recognition, but the moving forces which have made the modern world are simply ignored. Yet they are all Hellenic, all part and parcel of the Humanities in the true sense, and all of prime importance in modern education. Twin berries on one stem, grievous damage has been done to both in regarding the Humanities and Science in any other light than complemental. Perhaps the anomalous position of Science in our philosophical school is due to the necessary filtration, indeed the preservation, of our classical knowledge, through ecclesiastical channels. Of this the persistence of the Augustinian [127] questions until late in the eighteenth century is an interesting indication. The moulder of Western Christianity had not much use for Science, and the Greek spirit was stifled in the atmosphere of the Middle Ages. 'Content to be deceived, to live in a twilight of fiction, under clouds of false witnesses, inventing according to convenience, and glad to welcome the forger and the cheat'—such, Lord Acton [128] somewhere says, were the Middle Ages.

Frederic George *Kenyon* (1863–1952): English classical scholar who edited and translated classical works, including those by Aristotle. He was president of the Classical Association in 1913 and is best known as director of the British Museum. The "reports" were probably made to the British Academy, of which he was a founding member, a fellow, and president.

126. leaven: Osler emphasized its importance in "The Leaven of Science," delivered in 1894. For the definition of the word, see "The Leaven of Science," p. 153, n.

127. Saint *Augustine* (354–430): The greatest theologian in the early Christian Church. His doctrines reaffirmed and developed those of St. Paul. Osler is referring to Augustine's *Quaestiones in Heptateuchum* (Questions on the Heptateuch; that is, on the first seven books of the Bible), and his point is that Augustine there assumes the events recorded in those books are historical facts. For further information on Augustine, see "Chauvinism in Medicine," p. 248, n. 75.

128. John E. E. D. *Acton* (1834–1902): English historian and moralist who was Regius professor at Cambridge, where he formed a library of 59,000 volumes. The quoted phrase comes from *A Lecture on the Study of History* (London: Macmillan, 1895), pp. 10–11.

Strange, is it not, that one man alone, Roger Bacon,[129] mastered his environment and had a modern outlook![130]

The practical point for us here is that in the only school dealing with the philosophy of human thought, the sources of the new science that has made a new world are practically ignored. One gets even an impression of neglect in the Schools, or at any rate of scant treatment, of the Ionian philosophers, the very fathers of your fathers. Few 'Greats' men, I fear, could tell why Hippocrates is a living force to-day, or why a modern scientific physician would feel more at home with Erasistratus[131] and Herophilus[132] at Alexandria, or with Galen[133] at Pergamos, than at any period in our story up to, say, Harvey.[134] Except as a delineator of character, what does the Oxford scholar know of Theophrastus,[135] the founder of modern botany, and a living force to-day in one of the two departments of biology, and made accessible recently to English readers—perhaps indeed to Greek readers!—by Sir Arthur Hort.[136] Beggarly recognition or base indifference is meted out to the men whose minds have fertilized science in every department. The pulse of every student should beat faster as he reads the story of Archimedes, of Hero, of Aristarchus[137]—names not even mentioned in the

129. Roger *Bacon* (c.1214–1294): English philosopher and scientist who is sometimes referred to as "the Admirable Doctor." He invented the magnifying glass and an antecedent of gunpowder, and he spent almost twenty years of his life imprisoned because of his works.

130. Osler's original note reads: "How modern Bacon's outlook was may be judged from the following sentence: 'Experimental science has three great prerogatives over all other sciences—it verifies conclusions by direct experiment, it discovers truths which they could never reach, and it investigates the secrets of Nature and opens to us a knowledge of the past and of the future.'"

131. *Erasistratus* (3rd cent. B.C.): Greek anatomist of Antioch who worked on the distinction between the sensory and motor nerves. He is often referred to as the father of physiology. Of the several works he wrote on anatomy, practical medicine, and pharmacy, only the titles remain, but a large number of short fragments were preserved by Galen and other ancient medical writers.

132. *Herophilus* (4th–3rd cent. B.C.): Greek anatomist of Alexandria who was famous for the discovery of the nervous system. He is often referred to as the father of anatomy.

133. Claudius *Galen* (c.130–c.200): Greek physician and writer. See "Teaching and Thinking," pp. 181–182, n. 27.

134. William *Harvey* (1578–1657): English physician and anatomist who discovered the circulation of the blood. See "Teacher and Student," p. 116, n. 22.

135. *Theophrastus* (c.372–c.288 B.C.): Greek peripatetic philosopher and botanist who described human characteristics. A disciple of Aristotle, he continued the teachings of Aristotle after his master's death. The best known of his writings is the moral treatise *Characters,* which includes brief incisive sketches of various classes of people. He also wrote a *History of Plants* and *The Origins of Plants,* which during the Middle Ages were regarded as the great reference works on the subject.

136. Arthur Fenton *Hort* (1864–1935): Editor and translator of Theophrastus' *Enquiry into Plants* (London: W. Heinemann, 1916).

137. *Archimedes* (c.287–212 B.C.): Greek mathematician and physicist who discovered the principles of specific gravity and of the lever.

'Greats' papers in the past decade. Yet the methods of these men exorcised vagaries and superstitions from the human mind and pointed to a clear knowledge of the laws of Nature. It is surprising that some wag among the examiners has never relieved the grave monotony of the papers by such peripatetic [138] questions as 'How long a gnat lives,' 'To how many fathoms' depth the sunlight penetrates the sea,' and 'What an oyster's soul is like'—questions which indicate whence the modern Lucian [139] got his inspiration to chaff so successfully Boyle [140] and the Professors of Gresham College.[141]

May I dwell upon two instances of shocking neglect? It really is amusing in Oxford to assert neglect of 'the measurer of all Art and Science, whose is all that is best in the passing sublunary world,' as Richard de Bury calls 'the Prince of the Schooles.' [142] In Gulliver's voyage to Laputa [143] he paid a visit to the little island of Glubbdubdrib, whose Governor, you remember, had an Endorian command over the spirits,[144] such as Sir Oliver Lodge [145] or Sir Arthur Conan Doyle [146] might envy. When Aristotle and his commentators were summoned, to Gulliver's surprise they were strangers, for the reason that having so horribly mis-

―――

Hero of Alexandria (also *Heron*) (fl. c. 1st cent. A.D.): Greek naturalist and mathematician who discovered the formula for the area of the triangle. He also described siphons, water engines, and primitive forms of the steam engine, and invented several machines, among which was "Hero's fountain."

Aristarchus of Samos (late 3rd cent. B.C.): See p. 67, n. 16.

138. *peripatetic:* Pertaining to the Aristotelian school of philosophy, because Aristotle taught while walking in the Lyceum.

139. *Lucian* (c.125–c.200 A.D.): Greek satirist and poetand a skeptic who argued against old faiths, philosophies, and conventions. See also "Aequanimitas," p. 24, lines 4–8.

By the modern Lucian: Osler means Jonathan Swift (1667–1745), also a writer of prose satires, who described travels to imaginary countries in his *Gulliver's Travels* (1726). We can recognize his indebtedness to Lucian's *True Story.*

140. Charles *Boyle* (1676–1731): A friend of Jonathan Swift. For further information, see p. 94, n. 226.

141. Founded by Sir Thomas Gresham (c.1519–1579), the English financier who opened the college in 1596 in London. It was a forerunner of the University of London, which was founded in 1836 but remained separate, continuing lectures on divinity, astronomy, music, geometry, law, physic, and rhetoric.

142. *the Prince of the Schooles:* Osler is referring to Aristotle in the way that Richard *de Bury* (1281–1345), English classical scholar and founder of Durham College library at Oxford, refers to Aristotle as *princeps philosophorum*, "prince of philosophers." "Prologue," *Philobiblon*, ed. Antonio Altamura (Naples: Fausto Fiorentino, 1954), p. 71.

143. Jonathan Swift, *Gulliver's Travels*, chap. 8.

144. *an Endorian command:* 1 Samuel 28:7–14. Saul was taken to a woman in Endor who called up the spirit of Samuel for him.

145. Oliver *Lodge* (1851–1940): English physicist, and later psychic, who examined the nature of ether and of wireless telegraphy.

146. Arthur *Conan Doyle* (1859–1930): English detective story writer and physician, known especially for *The Adventures of Sherlock Holmes.* He was interested in the study of spiritualism and also wrote on this topic.

represented Aristotle's meaning to posterity, a consciousness of guilt and shame kept them far away from him in the lower world. Such shame, I fear, will make the shades of many classical dons of this University seek shelter with the commentators when they realize their neglect of one of the most fruitful of all the activities of the Master. In biology Aristotle speaks for the first time the language of modern science, and indeed he seems to have been first and foremost a biologist, and his natural history studies influenced profoundly his sociology, his psychology, and his philosophy in general. The beginner may be sent now to Professor D'Arcy Wentworth Thompson's [147] Herbert Spencer Lecture,[148] 1913, and he must be indeed a dull and muddy-mettled rascal [149] whose imagination is not fired by the enthusiastic—yet true—picture of the founder of modern biology, whose language is our language, whose methods and problems are our own, the man who knew a thousand varied forms of life, of plant, of bird, and animal, their outward structure, their metamorphosis, their early development; who studied the problems of heredity, of sex, of nutrition, of growth, of adaptation, and of the struggle for existence.[150] And the senior student, if capable of appreciating a biological discovery, I advise to study the account by Johannes Müller [151] (himself a pioneer in anatomy) of his rediscovery of Aristotle's remarkable discovery of a special mode of reproduction in one of the species of sharks.[152] For two thousand years the founder of the science of embryology had neither rival nor worthy follower. There is no reference, I believe, to the biological works in the Literae Humaniores papers for the past ten years, yet they form the very foundations of discoveries that have turned our philosophies topsy-turvy.

Nothing reveals the unfortunate break in Humanities more clearly than the treatment of the greatest nature-poet in literature, a man who had 'gazed on Nature's naked loveliness' [153] unabashed, the man who united, as no one else has

147. D'Arcy Wentworth *Thompson* (1860–1948): English zoologist and classical scholar.

148. Herbert *Spencer* (1820–1903): English philosopher whose philosophy was based on the doctrine of evolution. Spencer suggested that sciences should be classified as abstract, abstract-concrete, and concrete.

149. William Shakespeare, *Hamlet*, II, ii, 594. Onions, in his *Shakespeare Glossary*, defined *muddy-mettled* as "dull-spirited." An old sense of *muddy* is "gloomy, sullen."

150. Osler's original note reads: "Summarized from D'Arcy Wentworth Thompson." *On Aristotle as a Biologist* (the Herbert Spencer Lecture), (Oxford: Clarendon Press, 1913).

151. Johannes Peter *Müller* (1801–1858): German physiologist and a founder of modern physiology. He did research in anatomy, speech, hearing, sight, and glands and the quality of their secretions. He is known for Müller's capsule, (pronephric) ducts (canal), etc. Osler's original note reads: "*Über den Glatten Hai des Aristoteles*, Berlin, 1842."

152. Aristotle, *Historia Animalium*, book 3, chap. 1, 511a:5–11.

153. Charles Harold Herford, *The Poetry of Lucretius* (Manchester: The University Press, 1918), p. 15. The

ever done, the 'functions and temper and achievement of science and poetry'[154] (Herford). The golden work of Lucretius[155] is indeed recognized, and in Honour Moderations Books I–III and V are set as one of seven alternatives in section D; and scattered through the 'Greats' papers are set translations and snippets here and there; but anything like adequate consideration from the scientific side is to be sought in vain. Unmatched among the ancients or moderns is the vision by Lucretius of continuity in the workings of Nature—not less of *Le silence éternel de ces espaces infinis*[156] which so affrighted Pascal, than of 'the long limitless age of days, the age of all time that has gone by'—

longa diei
infinita aetas anteacti temporis omnis.[157]

And it is in a Latin poet[158] that we find up-to-date views of the origin of the world and of the origin of man. The description of the wild discordant storm of atoms (Book V) which led to the birth of the world might be transferred verbatim to the accounts of Poincaré[159] or of Arrhenius[160] of the growth of new celestial bodies in the Milky Way. What an insight into primitive man and the beginnings of civilization! He might have been a contemporary and friend, and doubtless was a tutor, of Tylor.[161] Book II, a manual of atomic physics with its marvellous conception of—

---

exact quotation is: "But here came a poet, and one of the greatest, who rent the veil asunder and bade men gaze upon the nature of things naked and unadorned."

154. Ibid., p. 25.

155. Titus *Lucretius* Carus (c.96–55 B.C.): Roman poet and philosopher. Author of *De Rerum Natura* (On the Nature of Things), which is an exposition of an Epicurean system of philosophy. Although not a scientist, he propounded theories of light, of the atomic constitution of matter, and of the origin of life, which anticipated discoveries in modern times.

156. *Le silence éternel de ces espaces infinis:* "The eternal silence of these infinite spaces." Blaise *Pascal, Pensées,* trans. A. J. Krailsheimer (Baltimore: Penguin Books, 1966), sect. 1, part 15 ("Transition from Knowledge of Man to Knowledge of God"), no. 201, p. 95.

157. The original Latin is taken from Lucretius' *De Rerum Natura,* book 1, line 558. Osler gives a good translation just before he quotes the Latin.

158. *Latin poet:* Lucretius. *Book V* refers to *De Rerum Natura.*

159. Jules Henri *Poincaré* (1854–1912): French mathematician and scientist who was professor of celestial mechanics at the Faculty of Science in Paris. He wrote *Les Méthodes nouvelles de la mécanique céleste* (The New Methods of Celestial Mechanics) (1892, 1893, 1899).

160. Svante August *Arrhenius* (1859–1927): Swedish physicist and chemist who established electrolytic dissociation theory. He applied the methods of physical chemistry to the study of toxins and anti-toxins. Author of *Worlds in the Making* (1908), in which he partly anticipated Einstein, arguing against Kelvin's theory of entropy that the universe is self-renewing.

161. Edward Burnett *Tylor* (1832–1917): English anthropologist and first professor of anthropology at Oxford. He wrote *Primitive Culture* (1871).

> the flaring atom streams
> and torrents of her myriad universe,[162]

can only be read appreciatively by pupils of Roentgen[163] or of J. J. Thomson.[164] The ring theory of magnetism advanced in Book VI has been reproduced of late by Parsons,[165] whose magnetons rotating as rings at high speed have the form and effect with which this disciple of Democritus[166] clothes his magnetic physics.

And may I here enter a protest? Of love-philtres that produce insanity we may read the truth in a chapter of that most pleasant manual of erotology, the *Anatomy of Melancholy*.[167] Of insanity of any type that leaves a mind capable in lucid intervals of writing such verses as *De Rerum Natura*[168] we know nothing. The sole value of the myth is its causal association with the poem of Tennyson.[169] Only exsuccous dons[170] who have never known the wiles and ways of the younger Aphrodite[171] would take the intensity of the feeling in Book IV as witness to anything but an accident which may happen to the wisest of the wise, when enthralled by Vivien[172] or some dark lady of the Sonnets![173]

In the School of Literae Humaniores the studies are based on classical lit-

162. Lucretius, *De Rerum Natura*, book 2.

163. Wilhelm Konrad *Roentgen* (1845–1923): German physicist and discoverer of X-rays in 1895.

164. Joseph John *Thomson* (1856–1940): English physicist who investigated the mass and charge of the electron, radioactivity, etc. He is considered the discoverer of the electron.

165. Charles Algernon *Parsons* (1854–1931): English engineer who developed the steam turbine, known as the Parsons Marine Turbine.

166. *Democritus* (c.460–c.370 B.C.): Greek philosopher known for his theory of atoms. See "Physic and Physicians as Depicted in Plato," p. 128, n. 3.

167. A long treatise full of miscellaneous learning by Robert Burton (1577–1640), an English clergyman. The exact reference is *Anatomy of Melancholy*, ed. Thomas C. Faulkner, Nicholas K. Kiessling, and Rhonda L. Blair (1621; Oxford: Oxford University Press, 1994), part 3, sect. 2, member 5, subsect. 4, pp. 240–242.

168. See p. 86, n. 155.

169. Alfred *Tennyson* constructed a poem, "Lucretius," from adapted passages of Lucretius' *De Rerum Natura*. Tennyson used an ancient tradition that Lucretius died by his own hand, haunted by phantoms of the gods he had rejected, after his wife unhinged his mind by giving him a love potion to improve his sexual prowess. As Osler says, there is no good reason to believe this story.

170. *exsuccous dons:* Sapless, dried-up university teachers.

171. *the younger Aphrodite:* The Greek goddess of erotic desire. For further information, see "The Master-Word in Medicine," p. 269, n. 83.

172. *Vivien:* An enchantress in Arthurian Romance.

173. *dark lady:* An unknown woman in William Shakespeare's "Sonnet 127–154." She is represented as first fascinating and then betraying both the poet and his young male friend by loving other men. The poet regards her as a bad influence on the younger man and regrets his own involvement with her, but cannnot break free. She is called "dark lady" because she has dark complexion and metaphorically dark morals.

erature and on history, 'but a large number of students approach philosophical study from other sides. Students of such subjects as mathematics, natural science, history, psychology, anthropology, or political economy, became naturally interested in philosophy, and their needs are at present very imperfectly provided for in this University.' This I quote from a Report to the Board of the Faculty of Arts made just before the (1914–18) war on a proposed new Honour School, the subject of which should be the principles of philosophy considered in their relation to the Sciences. That joint action of this kind should have been taken by the Boards of Arts and of Science indicates a widespread conviction that no man is cultivated up to the standard of his generation who has not an appreciation of how the greatest achievements of the human mind have been reached; and the practical question is how to introduce such studies into the course of liberal education, how to give the science school the leaven of an old philosophy, how to leaven the old philosophical school with the thoughts of science.[174]

It is important to recognize that there is nothing mysterious in the method of science, or apart from the ordinary routine of life. Science has been defined as the habit or faculty of observation. By such the child grows in knowledge, and in its daily exercise an adult lives and moves. Only a quantitative difference makes observation scientific—accuracy; in that way alone do we discover things as they really are. This is the essence of Plato's definition of science as 'the discovery of things as they really are,'[175] whether in the heavens above, in the earth beneath, or in the observer himself. As a mental operation, the scientific method is equally applicable to deciphering a bit of Beneventan script,[176] to the analysis of the Commission on Coal-mines, a study of the mechanism of the nose-dive, or of the colour scheme in tiger-beetles. To observation, with reasoned thought, the Greek added experiment (but never fully used it in biology), the instrument which has made science productive, and to which the modern world owes its civilization. Our everyday existence depends on the practical application of discoveries in pure science by men who had no other motives than a search for knowledge of Nature's laws, a disinterestedness which Burnet[177] claims to be the

174. Osler's original note reads: "Since I wrote this lecture Professor J. A. Stewart has sent me his just-published essay on *Oxford after the War and a Liberal Education,* in which he urges with all the weight of his learning and experience that the foundations of a liberal education in Oxford should be 'No Humane Letters without Natural Science and no Natural Science without Humane Letters.'"

John Alex *Stewart* (b.1846): Professor of Greek at Oxford.

175. Plato, *Charmides,* 166d.

176. *Beneventan script:* Characteristic medieval Italian writing developed from the Konan cursive script; also called Lombardic. Osler's point is that Beneventan script is notoriously hard for the untrained to read.

177. John *Burnet* (1863–1928): Professor of Greek at St. Andrews University in Scotland. He edited several

distinctive gift of Hellas to humanity. With the discovery of induced currents Faraday[178] had no thought of the dynamo, Crookes's[179] tubes were a plaything until Roentgen[180] turned them into practical use with the X-rays. Perkin[181] had no thought of transforming chemical industry when he discovered aniline dyes. Priestley[182] would have cursed the observation that an electrical charge produced nitrous acid had he foreseen that it would enable Germany to prolong the war, but he would have blessed the thought that it may make us independent of all outside sources for fertilizers.

The extraordinary development of modern science may be her undoing. Specialism, now a necessity, has fragmented the specialities themselves in a way that makes the outlook hazardous. The workers lose all sense of proportion in a maze of minutiae. Everywhere men are in small coteries intensely absorbed in subjects of deep interest, but of very limited scope. Chemistry, a century ago an appanage of the Chair of Medicine or even of Divinity, has now a dozen departments, each with its laboratory and literature, sometimes its own society. Applying themselves early to research, young men get into backwaters far from the main stream. They quickly lose the sense of proportion, become hypercritical, and the smaller the field, the greater the tendency to megalocephaly.[183] The study for fourteen years of the variations in the colour scheme of the 1,300 species of tiger-beetles scattered over the earth may sterilize a man into a sticker of pins and a paster of labels; on the other hand, he may be a modern biologist whose interest is in the experimental modification of types, and in the mysterious insulation of hereditary characters from the environment. Only in one direction does the modern specialist acknowledge his debt to the dead languages. Men of

---

works of Plato and Aristotle. Osler may have had in mind the introduction to his *Early Greek Philosophy* (1892; London: Adam & Charles Black, 1948), p. 25, where Burnet wrote: "It was just this great gift of curiosity . . . which enabled the Ionians to pick up and turn to their own use such scraps of knowledge as they could come by."

178. Michael *Faraday* (1791–1867): Author of *The Theory of the Earth* (1690–1691). See p. 000, n. 000.

179. William *Crookes* (1832–1919): English chemist and physicist who invented "Crookes' tube" as well as the radiometer.

180. Wilhelm Konrad *Roentgen* (1845–1923): See p. 87, n. 163.

181. William Henry *Perkin* (1838–1907): English chemist who invented synthetic dye.

182. Joseph *Priestley* (1733–1804): English theologian and chemist best known for his discovery of oxygen. He also discovered hydrochloric acid, nitric oxide, sulpher dioxide, and silicon tetrafluoride, among other compounds. He discovered how to make nitrous acid by electrolysis, and that enabled German scientists to make synthetic fertilizer during World War I, when the import of natural fertilizer was hampered by the British naval blockade of the coasts. Without the synthetic fertilizer, the Germans could not have grown so much food and would have been starved into submission sooner.

183. *megalocephaly*: A humorously pompous term for what is commonly called "a swelled head," meaning an over-high opinion of one's own abilities.

science pay homage, as do no others, to the god of words whose magic power is nowhere so manifest as in the plastic language of Greece. The only visit many students pay to Parnassus [184] is to get an intelligible label for a fact or form newly discovered. Turn the pages of such a dictionary of chemical terms as Morley and Muir,[185] and you meet in close-set columns countless names unknown a decade ago, and unintelligible to the specialist in another department unless familiar with Greek, and as meaningless as the Arabic jargon in such medieval collections as the *Synonyma* of Simon Januensis or the Pandects of Mathaeus Sylvaticus.[186] As *Punch* [187] put it the other day in a delightful poetical review of Professor West's volume:[188]

> Botany relies on Latin ever since Linnaeus' [189] days;
> Biologic nomenclature draws on Greek in countless ways;
> While in Medicine it is obvious you can never take your oath
> What an ailment means exactly if you haven't studied both.
> (17. iv. 19.)

Let me give a couple of examples.

Within the narrow compass of the primitive cell from which all living beings originate, onomatomania [190] runs riot. The process of mitosis has developed a special literature and language. Dealing not alone with the problems of heredity and of sex, but with the very dynamics of life, the mitotic complex is much more than a simple physiological process, and in the action and interaction of physical forces the cytologist hopes to find the key to the secret of life itself. And what a Grecian he has become! Listen to this account which Aristotle would understand much better than most of us.

The karyogranulomes, not the idiogranulomes or microsomenstratum in

---

184. *Parnassus:* A mountain in Central Greece that is considered to be a center of poetic or artistic activity because it was sacred to Apollo and the Muses in ancient times.

185. Osler is citing what was then a standard reference work, *Watts' Dictionary of Chemistry,* revised by M. M. Pattison Muir and H. Forster Morley, 4 vols. (London: Longmans, Green, 1889–1894).

186. Simon *Januensis* (also *Genuensis*) (d.1303): Italian medical writer who wrote *Synonyma* (1473) and *Clavis sanationis* (1474).

   Mathaeus *Sy(i)lvaticus* (fl. 1317): Italian medical writer and author of *Pandectae Medicinae* (1499).

187. *Punch:* A weekly satirical magazine published in England beginning in 1841.

188. Andrew Fleming *West* (1853–1943): Dean of Graduate Studies at Princeton University who edited the *Philobiblon.* Osler's original note reads: "*The Value of the Classics,* Princeton University Press, 1917."

189. Carolus *Linnaeus* (also Carl von *Linné*) (1707–1778): Swedish naturalist who was considered the father of botany. He adopted a binomial system of nomenclature that helped to make natural history more exact and intelligible.

190. *onomatomania:* Probably Osler's coinage, meaning "a mad obsession with naming things."

the protoplasm of the spermatogonia, unite into the idiosphaerosome, acrosoma of Lenhossék, a protean phase, as the idiosphaerosome differentiates into an idio-cryptosome and an idiocalyptosome, both surrounded by the idiosphaerotheca, the archoplasmic vesicle; but the idioectosome disappears in the metamorpho-sis of the spermatid into a sphere, the idiophtharosome. The separation of the calyptosome from the cryptosome antedates the transformation of the idio-sphaerotheca into the spermiocalyptrotheca.[191]

Or take a more practical if less Cratylean example.[192] In our precious cab-bage patches the holometabolous insecta are the hosts of parasitic polyembryonic hymenoptera, upon the prevalence of which rests the psychic and somatic stamina of our fellow-countrymen; for the larvae of *Pieris brassicae,* vulgarly cabbage butterfly, are parasitized by the *Apantales glomeratus,* which in turn has a hyperparasite, the *Mesochorus pallidus.*[193] It is tragic to think that the fate of a plant, the dietetic and pharmaceutical virtues of which have been so extolled by Cato,[194] and upon which two of my Plinian[195] colleagues of uncertain date, Chry-sippus[196] and Dieuches,[197] wrote monographs—it fills one with terror to think that a crop so dear to Hodge[198] (*et veris cymata!*[199] the Brussels sprouts of Colu-mella)[200] should depend on the deposition in the ovum of the *Pieris* of another polyembryonic egg. The cytoplasm or oöplasm of this forms a trophoamnion and develops into a polygerminal mass, a spherical morula, from which in turn

191. Osler's original note reads: "Made up from a recent number of the *American Journal of Anatomy,* xxiv, 1."

192. *Cratylean example:* Plato in his dialogue *Cratylus* describes him as believing that words in all lan-guages have naturally inherent meanings.

193. *Pieris brassicae:* The common cabbage pest that turns into the "cabbage white," a common butterfly. *Apantales glomeratus:* The parasite that lives on the cabbage butterfly, *pieris brassicae. Mesochorus pal-lidus:* The insect that lives on the parasite of the cabbage butterfly. The cabbage moth destroys cabbages unless it is eaten by the parasite.

194. Marcus Porcius *Cato* (the Elder) (234–149 B.C.): Roman statesman and writer and author of *De Agri-cultura* (On Agriculture) (158–156 B.C.). He was a model of severe morality and strict integrity.

195. *Pliny* (Latin name, Gaius Plinius Secundus; called Pliny the Elder) (23–79 A.D.): Roman naturalist and writer whose *Historia Naturalis* (Natural History), which deals with anthropology, zoology, botany, materia medica, mineralogy, painting, and sculpture contains many credulous errors.

196. *Chrysippus* (c.280–204 B.C.): Greek philosopher who systematized the Stoic doctrine and worked on the mathematical theory of combinations.

197. *Dieuches* (4th cent. B.C.): Greek physician.

198. *Hodge:* A familiar adaptation of "Roger," used as a typical name for the English rustic. In other words, the vegetable is widely eaten by ordinary country Englishmen. The name in this sense was originally taken from a character in William Stevenson's comedy *Gammer Gurton's Needle* (1575).

199. *veris cymata:* Spring cabbage.

200. Lucius Junius Moderatus *Columella* (1st cent. A.D.): Roman writer on agriculture and author of *De Re Rustica* (Of Country Matters).

develop a hundred or more larvae, which immediately proceed to eat up everything in and of the body of their host. Only in this way does Nature preserve the Selenas, the Leas, and the Crambes,[201] so dear to Cato and so necessary for the sustenance of our hard-working brawny-armed Brasserii.[202]

From over-specialization scientific men are in a more parlous state than are the Humanists from neglect of classical tradition. The salvation of science lies in a recognition of a new philosophy—the *scientia scientiarum*,[203] of which Plato speaks. 'Now when all these studies reach the point of intercommunion and connexion with one another and come to be considered in their mutual affinities, then I think, and not till then, will the pursuit of them have a value.'[204] Upon this synthetic process I hesitate to dwell; since like Dr. Johnson's[205] friend, Oliver Edwards,[206] I have never succeeded in mastering philosophy—'cheerfulness was always breaking in.'[207]

In the proposed Honour School the principles of philosophy are to be dealt with in relation to the sciences, and by the introduction of literary and historical studies, which George Sarton[208] advocates so warmly as the new Humanism,[209] the student will gain a knowledge of the evolution of modern scientific thought. But to limit the history to the modern period—Kepler[210] to the present time is suggested—would be a grave error. The scientific student should go to the sources and in some way be taught the connexion of Democritus[211] with Dalton,[212] of Archimedes[213] with Kelvin, of Aristarchus with Newton, of Galen

201. *the Selenas* and *the Leas:* Presumably also members of the cabbage family. *the Crambes:* Latin (plural) word for a kind of cabbage.

202. *Brasserii:* Latin word for cabbage is "brassica"; "brasserii" may mean people who subsist on cabbage.

203. *scientia scientiarum:* Latin phrase for the science of sciences (Plato, *Charmides,* 167b–c).

204. Plato, *Republic,* book 7, 531d.

205. Samuel *Johnson* (1709–1784): See "A Way of Life," p. 5, n. 14.

206. Oliver *Edwards* (1711–1791): College friend of Samuel Johnson (Pembroke College, Oxford) who practiced as a solicitor in chancery and then retired to a small farm.

207. It is chiefly for this statement that Oliver Edwards is remembered. It is recorded in James Boswell's, *Life of Samuel Johnson,* April 25, 1778.

208. Alfred Léon George *Sarton* (1884–1956): Harvard professor of the history of science. Author of *The History of Science and the New Humanism* (1937).

209. Osler's original note reads: "*Popular Science Monthly,* September, 1918, and *Scientia,* vol. xxiii, 3."

210. Johannes *Kepler* (1571–1630): German astronomer and mathematician as well as discoverer of "Kepler's laws," which revolutionized the study of astronomy by outlining basic facts concerning the movement of the planets around the sun (their elliptical orbits, distance from the sun, and speed of their revolutions).

211. *Democritus* (c.460–c.370 B.C.): See p. 87, n. 166.

212. John *Dalton* (1766–1844): See p. 70, n. 41.

213. *Archimedes* (c.287–212 B.C.): See p. 83, n. 137.

with John Hunter,[214] and of Plato and Aristotle with them all. And the glories of Greek science should be opened in a sympathetic way to 'Greats' men. Under new regulations at the public schools, a boy of sixteen or seventeen should have enough science to appreciate the position of Theophrastus [215] in Botany, and perhaps himself construct Hero's [216] fountain. Science will take a totally different position in this country when the knowledge of its advances is the possession of all educated men. The time too is ripe for the Bodleian [217] to become a *studium generale*,[218] with ten or more departments, each in charge of a special sub-librarian. When the beautiful rooms, over the portals of which are the mocking blue and gold inscriptions,[219] are once more alive with students, the task of teaching subjects on historical lines will be greatly lightened. What has been done with the Music-room, and with the Science-room through the liberality of Dr. and Mrs. Singer,[220] should be done for classics, history, literature, theology, &c., each section in charge of a sub-librarian who will be Doctor perplexorum [221] alike to professor, don, and undergraduate.

I wish time had permitted me to sketch even briefly the story of the evolution of science in this old seat of learning. A fortunate opportunity enables you to see two phases in its evolution. Through the kind permission of several of the Colleges, particularly Christ Church, Merton, St. John's, and Oriel, and with the co-operation of the Curators of the Bodleian and Dr. Cowley,[222] Mr. R. T.

214. William Thomson *Kelvin* (1824–1907): Scottish mathematician and physicist who was professor of natural philosophy at Glasgow for fifty-three years. He contributed much in almost every branch of the physical sciences, including theory of light, energy, the tides, heat, the trans-atlantic cable, the telephone, etc.

    Aristarchus of Samos (late 3rd cent. B.C.): See p. 67, n. 16.

    Isaac *Newton* (1642–1727): English mathematician and natural philosopher who formulated the laws of gravity and motion.

    Claudius *Galen* (c.130–c.200): Greek physician. See "Teaching and Thinking," p. 181, n. 27.

    John *Hunter* (1728–1793): Scottish anatomist and surgeon who entered St. George's Hospital in 1754 as a surgeon's pupil and later practiced in London. He began lecturing on surgery in 1773 and his approach to anatomy, physiology, and pathology was empirical. He gave an impetus to young people, including his student Edward Jenner.

215. *Theophrastus* (c.372–c.288 B.C.): See p. 83, n. 135.

216. *Hero* of Alexandria (fl. c.1st cent. A.D.): See p. 84, n. 137.

217. *the Bodleian:* The library of Oxford University. See p. 78, n. 100.

218. *stadium generale:* (Latin) "(place of) general study."

219. *the mocking blue and gold inscriptions:* See p. 78, n. 100.

220. Charles Joseph *Singer* (1876–1960) and Dorothea *Singer* (1882–1964): English historians of medicine and science who contributed much to improve the facilities for the study of the history of science.

221. *Doctor perplexorum:* Doctor (that is, teacher) of the perplexed and confused.

222. Arthur Ernest *Cowley* (1861–1931): Librarian at the Bodleian and orientalist who "inoculated him

Gunther[223] of Magdalen College has arranged a loan exhibition of the early scientific instruments and manuscripts. A series of quadrants and astrolabes shows how Arabian instruments, themselves retaining much of the older Greek models, have translated Alexandrian science into the Western world. Some were constructed for the latitude of Oxford, and one was associated with our astronomer-poet, Chaucer.[224]

For the first time the instruments and works of the early members of the Merton School of astronomer-physicians have been brought together. They belong to a group of men of the fourteenth century—Reed, Aschenden, Simon Bredon, Merle, Richard of Wallingford,[225] and others—whose labours made Oxford the leading scientific University of the world.

Little remains of the scientific apparatus of the early period of the Royal Society, but through the kindness of the Dean and governing body of Christ Church, the entire contents of the cabinet of philosophical apparatus of the Earl of Orrery,[226] who flourished some thirty years after the foundation of the Society, are on exhibit, and the actual astronomical model, the 'Orrery,' made for him and called after his name.

The story of the free cities of Greece shows how a love of the higher and brighter things in life may thrive in a democracy. Whether such love may develop in a civilization based on a philosophy of force is the present problem of the Western

---

(Osler) with a desire for some ancient manuscripts which ultimately found their way into his library." (Cushing, vol. 2, p. 256.)

223. Robert William Theodore *Gunther* (1869–1940): English zoologist and antiquary.

224. Geoffrey *Chaucer* (c.1340–1400): English poet referred to as "the father of English poetry"; author of the well-known *Canterbury Tales*. His interest and knowledge in astronomy appears in many of his works and is especially shown in "The Miller's Tale." He also wrote a prose treatise on the use of the astrolabe.

225. William *Reed* (also *Rede* or *Reade*) (d.1385): English bishop, mathematician, and astronomer who established Merton College Library in 1375.

John *Aschenden* (date unknown): English author of a compendium on astrology.

Simon *Bredon* (died after 1368): English mathematician, astronomer, and physician who wrote on trigonometry. He was fellow of Balliol College, then of Merton College, Oxford.

William *Merle* (also *Morley*) (d.1347): English meteorologist who wrote the oldest systematic record of the weather. He was a fellow of Merton College, Oxford.

Richard of *Wallingford* (c.1292–1336): Abbot of St. Albans and a fellow of Merton College. He devised the Albion clock, which showed the courses of the sun, moon, and planets according to Ptolemaic astronomy.

226. Charles *Boyle* (1676–1731): 4th earl of Orrery, educated at Christ Church, Oxford. He was a patron of George Graham (d.1751), who invented the "orrery," a mechanism representing the motions of the planets about the sun by means of clockwork.

world. To-day there are doubts, even thoughts of despair, but neither man nor nation is to be judged by the behaviour in a paroxysm of delirium. Lavoisier[227] perished in the Revolution, and the Archbishop of Paris[228] was butchered at the altar by the Commune, yet France was not wrecked; and Russia may survive the starvation of such scholars as Danielevski[229] and Smirnov,[230] and the massacre of Botkin.[231] To have intelligent freemen of the Greek type with a stake in the State (not mere chattels from whose daily life the shadow of the workhouse never lifts), to have the men and women who could love the light put in surroundings in which the light may reach them, to encourage in all a sense of brotherhood reaching the standard of the Good Samaritan[232] — surely the realization in a democracy of such reasonable ambitions should be compatible with the control by science of the forces of Nature for the common good, and a love of all that is best in religion, in art, and in literature.

Amid the smoke and squalor of a modern industrial city, after the bread-and-butter struggle of the day, 'the Discobolus has no gospel.'[233] Our puritanized culture has been known to call the Antinous[234] vulgar. Copies of these two

227. Antoine Laurent *Lavoisier* (1743–1794): French chemist and pioneer in modern chemistry who later was guillotined. He was condemned by a tribunal that answered a plea to save him with the reply, "we need no more scientists in France."

228. Monseigneur Georges *Darboy* (1813–1871): At the Vatican Council of 1870 he opposed the definition of papal infallibility, but accepted the decree when passed by a majority. He was shot at La Roquette on May 24, 1871.

229. Nikolai Ia. *Danilevsky* (1822–1885): Russian philosopher who applied his knowledge of natural science, especially biology, to his view of violence. According to him, violence biologically intrinsic to European culture spurred wars, in particular the French Revolution. His philosophy also advocated nationalism and racism.

230. Probably S. A. *Smirnov* (date unknown): Russian physician and director of the Water Authority (1860s). Or, possibly, Vasílii Dmitrievich *Smirnov* (1846–1922): Russian orientalist who was professor in the faculty of Oriental languages at the University of St. Petersburg, and specialist in the history and literature of Turkey.

231. Eugene *Botkin* (d.1918): A house surgeon of the Russian Emperor who was murdered with the emperor and his family. Osler would not have approved of any of these murders, and certainly not of those of Nicholas' children.

232. Luke 10:30–37. A person who feels for the sufferings of others and helps people in distress.

233. Samuel Butler, "Seven Sonnets and a Psalm of Montreal," line 1. In the poem an old man in Montreal claims that the plaster cast of the Discobolus (the discus thrower) is vulgar, immoral, and pointless; hence "has no gospel." The exact quotation is: "The Discobolus is put here because he is vulgar, He has neither vest nor pants with which to cover his limbs: I, Sir, am a person of most respectable connections—My brother-in-law is haberdasher to Mr. Spurgeon."

234. *Antinous* (d.130 A.D.): The beautiful companion of the Roman Emperor Hadrian (76–138 A.D.). After his untimely death, Hadrian had him enrolled among the gods and erected statues and built temples in his honor.

statues, you may remember, Samuel Butler found stored away in the lumber-room of the Natural History Museum, Montreal, with skins, plants, snakes, and insects, and in their midst, stuffing an owl, sat 'the brother-in-law of the haber-dasher of Mr. Spurgeon.'[235] Against the old man[236] who thus blasphemed beauty, Butler broke into those memorable verses with the refrain 'O God! O Montreal!'[237]

Let us not be discouraged. The direction of our vision is everything, and after weltering four years in chaos poor stricken humanity still nurses the unconquerable hope of an ideal state 'whose citizens are happy . . . absolutely wise, all of them brave, just and self-controlled . . . all at peace and unity, and in the enjoyment of legality, equality, liberty, and all other good things.'[238] Lucian's winning picture of this 'Universal Happiness' might have been sketched by a Round Table pen[239] or some youthful secretary to the League of Nations.[240] That such hope persists is a witness to the power of ideals to captivate the mind; and the reality may be nearer than any of us dare dream. If survived, a terrible infection, such as confluent small-pox, seems to benefit the general health. Perhaps such an attack through which we have passed may benefit the body cosmic. After discussing the various forms of government, Plato concludes that 'States are as the men are, they grow out of human characters'[241] (*Rep.* VIII), and then, as the dream-republic approached completion, he realized that after all the true State is within, of which each one of us is the founder, and patterned on an ideal the exis-

235. *Mr. Spurgeon:* One of the haberdasher's customers, and presumably a wealthy "philistine" who made money in commerce. It shows that he is only concerned with commerce, not with beauty.

236. Osler's original note reads: "I knew him well—a dear old Cornishman named Passmore."

237. Samuel Butler, "Seven Sonnets and a Psalm of Montreal."

238. *Lucian* (c.125–c.200 A.D.): Greek satirist and poet. We cannot find the exact quote, but the reference seems to be to "A True Story," book 2, where Lucian claims to have voyaged out into the Atlantic to the Island of Rhadamanthus where the souls of the virtuous dead lead a happy and carefree existence. See Lucian's *Works,* trans. A. M. Harman (London: Heinemann; New York: Macmillan, 1913), vol. 1, pp. 308–333.

239. *Round Table:* The original name came from the round table at which King Arthur sat with his knights, but Osler here is referring to conferences about the state and future of the British Empire, whose proceedings were reported in *The Round Table,* along with proposals for some kind of federal government for the Empire. Osler is thus using it as an example of a hopeful, utopian attempt that is unlikely to work perfectly.

240. An international organization that attempted to promote cooperation and peace between nations. It was formed at the Paris Peace Conference in 1919 and began to function in January, 1920. It ended in 1946 when it was superseded by the United Nations.

241. Plato, *Republic,* book 8, 544d–e. Osler is summarizing the following: "Do you know, I said, that governments vary as the dispositions of men vary, and that there must be as many of the one as there are of the other? Or do you suppose that States spring from 'oak and rock,' and not from the human natures which are in them?"

tence of which matters not a whit. Is not the need of this individual reconstruction the Greek message to modern democracy? and with it is blended the note of individual service to the community on which Professor Gilbert Murray[242] has so wisely dwelt.

With the hot blasts of hate still on our cheeks, it may seem a mockery to speak of this as the saving asset in our future; but is it not the very marrow of the teaching in which we have been brought up? At last the gospel of the right to live, and the right to live healthy, happy lives, has sunk deep into the hearts of the people; and before the (1914–18) war, so great was the work of science in preventing untimely death that the day of Isaiah seemed at hand 'when a man's life should be more precious than fine gold, even a man than the gold of Ophir.'[243] There is a sentence in the writings of the Father of Medicine upon which all commentators have lingered 'ἢν γὰρ παρῇ φιλανθρωπίη, πάρεστι καὶ φιλοτεχνίη'[244]—the love of humanity associated with the love of his craft!—philanthropia and philotechnia—the joy of working joined in each one to a true love of his brother. Memorable sentence indeed! in which for the first time was coined the magic word *philanthropy*, and conveying the subtle suggestion that perhaps in this combination the longings of humanity may find their solution, and Wisdom—philosophia—at last be justified of her children.[245]

242. George Gilbert *Murray* (1866–1957): Regius professor of Greek at Oxford and distinguished interpreter of Greek ideas who propounded that for the ideal State we must each strive for individual self-improvement and service to others. He wrote *The Rise of the Greek Epic* (1907).

243. Isaiah 13:12. Ophir is a land mentioned several times in the Old Testament as the source of gold.

244. (Greek) "If love of humanity is present, love of craft is also present" (Hippocrates, *Precepts*, vi, 6). Osler's original note reads: "*Œuvres complètes d'Hippocrate,* par E. Littré, ix, 258."

245. *Wisdom—philosophia—at last be justified of her children:* Matthew 11:19.

5

DOCTOR AND NURSE

There are men and classes of men that stand above the common herd: the soldier, the sailor, and the shepherd not infrequently; the artist rarely; rarelier still, the clergyman; the physician almost as a rule. He is the flower (such as it is) of our civilization; and when that stage of man is done with, and only to be marvelled at in history, he will be thought to have shared as little as any in the defects of the period, and most notably exhibited the virtues of the race. Generosity he has, such as is possible to those who practise an art, never to those who drive a trade; discretion, tested by a hundred secrets; tact, tried in a thousand embarrassments; and what are more important, Heraclean cheerfulness and courage. So that he brings air and cheer into the sick room, and often enough, though not so often as he wishes, brings healing.

ROBERT LOUIS STEVENSON, preface to *Underwoods.*

Think not Silence the wisdom of Fools, but, if rightly timed, the honour of wise Men, who have not the Infirmity, but the Virtue of Taciturnity, and speak not out of the abundance, but the well-weighed thoughts of their Hearts. Such Silence may be Eloquence, and speak thy worth above the power of Words.

SIR THOMAS BROWNE, *Christian Morals*

THIS ADDRESS WAS DELIVERED to the graduates of the first class at the Johns Hopkins Training School for Nurses in 1891. It must be read in light of the views of women in its day. Only thirty-five schools then trained nurses.

Osler emphasizes the unceasing need for medical practitioners as "inevitable stage accessories" in the great drama of human suffering. But he points out that nurses must realize that they are also viewed as an unwelcome reminder of a patient's mortality. For generations, women have tended the sick and wounded. The profession has been shaped both by religious teaching of "love thy neighbor" and by war, as Florence Nightingale led nursing to its modern position.

Osler urges nurses to be hospitable and nonjudgemental. He stresses the importance of medical research; much suffering is due to ignorance of nature's laws, rather than to sins.

Osler maintains that nurses' training (then two years) builds character and widens their sympathies, making them better human beings. He predicts that, as a group, the graduates will have useful lives and be happy, because happiness is "absorption in some vocation that satisfies the soul."

Giving copies of this speech to nurses at graduation became a tradition at Johns Hopkins. It is interesting to note that one nurse from this first graduating class, Mary Adelaide Nutting,[1] became a national leader in nursing education, as head of this Nursing School and later of Columbia.

1. Helen E. Marshall, *Mary Adelaide Nutting, Pioneer of Modern Nursing* (Baltimore: Johns Hopkins University Press, 1972), p. 48.

DOCTOR AND NURSE

THERE ARE INDIVIDUALS—doctors and nurses, for example—whose very existence is a constant reminder of our frailties; and considering the notoriously irritating character of such people, I often wonder that the world deals so gently with them. The presence of the parson suggests dim possibilities, not the grim realities conjured up by the names of the persons just mentioned; the lawyer never worries us—in this way, and we can imagine in the future a social condition in which neither divinity nor law shall have a place—when all shall be friends and each one a priest, when the meek shall possess the earth;[2] but we cannot picture a time when Birth and Life and Death shall be separated from the "grizzly troop"[3] which we dread so much and which is ever associated in our minds with "physician and nurse."

Dread! Yes, but mercifully for us in a vague and misty way. Like schoolboys we play among the shadows cast by the turrets of the temple of oblivion, towards which we travel, regardless of what awaits us in the vale of years beneath.[4] Suffering and disease are ever before us, but life is very pleasant; and the

An address delivered to the first class of graduates from the Training School for Nurses at Johns Hopkins Hospital, June 4, 1891.

2. Matthew 5:5. The exact quotation is: "Blessed are the meek: for they shall inherit the earth."

3. Thomas Gray, "Ode on a Distant Prospect of Eton College," stanza 9. The exact quotation is:

> Lo, in the vale of years beneath
> A griesly troop are seen,
> The painful family of Death,
> More hideous than their Queen."

4. Ibid., stanza 6–9.

motto of the world, when well, is "forward with the dance."[5] Fondly imagining that we are in a happy valley, we deal with ourselves as the King did with the Gautama,[6] and hide away everything that suggests our fate. Perhaps we are wise. Who knows? Mercifully, the tragedy of life, though seen, is not realized. It is so close that we lose all sense of its proportions. And better so; for, as George Eliot has said, "if we had a keen vision and feeling of all ordinary human life, it would be like hearing the grass grow, or the squirrel's heart beat, and we should die of that roar which lies on the other side of silence."[7]

With many, however, it is a wilful blindness, a sort of fool's paradise,[8] not destroyed by a thought, but by the stern exigencies of life, when the "ministers of human fate"[9] drag us, or—worse still—those near and dear to us, upon the stage. Then, we become acutely conscious of the drama of human suffering, and of those inevitable stage accessories—doctor and nurse.

If, Members of the Graduating Class, the medical profession, composed chiefly of men, has absorbed a larger share of attention and regard, you have, at least, the satisfaction of feeling that yours is the older, and, as older, the more honourable calling. In one of the lost books of Solomon, a touching picture is given of Eve, then an early grandmother, bending over the little Enoch,[10] and showing Mahala how to soothe his sufferings and to allay his pains. Woman, "the link among the days,"[11] and so trained in a bitter school, has, in succes-

---

5. This is a catch phrase meaning "life is too good to brood seriously." Osler may have been thinking of a line of a poem by George Gordon Byron, "On with the dance! let joy be unconfined" ("Childe Harold's Pilgrimage," canto 3, stanza 22).

6. Gautama Buddha (c.563–c.483 B.C.): Indian philosopher and founder of Buddhism. According to various biographies, when Gautama was born a prophet foretold that he would retire from the world. His father, worried about the prophecy, gave him luxury and indulgence and also hid from him all ugly things, including human sorrows and sufferings, in a vain effort to hold on to him.

7. George Eliot, *Middlemarch,* ed. Gordon S. Haight (1871; Boston: Houghton Mifflin, 1968), book 2, chap. 20, p. 144.

8. A proverbial expression, meaning "a state of illusive happiness."

9. Thomas Gray, "Ode on a Distant Prospect of Eton College," stanza 6. The exact quotation is:

> Yet see how all around 'em wait
> The Ministers of human fate,
> And black Misfortune's baleful train!

10. Enoch is the grandson of Adam and Eve. It is possible Osler invented this episode because it was not found in *Apocrypha and Pseudepigrapha of the Old Testament.*

11. Alfred Tennyson, "In Memoriam A.H.H.," part 40, stanza 4, line 3, tells about a mother's role. The exact quotation is:

> Her office there to rear, to teach,
> Becoming as is meet and fit
> A link among the days, to knit
> The generations each with each."

sive generations, played the part of Mahala to the little Enoch,[12] of Elaine to the wounded Lancelot.[13] It seems a far cry from the plain of Mesopotamia [14] and the lists of Camelot [15] to the Johns Hopkins Hospital, but the spirit which makes this scene possible is the same, tempered through the ages, by the benign influence of Christianity. Among the ancients, many had risen to the idea of forgiveness of enemies, of patience under wrong doing, and even of the brotherhood of man; but the spirit of Love only received its incarnation with the ever memorable reply to the ever memorable question, Who is my neighbour? [16]—a reply which has changed the attitude of the world. Nowhere in ancient history, sacred or profane, do we find pictures of devoted heroism in women such as dot the annals of the Catholic Church, or such as can be paralleled in our own century. Tender maternal affection, touching filial piety were there; but the spirit abroad was that of Deborah not Rizpah, of Jael not Dorcas.[17]

In the gradual division of labour, by which civilization has emerged from barbarism, the doctor and the nurse have been evolved, as useful accessories in the incessant warfare in which man is engaged. The history of the race is a grim record of passions and ambitions, of weaknesses and vanities, a record, too often, of barbaric inhumanity, and even to-day, when philosophers would have us believe his thoughts had widened, he is ready as of old to shut the gates of mercy, and to let loose the dogs of war.[18] It was in one of these attacks of

12. See note 10.

13. Alfred Tennyson, "Lancelot and Elaine," in *The Idylls of the King*, lines 773–872.

14. Location of the biblical plain of Shinar (or Chaldea); it is presumed to be where Enoch dwelt.

15. Legendary court of King Arthur of Britain, where the Round Table was situated. *Lists* here means "a stadium for knightly jousting."

16. Luke 10:29–37. Jesus answered the question with the parable of the Good Samaritan who helped a stranger.

17. Osler contrasts the militant women Deborah and Jael with the benevolent Rizpah and Dorcas. All of these women were inspired by religious zeal, but to very different ends.

Deborah: A "prophetess" and leader of Israel who roused the people to defeat the Canaanites (Judges 4:4–16).

Rizpah: King David of Israel handed over seven sons of his predecessor and rival, King Saul, to the Gibeonites, who hanged them and, contrary to the law of Moses, left the corpses hanging to be picked clean by the birds and beasts. Rizpah, the mother of two of the dead men, camped by the corpses and chased all scavengers away until, moved by her piety, David seems to have relented and let the bodies be taken down and given honorable burial (2 Samuel 21:1–14). Leaving dead men hanging was thought to offend God and bring a curse on the land (Deuteronomy 21:22–23).

Jael: Heber's wife who treacherously killed Sisera, a defeated Canaanite general to whom she had offered shelter (Judges 4:17–22).

Dorcas: A Christian woman at Joppa, "full of good works and acts of charity." After her death she was restored to life by St. Peter's prayer (Acts 9:36–41).

18. *let loose the dogs of war:* William Shakespeare, *Julius Caesar*, III, i, 269–273. The exact quotation is:

race-mania[19] that your profession, until then unsettled and ill-defined, took, under Florence Nightingale—ever blessed be her name—its modern position.

Individually, man, the unit, the microcosm, is fast bound in chains of atavism,[20] inheriting legacies of feeble will and strong desires, taints of blood and brain. What wonder, then, that many, sore let and hindered in running the race, fall by the way, and need a shelter in which to recruit[21] or to die, a hospital, in which there shall be no harsh comments on conduct, but only, so far as is possible, love and peace and rest? Here, we learn to scan gently our brother man, judging not, asking no questions, but meting out to all alike a hospitality worthy of the *Hôtel Dieu*,[22] and deeming ourselves honoured in being allowed to act as its dispensers. Here, too, are daily before our eyes the problems which have ever perplexed the human mind; problems not presented in the dead abstract of books, but in the living concrete of some poor fellow in his last round, fighting a brave fight, but sadly weighted, and going to his account "unhousell'd, disappointed, unanel'd, no reckoning made."[23] As we whisper to each other over his bed that the battle is decided and Euthanasia[24] alone remains, have I not heard in reply to that muttered proverb, so often on the lips of the physician, "the fathers have eaten sour grapes,"[25] your answer, in clear accents—the comforting words of the prayer of Stephen?[26]

But our work would be much restricted were it not for man's outside adversary—Nature, the great Moloch,[27] which exacts a frightful tax of human blood, sparing neither young nor old; taking the child from the cradle, the mother from

All pity choked with custom of fell deeds.
And Caesar's spirit ranging for revenge, . . .
Cry 'Havoc,' and let slip the dogs of war."

19. Osler refers to the Crimean War (1853–1856).

20. *atavism:* Reversion or genetic throwback in plants and animals to traits of past generations

21. *recruit:* Recuperate.

22. A huge medieval hospital in Paris.

23. William Shakespeare, *Hamlet*, I, v, 77–78.

24. *Euthanasia* here means "a gentle and easy death," not the act of putting a person to death painlessly.

25. Ezekiel 18:2. The exact quotation is: "The word of the Lord came unto me again, saying, What mean ye, that ye use this proverb concerning the land of Israel, saying, The fathers have eaten sour grapes, and the children's teeth are set on edge?" Osler maintains that doctors tend to blame patients for their plights, as the Jewish exiles blamed their misfortunes on their fathers.

26. The Acts 7:59–60. The exact quotation is: "And they stoned Stephen, calling upon God, and saying, Lord Jesus, receive my spirit. And he kneeled down, and cried with a loud voice, Lord, lay not this sin to their charge."

27. *Moloch* (also *Molech*): A god worshipped by the people of Judah, requiring sacrifice of children (Leviticus 18:21, 2 Kings 23:10, Jeremiah 32:35).

28. The idea that sickness is a punishment for sin was formerly a common Christian teaching; for ex-

her babe, and the father from the family. Is it strange that man, unable to dissociate a personal element from such work, has incarnated an evil principle—the devil? If we have now so far outgrown this idea as to hesitate to suggest, in seasons of epidemic peril, that "it is for our sins we suffer"[28]—when we know the drainage is bad; if we no longer mock the heart prostrate in the grief of loss with the words "whom the Lord loveth He chasteneth"[29]—when we know the milk should have been sterilized—if, I say, we have, in a measure, become emancipated from such teachings, we have not yet risen to a true conception of Nature. Cruel, in the sense of being inexorable, she may be called, but we can no more upbraid her great laws than we can the lesser laws of the state, which are a terror only to evildoers. The pity is that we do not know them all; in our ignorance we err daily, and pay a blood penalty.[30] Fortunately it is now a great and growing function of the medical profession to search out the laws about epidemics, and these outside enemies of man, and to teach to you, the public—dull, stupid pupils you are, too, as a rule—the ways of Nature, that you may walk therein and prosper.

It would be interesting, Members of the Graduating Class, to cast your horoscopes. To do so collectively you would not like; to do so individually—I dare not; but it is safe to predict certain things of you, as a whole. You will be better women for the life which you have led here. But what I mean by "better women" is that the eyes of your souls have been opened, the range of your sympathies has been widened, and your characters have been moulded by the events in which you have been participators during the past two years.

Practically there should be for each of you a busy, useful, and happy life; more you cannot expect; a greater blessing the world cannot bestow. Busy you will certainly be, as the demand is great, both in private and public, for women with your training. Useful your lives must be, as you will care for those who cannot care for themselves, and who need about them, in the day of tribulation, gentle hands and tender hearts. And happy lives shall be yours, because busy and useful; having been initiated into the great secret—that happiness lies in the absorption in some vocation which satisfies the soul; that we are here to add what we can *to*, not to get what we can *from*, life.[31]

---

ample, the prayer of a suffering penitent reads: "There is no soundness in my flesh because of thine anger; neither is there any rest [or, health] in my bones because of my sin" (Psalm 38:3). Cf. Rudyard Kipling, "Natural Theology," lines 17–20.

29. Hebrews 12:6.

30. Leviticus 4–5.

31. According to *Bartlett's Familiar Quotations* (1955 ed.) Osler originated this, which has been frequently quoted by others.

And, finally, remember what we are — useful supernumeraries in the battle, simply stage accessories in the drama, playing minor, but essential, parts at the exits and entrances, or picking up, here and there, a strutter, who may have tripped upon the stage. You have been much by the dark river — so near to us all — and have seen so many embark, that the dread of the old boatman[32] has almost disappeared, and

> When the Angel of the darker Drink[33]
> At last shall find you by the river brink,
> And offering his cup, invite your soul
> Forth to your lips to quaff — you shall not shrink:[34]

your passport shall be the blessing of Him in whose footsteps you have trodden, unto whose sick you have ministered, and for whose children you have cared.

32. In Greek mythology the old boatman, Charon, ferried the souls of the dead across the river Styx, to Hades or Hell.

33. According to an Oriental legend "the Angel of the darker Drink" refers to Azrael who accomplished his mission by holding to the nostril an apple from the Tree of Life. In Muslim tradition Azrael is the angel of death, and according to Jewish and Islamic angelology he is the angel who separates the soul from the body at the time of death.

34. *The Rubáiyát of Omar Khayyám,* 3rd ed., trans. Edward FitzGerald (1872), quatrain 43.

6

TEACHER AND STUDENT

A University consists, and has ever consisted,
in demand and supply in wants which it alone can
satisfy and which it does satisfy, in the communication
of knowledge, and the relation and bond which exists between
the teacher and the taught. Its constituting, animating principle is
this moral attraction of one class of persons to another; which is prior
in its nature, nay commonly in its history, to any other tie whatever;
so that, where this is wanting, a University is alive only in name, and
has lost its true essence, whatever be the advantages, whether
of position or of affluence, with which the civil power
or private benefactors contrive to encircle it.
JOHN HENRY NEWMAN, "Free Trade
in Knowledge: The Sophists"

It would seem, Adeimantus, that the direction in which
education starts a man will determine his future life.
PLATO, *Republic*

A "REVOLUTION" IN TEACHING medicine is the subject of this address. It was
given in 1892 at the University of Minnesota, one of the first state-supported
medical schools. Osler praises the trend of connecting medical schools with
universities because it improves faculty standards, teaching, and equipment.
Furthermore, it lessens rivalries between schools and helps eliminate marginal
medical schools.

Early medical education in the United States lagged far behind German
schools in teaching laboratory science. This lag was due to the frontier conditions, the lack of money for equipment, and the lack of scientifically trained
faculty. Osler urges giving a high priority to developing *scientific* medical education.

Scientific education requires enthusiastic professors with practical knowledge. Research is necessary for new knowledge; teachers must be aware of the work of colleagues all over the world. Osler also stresses the need for clinical instruction in hospitals. He urges professors who are not receptive to new ideas to retire. Medicine is a "high calling combining intellectual and moral interests and offering novelty, utility, and charity."

Osler advises medical students to cultivate three habits to help achieve success, in medical school and, later, in their practice. First, cultivate the *art of detachment* or *self-discipline* in work. However, outside interests must balance this renunciation of idleness and the pursuit of pleasure. Second, in order to accomplish much, cultivate *system*—the orderly arrangement of work, study, and observations. Third, cultivate *thoroughness*, especially to understand the underlying scientific principles of medicine. Only thoroughness can prevent charlatanism.

Beyond these three habits, Osler advises *humility* and a *reverence for truth*. Doctors must avoid overconfidence and self-deception, that is, not admitting their mistakes. Osler urges students to have high ideals and the zeal to surmount obstacles. He admonishes them to strive for serenity, charity, and peace of mind.

TEACHER AND STUDENT

I

TRULY IT MAY BE SAID to-day that in the methods of teaching medicine the old order changeth, giving place to new,[1] and to this revolution let me briefly refer, since it has an immediate bearing on the main point I wish to make in the first portion of my address. The medical schools of the country have been either independent, University, or State Institutions. The first class, by far the most numerous, have in title University affiliations, but are actually devoid of organic union with seats of learning. Necessary as these bodies have been in the past,[2] it is a cause for sincere congratulation that the number is steadily diminishing. Admirable in certain respects—adorned too in many instances by the names of men who bore the burden and heat of the day of small things, and have passed to their rest amid our honoured dead—the truth must be acknowledged that the lamentable state of medical education in this country twenty years ago was the direct result of the inherent viciousness of a system they fostered.[3] Something in the scheme gradually deadened in the professors

An address delivered at the opening of the new medical buildings of the University of Minnesota, October 4, 1892.

1. Alfred Tennyson, "Morte d'Arthur," line 291. It means that appreciation and creation of the new was the spirit of the day. Tennyson wrote "yielding (not 'giving') place to new."

2. With the opening of the West and the wave of immigration, over four hundred medical schools, many inferior, were established in the United States Osler deplored the situation of poorly trained physicians and demanded reform.

3. Henry E. Sigerist (1891–1957) writes about such institutions as follows: "Instruction was, as may be imagined, quite insufficient. There was a complete lack of medical supplies. The schools were without funds. The only income was derived from the tuition fees and these were for the most part divided among

all sense of the responsibility until they professed to teach (mark the word), in less than two years, one of the most difficult arts in the world to acquire. Fellow teachers in medicine, believe me that when fifty or sixty years hence some historian traces the development of the profession in this country, he will dwell on the notable achievements, on the great discoveries, and on the unwearied devotion of its members, but he will pass judgment — yes, severe judgment — on the absence of the sense of responsibility which permitted a criminal laxity in medical education unknown before in our annals. But an awakening has come, and there is sounding the knell of doom for the medical college, responsible neither to the public nor the profession.

The schools with close university connexions have been the most progressive and thorough in this country. The revolution referred to began some twenty years ago with the appearance of the President of a well-known University[4] at a meeting of its medical faculty with a peremptory command to set their house in order.[5] Universities which teach only the Liberal Arts remain to-day, as in the middle ages, Scholæ minores,[6] lacking the technical faculties which make the Scholæ majores. The advantages of this most natural union are manifold and reciprocal. The professors in a University medical school have not that independence of which I have spoken, but are under an influence which tends constantly to keep them at a high level: they are urged by emulation with the other faculties to improve the standard of work, and so are given a strong stimulus to further development.

------

the professors . . . the laboratories non-existent. . . . The majority of schools had no connection with a university. . . . Nor were most of them connected with hospitals, so that their instruction was limited to theory. The time required was now as a rule two years, . . . the second year was nothing but a repetition of the first, and besides, in many places the academic year lasted only sixteen to twenty weeks. No previous training was required of the students." *American Medicine,* trans. Hildegard Nagel (New York: W. W. Norton, Inc., 1934), pp. 132–33.

4. Charles William *Eliot* (1834–1926): President of Harvard (1869–1909). His efforts to raise the standards of university education included the reorganization of the medical school.

5. Oliver Wendell Holmes wrote in a letter to his friend John L. Motley (April 3, 1870): "Firstly, then, our new President, Eliot, has turned the whole University over like a flapjack. There never was such a *bouleversement* as that in our Medical Faculty. The Corporation has taken the whole management of it out of our hands and changed everything. We are paid salaries, which I rather like, though I doubt if we gain in pocket by it. We have, partly in consequence of outside pressure, remodelled our whole course of instruction. Consequently we have a smaller class, but better students." John T. Morse, *Life and Letters of O. W. Holmes* (Boston: Houghton, Mifflin, 1896), vol. 2, pp. 187–91.

6. *Scholæ minores* and *Scholæ majores:* A medieval division. Generally speaking, the curriculum in the Middle Ages comprised the *trivium,* or lower studies (grammar, rhetoric, and dialectics), and the *quadrivium,* or higher studies (arithmetic, geometry, music, and astronomy), the whole making up what were known as the Seven Liberal Arts. Osler is advocating a return to something like the medieval system, under which a student had to obtain his arts degree before he was allowed to study medicine.

To anyone who has watched the growth of the new ideas in education it is evident that the most solid advances in method of teaching, the improved equipment, clinical and laboratory, and the kindlier spirit of generous rivalry—which has replaced the former debased method of counting heads as a test of merit—all these advantages have come from a tightening of the bonds between the medical school and the University.

And lastly there are the State schools, of which this college is one of the few examples. It has been a characteristic of American Institutions to foster private industries and to permit private corporations to meet any demands on the part of the public. This idea carried to extreme allowed the unrestricted manufacture—note the term—of doctors, quite regardless of the qualifications usually thought necessary in civilized communities—of physicians who may never have been inside a hospital ward, and who had, after graduation, to learn medicine somewhat in the fashion of the Chinese doctors who recognized the course of the arteries of the body, by noting just where the blood spurted when the acupuncture needle was inserted. So far as I know, State authorities have never interfered with any legally instituted medical school, however poorly equipped for its work, however lax the qualifications for license. Not only has this policy of non-intervention been carried to excess, but in many States a few physicians in any town could get a charter for a school without giving guarantees that laboratory or clinical facilities would be available. This anomalous condition is rapidly changing, owing partly to a revival of loyalty to higher ideals within the medical profession, and partly to a growing appreciation in the public of the value of physicians thoroughly educated in modern methods. A practical acknowledgment of this is found in the recognition in three States at least of medicine as one of the technical branches to be taught in the University supported by the people at large.

But it is a secondary matter, after all, whether a school is under State or University control, whether the endowments are great or small, the equipments palatial or humble; the fate of an institution rests not on these; the inherent, vital element, which transcends all material interests, which may give to a school glory and renown in their absence, and lacking which, all the "pride, pomp and circumstance"[7] are vain—this vitalizing element, I say, lies in the men who work in its halls, and in the ideals which they cherish and teach. There is a passage in one of John Henry Newman's *Historical Sketches* which expresses this feeling in terse and beautiful language: "I say then, that the personal influence of the teacher is able in some sort to dispense with an academical system, but that sys-

---

7. William Shakespeare, *Othello*, III, iii, 354.

tem cannot in any way dispense with personal influence. With influence there is life, without it there is none; if influence is deprived of its due position, it will not by those means be got rid of, it will only break out irregularly, dangerously. An academical system without the personal influence of teachers upon pupils, is an Arctic winter; it will create an ice-bound, petrified, cast-iron University, and nothing else."[8]

Naturally from this standpoint the selection of teachers is the function of highest importance in the Regents of a University. Owing to local conditions the choice of men for certain of the chairs is restricted to residents in the University town, as the salaries in most schools of this country have to be supplemented by outside work. But in all departments this principle should be acknowledged and acted upon by trustees and faculties, and supported by public opinion — that the very best men available should receive appointments. It is gratifying to note the broad liberality displayed by American colleges in welcoming from all parts teachers who may have shown any special fitness, emulating in this respect the liberality of the Athenians, in whose porticoes and lecture halls the stranger was greeted as a citizen[9] and judged by his mental gifts alone. Not the least by any means of the object lessons taught by a great University is that literature and science know no country, and, as has been well said, acknowledge "no sovereignty but that of the mind, and no nobility but that of genius."[10] But it is difficult in this matter to guide public opinion, and the Regents have often to combat a provincialism which is as fatal to the highest development of a University as is the shibboleth of a sectarian institution.[11]

8. John Henry Newman, "Discipline and Influence," in *Historical Sketches*, (1872–73; Westminister, Md.: Christian Classics, 1970), vol. 3, chap. 6, p. 74.

9. The Athenians had a long tradition of accepting talented foreigners, among whom were Aristotle and several other physicians. Toxaris, a Scythian, for example, was ranked among the Heroes of Athens and called "the Foreign Physician," after his deification. Lucian, "The Scythian," in *The Dialogues of Lucian* (London: Private Printing, 1930), p. 102.

10. John Henry Newman, "Site of a University," in *Historical Sketches*, (1872–73; Westminister, Md.: Christian Classics, 1970), vol. 3, chap. 3, p. 18.

11. Judges 12:4–6. The Ephraimites were identified by their inability to pronounce "sh" the way other Hebrews did. From this, "shibboleth" has come to mean any test word or notion that betrays the user's party or principles and, by extension, any doctrine once held to be essential but now generally abandoned as old-fashioned and discredited. Osler was probably thinking particularly of the long controversy in Ontario (strongest in the 1830s and 1840s) between those who wished the provincial university to be connected with the Church of England and those who wished it to be nonsectarian. His father was concerned with this.

II

To paraphrase the words of Matthew Arnold, the function of the teacher is to teach and to propagate the best that is known and taught in the world.[12] To teach the current knowledge of the subject he professes—sifting, analyzing, assorting, laying down principles. To propagate, i.e., to multiply, facts on which to base principles—experimenting, searching, testing. The best that is known and taught in the world—nothing less can satisfy a teacher worthy of the name, and upon us of the medical faculties lies a bounden duty in this respect, since our Art,[13] co-ordinate with human suffering, is cosmopolitan.

There are two aspects in which we may view the teacher—as a worker and instructor in science, and as practitioner and professor of the art; and these correspond to the natural division of the faculty into the medical school proper and the hospital.

In this eminently practical country the teacher of science has not yet received full recognition, owing in part to the great expense connected with his work, and in part to carelessness or ignorance in the public as to the real strength of a nation. To equip and maintain separate laboratories in Anatomy, Physiology, Chemistry (physiological and pharmacological), Pathology and Hygiene, and to employ skilled teachers, who shall spend all their time in study and instruction, require a capital not to-day at the command of any medical school in the land. There are fortunate ones with two or three departments well organized, not one with all. In contrast, Bavaria,[14] a kingdom of the German Empire, with an area less than this State, and a population of five and a half millions, supports in its three University towns flourishing medical schools with extensive laboratories, many of which are presided over by men of world-wide reputation, the steps of whose doors are worn in many cases by students who have crossed the Atlantic; seeking the wisdom of methods and the virtue of inspiration not easily accessible at home. But there were professors in Bavarian medical schools before Marquette and Joliet had launched their canoes on the great stream which the intrepid La Salle had discovered, before Du Lhut met Father Hennepin[15] below

12. Matthew Arnold, "The Function of Criticism at the Present Time," *Lectures and Essays in Criticism* (1865), *The Complete Prose Works of Matthew Arnold,* ed. R. H. Super (Ann Arbor: The University of Michigan Press, 1962), vol. 3 p. 283. The exact quotation is: "I am bound by my own definition of criticism: *a disinterested endeavour to learn and propagate the best that is known and thought in the world.*" Osler, in order to explain the function of the teacher instead of the definition of criticism, is paraphrasing such words as "learn" into "teach" and "thought" into "taught."

13. Osler maintains that medicine is an art.

14. A state in southern Germany.

15. French explorers in North America.

the falls of St. Anthony; and justice compels us to acknowledge that while winning an empire from the back-woods the people of this land had more urgent needs than laboratories of research. All has now changed. In this State, for example, the phenomenal growth of which has repeated the growth of the nation, the wilderness has been made to blossom as the rose, and the evidences of wealth and prosperity on every side almost constrain one to break out into the now old song, "Happy is that people that is in such a case."[16]

But in the enormous development of material interests there is danger lest we miss altogether the secret of a nation's life, the true test of which is to be found in its intellectual and moral standards. There is no more potent antidote to the corroding influence of mammon[17] than the presence in a community of a body of men devoted to science, living for investigation and caring nothing for the lust of the eyes and the pride of life. We forget that the measure of the value of a nation to the world is neither the bushel nor the barrel, but *mind;* and that wheat and pork, though useful and necessary, are but dross in comparison with those intellectual products which alone are imperishable. The kindly fruits of the earth[18] are easily grown; the finer fruits of the mind are of slower development and require prolonged culture.

Each one of the scientific branches to which I have referred has been so specialized that even to teach it takes more time than can be given by a single Professor, while the laboratory classes also demand skilled assistance. The aim of a school should be to have these departments in the charge of men who have, first, *enthusiasm,* that deep love of a subject, that desire to teach and extend it without which all instruction becomes cold and lifeless; secondly, *a full personal knowledge of the branch taught;* not a second-hand information derived from books, but the living experience derived from experimental and practical work in the best laboratories. This type of instructor is fortunately not rare in American

---

Jacques *Marquette* (1637–1675): Jesuit missionary who with Jolliet explored the Wisconsin and Mississippi rivers.

Louis *Joliet* (also *Jolliet*) (1645–1700): Discoverer of the Mississippi River in 1673.

Robert Cavelier de *La Salle* (1643–1687): Pioneer settler, explorer, and trader who descended the Mississippi River to the Gulf of Mexico, claiming the whole valley for Louis XIV and naming the region Louisiana.

Daniel Greysolon *Du Lhut* (also *Duluth* or *Dulhut*) (1636–1710): Explorer who made many trips into the Lake Superior region, establishing French control over the northern country. The modern city of Duluth, Minnesota, is named after him.

Louis Johannes *Hennepin* (1640–c.1701): Roman Catholic friar who accompanied La Salle through the Great Lakes and discovered St. Anthony's Falls on the Mississippi in 1680.

16. Psalm 144:15.

17. *mammon:* Riches or material wealth, personified as a spirit of evil (Matthew 6:24; Luke 16:9, 11, 13).

18. *the kindly fruits of the earth:* The Litany, in the *Book of Common Prayer. Kindly* here means "natural."

schools. The well-grounded students who have pursued their studies in England and on the Continent have added depth and breadth to our professional scholarship, and their critical faculties have been sharpened to discern what is best in the world of medicine. It is particularly in these branches that we need teachers of wide learning, whose standards of work are the highest known, and whose methods are those of the masters in lsrael.[19] Thirdly, men are required who have a *sense of obligation*, that feeling which impels a teacher to be also a contributor, and to add to the stores from which he so freely draws. And precisely here is the necessity to know the best that is taught in this branch, the world over. The investigator, to be successful, must start abreast of the knowledge of the day, and he differs from the teacher, who, living in the present, expounds only what is current, in that his thoughts must be in the future, and his ways and work in advance of the day in which he lives. Thus, unless a bacteriologist has studied methods thoroughly, and is familiar with the extraordinarily complex flora associated with healthy and diseased conditions, and keeps in touch with every laboratory of research at home and abroad, he will in attempting original work, find himself exploring ground already well-known, and will probably burden an already over-laden literature with faulty and crude observations. To avoid mistakes, he must know what is going on in the laboratories of England, France and Germany, as well as in those of his own country, and he must receive and read six or ten journals devoted to the subject. The same need for wide and accurate study holds good in all branches.

Thoroughly equipped laboratories, in charge of men, thoroughly equipped as teachers and investigators, is the most pressing want to-day in the medical schools of this country.

The teacher as a professor and practitioner of his art is more favoured than his brother, of whom I have been speaking; he is more common, too, and less interesting; though in the eyes of "the fool multitude who choose by show"[20] more important. And from the standpoint of medicine as an art for the prevention and cure of disease, the man who translates the hieroglyphics of science into the plain language of healing is certainly the more useful. He is more favoured inasmuch as the laboratory in which he works, the hospital, is a necessity in every centre of population. The same obligation rests on him to know and to teach the

---

19. Osler probably refers to the early scribes mentioned in *The Wisdom of Jesus the Son of Sirach* (Ecclesiasticus 38:24–34, 39:1–11). Sirach was one of the scribes who had a school in Jerusalem and taught that "wisdom" refers to both practical matters and research in the scriptures and sciences. There is also a reference to John 3:10, where Jesus asks Nicodemus "art thou a master of Israel, and knowest not these things?"

20. William Shakespeare, *Merchant of Venice*, II, ix, 26.

best that is known and taught in the world—on the surgeon the obligation to know thoroughly the scientific principles on which his art is based, to be a master in the technique of his handicraft, ever studying, modifying, improving;—on the physician, the obligation to study the natural history of diseases and the means for their prevention, to know the true value of regimen, diet and drugs in their treatment, ever testing, devising, thinking;—and upon both, to teach to their students habits of reliance, and to be to them examples of gentleness, forbearance and courtesy in dealing with their suffering brethren.

I would fain dwell upon many other points in the relation of the hospital to the medical school—on the necessity of ample, full and prolonged clinical instruction, and on the importance of bringing the student and the patient into close contact, not through the cloudy knowledge of the amphitheatre, but by means of the accurate, critical knowledge of the wards; on the propriety of encouraging the younger men as instructors and helpers in ward work; and on the duty of hospital physicians and surgeons to contribute to the advance of their art—but I pass on with an allusion to a very delicate matter in college faculties.

From one who, like themselves, has passed *la crise de quarante ans*,[21] the seniors present will pardon a few plain remarks upon the disadvantages to a school of having too many men of mature, not to say riper, years. Insensibly, in the fifth and sixth decades, there begins to creep over most of us a change, noted physically among other ways in the silvering of the hair and that lessening of elasticity, which impels a man to open rather than to vault a five-barred gate. It comes to all sooner or later; to some it is only too painfully evident, to others it comes unconsciously, with no pace perceived. And with most of us this physical change has its mental equivalent, not necessarily accompanied by loss of the powers of application or of judgment; on the contrary, often the mind grows clearer and the memory more retentive, but the change is seen in a weakened receptivity and in an inability to adapt oneself to an altered intellectual environment. It is this loss of mental elasticity which makes men over forty so slow to receive new truths. Harvey complained in his day that few men above this critical age seemed able to accept the doctrine of the circulation of the blood,[22] and in our own time it is interesting to note how the theory of the bacterial origin of

21. *la crise de quarante ans:* A French idiom meaning the crisis of forty years. Osler regards the age forty as a critical age. He later discussed the comparative uselessness of men over forty years of age in his 1905 speech. See "The Fixed Period," p. 294, n. 20.

22. William Harvey (1578–1657): English physician and anatomist who discovered the circulation of the blood. He later wrote: "These views [the circulation of the blood], as usual, pleased some more, others less; some chid and calumniated me, . . ." "Motion of the Heart and Blood in Animals," *The Works of William Harvey,* trans. Robert Willis (Philadelphia: University of Pennsylvania Press, 1989), chap. 1, "The Author's Motive for Writing," p. 20.

certain diseases has had, as other truths, to grow to acceptance with the generation in which it was announced. The only safeguard in the teacher against this
lamentable condition is to live in, and with the third decade, in company with
the younger, more receptive and progressive minds.

There is no sadder picture than the Professor who has outgrown his usefulness, and, the only one unconscious of the fact, insists, with a praiseworthy
zeal, upon the performance of duties for which the circumstances of the time
have rendered him unfit. When a man nor wax nor honey can bring home, he
should, in the interests of an institution, be dissolved from the hive to give more
labourers room; though it is not every teacher who will echo the sentiment—

> Let me not live . . .
> After my flame lacks oil, to be the snuff
> Of younger spirits whose apprehensive senses
> All but new things disdain.[23]

As we travel farther from the East, our salvation lies in keeping our faces toward
the rising sun, and in letting the fates drag us, like Cacus[24] his oxen, backward
into the cave of oblivion.

III

Students of Medicine, Apprentices of the Guild, with whom are the promises,
and in whom centre our hopes—let me congratulate you on the choice of calling which offers a combination of intellectual and moral interests found in no
other profession, and not met with at all in the common pursuits of life—a combination which, in the words of Sir James Paget,[25] "offers the most complete and
constant union of those three qualities which have the greatest charm for pure
and active minds—novelty, utility, and charity."[26] But I am not here to laud our
profession; your presence here on these benches is a guarantee that such praise

23. William Shakespeare, *All's Well that Ends Well*, I, ii, 58–61.

24. A fire-breathing Roman giant, and in some versions of the myth, son of Vulcan. He stole some of
the cattle of the sun god, which Heracles had been set to guard, and drove them backward into his cave,
to avoid detection. Osler probably found this in Thomas Browne's "A Letter to a Friend," *Sir Thomas
Browne's Works*, ed. Simon Wilkin (London: William Pickering, 1835), vol. 4, p. 50.

25. James *Paget* (1814–1899): English surgeon, one of the founders of the modern science of pathology,
specializing in tumors and bone diseases. He was vice-chancellor of the University of London and president of the Royal College of Surgeons.

26. The publications of James Paget include: *Lectures on Surgical Pathology* (London: Longmans, 1853)
and *Clinical Lectures* (New York: Appleton, 1875). The exact quote in the books surveyed has not been
located.

is superfluous. Rather allow me, in the time remaining at my disposal, to talk of the influences which may make you good students—now in the days of your pupilage, and hereafter when you enter upon the more serious duties of life.

In the first place, acquire early the *Art of Detachment*,[27] by which I mean the faculty of isolating yourselves from the pursuits and pleasures incident to youth. By nature man is the incarnation of idleness, which quality alone, amid the ruined remnants of Edenic characters,[28] remains in all its primitive intensity. Occasionally we do find an individual who takes to toil as others to pleasure, but the majority of us have to wrestle hard with the original Adam, and find it no easy matter to scorn delights and live laborious days. Of special importance is this gift to those of you who reside for the first time in a large city, the many attractions of which offer a serious obstacle to its acquisition. The discipline necessary to secure this art brings in its train habits of self-control and forms a valuable introduction to the sterner realities of life.

I need scarcely warn you against too close attention to your studies. I have yet to meet a medical student, the hey-day in whose blood had been quite tamed in his college days; but if you think I have placed too much stress upon isolation in putting the Art of Detachment first in order amongst the *desiderata*[29] let me temper the hard saying by telling you how with "labors assiduous due pleasures to mix."[30] Ask of any active business man or a leader in a profession the secret which enables him to accomplish much work, and he will reply in one word, *system;* or as I shall term it, the *Virtue of Method,* the harness without which only the horses of genius travel. There are two aspects of this subject; the first relates to the orderly arrangement of your work, which is to some extent enforced by the roster of demonstrations and lectures, but this you would do well to supplement in private study by a schedule in which each hour finds its allotted duty. Thus faithfully followed day by day system may become at last engrained in the most shiftless nature, and at the end of a semester a youth of moderate ability may find himself far in advance of the student who works spasmodically, and trusts to *cramming.* Priceless as this virtue is now in the time of your probation, it becomes in the practising physician an incalculable blessing. The incessant and irregular demands upon a busy doctor make it very difficult to retain, but the

27. Osler again stresses the importance of this art in his address in 1902 to the Canadian Medical Association. See "Chauvinism in Medicine," p. 229.

28. *Characters* is here equivalent to "characteristics." Eden was the Paradise of God, where Adam and Eve, the ancestors of the human race, lived before they fell by disobeying God's commandment.

29. *desiderata:* (Latin) plural form of "desideratum," which means a thing which is needed or wanted.

30. *labors assiduous due pleasures to mix:* Probably this derives from Milton's oration to students, which reads: "The alternation of labor and pleasure is wont to banish the weariness of satiety." John Milton, "Prolusions 6," in *The Works of John Milton* (New York: Columbia University Press, 1931), vol. 12, p. 205.

public in this matter can be educated, and the men who practise with system, allotting a definite time of the day to certain work, accomplish much more and have at any rate a little leisure; while those who are unmethodical never catch up with the day's duties and worry themselves, their *confrères*,[31] and their patients.

The other aspect of method has a deeper significance, hard for you to reach, not consoling when attained, since it lays bare our weaknesses. The practice of medicine is an art, based on science. Working with science, in science, for science, it has not reached, perhaps never will, the dignity of a complete science, with exact laws, like astronomy or engineering. Is there then no science of medicine? Yes, but in parts only, such as anatomy and physiology, and the extraordinary development of these branches during the present century has been due to the cultivation of method, by which we have reached some degree of exactness, some certainty of truth. Thus we can weigh the secretions in the balance and measure the work of the heart in foot-pounds. The deep secrets of generation have been revealed and the sesame of evolution has given us fairy tales of science more enchanting than the Arabian Nights' entertainment. With this great increase in our knowledge of the laws governing the processes of life, has been a corresponding, not less remarkable, advance in all that relates to life in disorder, that is, disease. The mysteries of heredity are less mysterious, the operating room has been twice over robbed of its terrors; the laws of epidemics are known, and the miracle of the threshing floor of Araunah the Jebusite,[32] may be repeated in any town out of Bumbledom. All this change has come about by the observation of facts, by their classification, and by the founding upon them of general laws. Emulating the persistence and care of Darwin, we must collect facts with open-minded watchfulness, unbiased by crotchets [33] or notions; fact on fact, instance on instance, experiment on experiment, facts which fitly joined together by some master who grasps the idea of their relationship may establish a general principle. But in the practice of medicine, where our strength should be lies our great weakness. Our study is man, as the subject of accidents or diseases. Were he always, inside and outside, cast in the same mould, instead of differing from his fellow man as much in constitution and in his reaction to stimulus as in feature, we should ere this have reached some settled principles in our art. And not only are the reactions themselves variable, but we, the doctors, are so fallible, ever beset with the common and fatal facility of reaching conclusions

31. *confrères:* (French) colleagues.

32. 2 Samuel 24:18–25. The angel who was causing the plague stayed his hand, at God's command, at the threshing-floor of Araunah, and thus Jerusalem was spared from the plague. In gratitude, David bought the site and built an altar there to the Lord.

33. *crotchets:* Whimsical notions or eccentric personal preferences

from superficial observations, and constantly misled by the ease with which our minds fall into the ruts of one or two experiences.

And thirdly add to the Virtue of Method, the *Quality of Thoroughness,* an element of such importance that I had thought of making it the only subject of my remarks. Unfortunately, in the present arrangement of the curriculum, few of you as students can hope to obtain more than a measure of it, but all can learn its value now, and ultimately with patience become living examples of its benefit. Let me tell you briefly what it means. A knowledge of the fundamental sciences upon which our art is based—chemistry, anatomy, and physiology—not a smattering, but a full and deep acquaintance, not with all the facts, that is impossible, but with the great principles based upon them. You should, as students, become familiar with the methods by which advances in knowledge are made, and in the laboratory see clearly the paths the great masters have trodden, though you yourselves cannot walk therein. With a good preliminary training and a due apportioning of time you can reach in these three essential studies a degree of accuracy which is the true preparation for your life duties. It means such a knowledge of diseases and of the emergencies of life and of the means for their alleviation, that you are safe and trustworthy guides for your fellowmen. You cannot of course in the brief years of pupilage so grasp the details of the various branches that you can surely recognize and successfully treat all cases. But here if you have mastered certain principles is at any rate one benefit of thoroughness—you will avoid the sloughs of charlatanism. Napoleon, according to Sainte Beuve,[34] one day said when somebody was spoken of in his presence as a charlatan, "Charlatan as much as you please, but where is there not charlatanism?"[35] Now, thoroughness is the sole preventive of this widespread malady, which in medicine is not met with only outside of the profession. Matthew Arnold, who quotes the above from Sainte Beuve, defines charlatanism as the "confusing or obliterating the distinctions between excellent and inferior, sound and unsound, or only half sound, true and untrue or half true."[36] The higher the standard of education in a profession the less marked will be the charlatanism, whereas no greater incentive to its development can be found than in sending out from our colleges men who have not had mental training sufficient to enable them to judge between the excellent and the inferior, the sound and the unsound, the true and

34. Charles Augustin *Sainte-Beuve* (1804–1869): French writer who studied medicine.

35. Matthew *Arnold,* "The Study of Poetry," in *English Literature and Irish Politics, The Complete Prose Works of Matthew Arnold,* ed. R. H. Super (1882; Ann Arbor: The University of Michigan Press, 1973), vol. 9 p. 162. The reference for Sainte-Beuve is *Les Cahiers de Sainte-Beuve,* ed. J. Troubat (Paris: A. Lemerre, 1876), p. 51.

36. Ibid.

the half true. And if we of the household are not free from the seductions of this vice, what of the people among whom we work? From the days of the sage of Endor,[37] even the rulers have loved to dabble in it, while the public of all ages have ever revelled in its methods—to-day, as in the time of the Father of Medicine,[38] one of whose contemporaries (Plato) thus sketches the world old trait: "And what a delightful life they lead! they are always doctoring and increasing and complicating their disorders and always fancying they will be cured by any nostrum which anybody advises them to try."[39]

The Art of Detachment, the Virtue of Method, and the Quality of Thoroughness may make you students, in the true sense of the word, successful practitioners, or even great investigators; but your characters may still lack that which can alone give permanence to powers—the *Grace of Humility*. As the divine Italian[40] at the very entrance to Purgatory was led by his gentle Master to the banks of the island and girt with a rush, indicating thereby that he had cast off all pride and self-conceit, and was prepared for his perilous ascent to the realms above, so should you, now at the outset of your journey take the reed of humility in your hands, in token that you appreciate the length of the way, the difficulties to be overcome, and the fallibility of the faculties upon which you depend.

In these days of aggressive self-assertion, when the stress of competition is so keen and the desire to make the most of oneself so universal, it may seem a little old-fashioned to preach the necessity of this virtue, but I insist for its own sake, and for the sake of what it brings, that a due humility should take the place of honour on the list. For its own sake, since with it comes not only a reverence for truth, but also a proper estimation of the difficulties encountered in our search for it. More perhaps than any other professional man, the doctor has a curious–shall I say morbid?—sensitiveness to (what he regards) personal error. In a way this is right; but it is too often accompanied by a *cocksureness* of opinion which, if encouraged, leads him to so lively a conceit that the mere suggestion of mistake under any circumstances is regarded as a reflection on his honour,

37. 1 Samuel 28:7. King Saul consulted a medium at Endor to call up the spirit of Samuel to ask his advice on fighting the Philistines. His defeat and death were foretold.

38. Hippocrates (c.460–c.375 B.C.): Ancient Greek physician who taught scientific medicine at the famous temple of Asclepius at Cos. Osler refers to the Hippocratic Oath as a guideline for the medical students. See "The Master-Word in Medicine," p. 274.

39. Plato, *Republic*, book 4, 426.

40. The divine Italian refers to Dante Alighieri (1265–1321), an Italian poet and author of *La Divina Commedia*. His "gentle master" was Virgil (70–19 B.C.), a Roman poet and author of *The Aeneid*, whom Dante represented as his guide through hell and purgatory. "Purgatory," *La Divina Commedia* (1307–1321), canto 1.

a reflection equally resented whether of lay or of professional origin. Start out with the conviction that absolute truth is hard to reach in matters relating to our fellow creatures, healthy or diseased, that slips in observation are inevitable even with the best trained faculties, that errors in judgment must occur in the practice of an art which consists largely of balancing probabilities; — start, I say, with this attitude in mind, and mistakes will be acknowledged and regretted; but instead of a slow process of self-deception, with ever increasing inability to recognize truth, you will draw from your errors the very lessons which may enable you to avoid their repetition.

And, for the sake of what it brings, this grace of humility is a precious gift. When to the sessions of sweet silent thought you summon up the remembrance[41] of your own imperfections, the faults of your brothers will seem less grievous, and, in the quaint language of Sir Thomas Browne, you will "allow one eye for what is laudable in them."[42] The wrangling and unseemly disputes which have too often disgraced our profession arise, in a great majority of cases, on the one hand, from this morbid sensitiveness to the confession of error, and, on the other, from a lack of brotherly consideration, and a convenient forgetfulness of our own failings. Take to heart the words of the son of Sirach, winged words[43] to the sensitive souls of the sons of Esculapius: "Admonish a friend, it may be he has not done it; and if he have done it, that he do it no more. Admonish thy friend, it may be he hath not said it; and if he have, that he speak it not again. Admonish a friend, for many times it is a slander, and believe not every tale."[44] Yes, many times it is a slander, and believe not every tale.

The truth that lowliness is young ambition's ladder is hard to grasp, and when accepted harder to maintain. It is so difficult to be still amidst bustle, to be quiet amidst noise; yet, "*es bildet ein Talent sich in der Stille*"[45] alone, in the calm life necessary to continuous work for a high purpose. The spirit abroad at present in this country is not favourable to this Teutonic view, which galls the quick apprehension and dampens the enthusiasm of the young American. All

---

41. *When to the sessions of sweet silent thought you summon up the remembrance:* William Shakespeare, "Sonnet 30," lines 1–2. The exact quotation is:

> When to the sessions of sweet silent thought
> I summon up remembrance of things past,
> I sigh the lack of many a thing I sought,
> And with old woes new wail my dear time's waste.

42. Thomas Browne, *Christian Morals* (1716), part 1, sect. 28.

43. *winged words:* A frequent formula in the poems of Homer (fl. before 700 B.C.), which means words that deliver messages speedily. *Iliad,* book 1, line 201, etc.

44. *The Wisdom of Jesus the Son of Sirach:* (Ecclesiasticus, a book of the Apocrypha), Sirach 19:13.

45. (German) "A talent forms itself in stillness." Goethe, *Torquato Tasso* (1790), I, ii, 54.

the same, it is true, and irksome at first though the discipline may be, there will come a time when the very fetters in which you chafed shall be a strong defence, and your chains a robe of glory.

Sitting in Lincoln Cathedral[46] and gazing at one of the loveliest of human works—for such the angel Choir has been said to be—there arose within me, obliterating for the moment the thousand heraldries and twilight saints and dim emblazonings, a strong sense of reverence for the minds which had conceived and the hands which had executed such things of beauty. What manner of men were they who could, in those (to us) dark days, build such transcendent monuments? What was the secret of their art? By what spirit were they moved? Absorbed in thought, I did not hear the beginning of the music, and then, as a response to my reverie and arousing me from it, rang out the clear voice of the boy leading the antiphon,[47] "That thy power, thy glory and mightiness of thy kingdom might be known unto men."[48] Here was the answer. Moving in a world not realized, these men sought, however feebly, to express in glorious structures their conceptions of the beauty of holiness, and these works, our wonder, are but the outward and visible signs of the ideals which animated them.

To us in very different days life offers nearly the same problems, but the conditions have changed, and, as has happened before in the world's history, great material prosperity has weakened the influence of ideals, and blurred the eternal difference between means and end. Still, the ideal State, the ideal Life, the ideal Church[49]—what they are and how best to realize them—such dreams continue to haunt the minds of men, and who can doubt that their contemplation greatly assists the upward progress of our race? We, too, as a profession, have cherished standards, some of which, in words sadly disproportionate to my subject, I have attempted to portray.

My message is chiefly to you, Students of Medicine, since with the ideals entertained now your future is indissolubly bound. The choice lies open, the paths are plain before you. Always seek your own interests, make of a high and sacred calling a sordid business, regard your fellow creatures as so many tools of trade, and, if your heart's desire is for riches, they may be yours; but you will have bartered away the birthright of a noble heritage, traduced the physi-

46. Thirteenth-century English gothic cathedral noted for the sculptures of angels in its choir.

47. *Antiphon* is a classical form of "anthem," meaning a piece of church music rendered by the choir without the help of the congregation.

48. Psalm 145:12, in the version in *Book of Common Prayer*. What Osler heard was probably not actually an anthem but the appointed psalm for Morning Prayer on the thirtieth day of the month.

49. The underlying idea is the theme of Plato's *Republic:* the most nearly perfect political system, and the purest teaching about the gods, as the means of shaping mankind to live as well and nobly as possible.

cian's well-deserved title of the Friend of Man, and falsified the best traditions of an ancient and honourable Guild. On the other hand, I have tried to indicate some of the ideals which you may reasonably cherish. No matter though they are paradoxical in comparison with the ordinary conditions in which you work, they will have, if encouraged, an ennobling influence, even if it be for you only to say with Rabbi Ben Ezra, "what I aspired to be and was not, comforts me."[50] And though this course does not necessarily bring position or renown, consistently followed it will at any rate give to your youth an exhilarating zeal and a cheerfulness which will enable you to surmount all obstacles—to your maturity a serene judgment of men and things, and that broad charity without which all else is nought—to your old age that greatest of blessings, peace of mind, a realization, maybe, of the prayer of Socrates for the beauty in the inward soul and for unity of the outer and the inner man;[51] perhaps, of the promise of St. Bernard, "*pax sine crimine, pax sine turbine, pax sine rixa.*"[52]

50. Robert Browning, "Rabbi Ben Ezra," stanza 7, lines 4–5. Browning presents ideas from Rabbi Abenezra or "Ben Ezra" (1092–1167), a great Jewish poet, philosopher, and physician who wandered Europe, Asia, and Africa in pursuit of knowledge. The first stanza runs as follows:

> Grow old along with me!
> The best is yet to be,
> The last of life, for which the first was made:
> Our times are in His Hand
> Who saith, 'A whole I planned,
> Youth shows but half; trust God: see all, nor be afraid!'

51. Socrates, in Plato, *Phaedrus*, 279b–c.

52. *pax sine crimine, pax sine turbine, pax sine rixa:* (Latin) peace without crime, peace without disturbance, peace without strife. Bernard of Cluny (or, of Morlaix), *De Contemptu Mundi*, ed. H. C. Hoskier (London: B. Quaritch, 1929), 1ine 119, p. 5.

7

PHYSIC AND PHYSICIANS AS
DEPICTED IN PLATO

To one small people . . . it was given to create the principle of Progress. That people was the Greek. Except the blind forces of Nature, nothing moves in this world which is not Greek in its origin.

SIR HENRY MAINE, *Village Communities*

From the lifeless background of an unprogressive world—Egypt, Syria, frozen Scythia—a world in which the unconscious social aggregate had been everything, the conscious individual, his capacity and rights, almost nothing, the Greek had stepped forth, like the young prince in the fable, to set things going.

WALTER PATER, *Plato and Platonism*

These (years of vague, restless speculation) had now lasted long enough, and it was time for the *Meisterjahre* of quiet, methodical research to succeed if science was to acquire steady and sedentary habits instead of losing itself in a maze of phantasies, revolving in idle circles. It is the undying glory of the medical school of Cos that it introduced this innovation in the domain of its art, and thus exercised the most beneficial influence on the whole intellectual life of mankind. "Fiction to the right! Reality to the left!" was the battle-cry of this school in the war they were the first to wage against the excesses and defects of the nature-philosophy. Nor could it have found any more suitable champions, for the serious and noble calling of the physician, which brings him every day and every hour in close communion with nature, in the exercise of which mistakes in theory engender the most fatal practical consequences, has served in all ages as a nursery of the most genuine and incorruptible sense of truth. The best physicians must be the best observers, but the man who sees keenly, who hears clearly, and whose senses, powerful at the start, are sharpened and refined by constant exercise, will only in exceptional instances be a visionary or a dreamer.

THEODOR GOMPERZ, *Greek Thinkers*

THIS ADDRESS ON EARLY Greek medicine was delivered to the Johns Hopkins Hospital Historical Club in 1892. The writings of the philosopher Plato reveal much about physicians of ancient Greece, their role in society, and the relationships among medicine, physical fitness, and theology. Plato defined medicine as that "which considers the constitution of the patient and has principles of action and reasons in each case."

Plato's *Dialogues* tell us that medicine of that time stressed treating the body and the soul as a whole. In the *Timæus*, Plato sets forth his view that the body is composed of various triangles, combining to make marrow, blood, bile, and bones. Disease results when one of these humors, often bile, is out of place. Although his theories of respiration and digestion seemed strange by Osler's time, Plato knew that blood circulated and nourished the system. In his theory of aging, the triangles of the marrow weaken until they no longer assimilate food, and then they release the soul in death.

Plato discusses psychology in terms of conflicts of spirit, reason, and appetites. In one dialogue, the mind is compared to a block of wax that holds impressions and, in another, to a cage into which various birds of knowledge are placed as they are caught. He also discusses beneficial or "divine" madness, which gives us prophecy, poetry, inspiration, and love (*Phædrus*). Vice is considered to be involuntary, caused by bad education or disease. Mental illness can be avoided by maintaining a balance between mind and body; treatments are based on exercise and diet, rather than on medicines.

Plato's writings contain many other references to the lives of doctors, both private practitioners and the distinguished, elected state physicians. Although physicians were considered socially elite, Plato only ranks them fourth among the professions (with philosophers first—and tyrants, ninth).

Probably Plato's most shocking advice is that *physicians should experience all manners of diseases themselves!* (*The Republic*). Plato often used medical analogies; Socrates described himself as a midwife diagnosing whether men are pregnant with truth or folly. Much medical detail is given about Socrates' poisoning, and his final toast is to Aesculapius, the god of healing. Osler praises the freshness of Plato's writing and its continuing interest to his fellow physicians.

PHYSIC & PHYSICIANS AS DEPICTED IN PLATO

O UR HISTORICAL CLUB HAD under consideration last winter the sub-ject of Greek Medicine. After introductory remarks and a de-scription of the Æsculapian temples[1] and worship by Dr. Welch,[2] we proceeded to a systematic study of the Hippocratic writings, taking up in order, as found in them, medicine, hygiene, surgery, and gynæ-cology. Among much of interest which we gleaned, not the least important was the knowledge that as an art, medicine had made, even before Hippocrates, great progress, as much almost as was possible without a basis in the sciences of anatomy and physiology. Minds inquisitive, acute, and independent had been studying the problems of nature and of man; and several among the pre-Socratic philosophers had been distinguished physicians, notably, Pythagoras, Empedo-cles, and Democritus.[3] Unfortunately we know but little of their views, or even

A paper read at the meeting of the Johns Hopkins Hospital Historical Club, December 14, 1892, and printed in 1893. Notes about Plato's passages are from *The Dialogues of Plato*, 4th ed., trans. Benjamin Jowett (1871; Oxford: the Clarendon Press, 1953), unless otherwise stated. *Physic* is an archaic term for the art and skill of healing, or more specifically, treating patients with medicine.

1. There were temples and shrines to Æsculapius (Asclepius), god of healing, throughout Greece, of which the most famous was at Epidaurus where miraculous healings were recorded.

2. William Henry *Welch* (1850–1934): American pathologist and professor at Johns Hopkins University. He was an eminent authority on bacteriology and pathology and the first professor at Johns Hopkins of the history of medicine.

3. *Pythagoras* (c.582–c.500 B.C.): Greek philosopher and mathematician, to whom are ascribed the doc-trine of metempsychosis (the passage of the soul from one body to another) and the teaching that earthly life is only a purification of the soul. He and his disciples (Pythagoreans) are known to have made con-siderable advances in geometry.

of the subjects in medicine on which they wrote. In the case of Democritus, however, Diogenes Laërtius[4] has preserved a list of his medical writings, which intensifies the regret at the loss of the works of this great man, the title of one of whose essays, "On Those who are Attacked with Cough after Illness," indicates a critical observation of disease, which Daremberg[5] seems unwilling to allow to the pre-Hippocratic philosopher-physicians.

We gathered also that in the golden age of Greece, medicine had, as to-day, a triple relationship, with science, with gymnastics, and with theology. We can imagine an Athenian father of the early fourth century worried about the enfeebled health of one of his growing lads, asking the advice of Hippocrates about a suspicious cough, or sending him to the palæstra of Taureas[6] for a systematic course in gymnastics; or, as Socrates advised, "when human skill was exhausted,"[7] asking the assistance of the divine Apollo,[8] through his son, the "hero-physician," Æsculapius, at his temple in Epidaurus[9] or at Athens itself. Could the Greek live over his parental troubles at the end of the nineteenth century, he would get a more exact diagnosis and a more rational treatment; but he might travel far to find so eminent a "professor" of gymnastic as Miccus[10] for his boy, and in Christian science[11] or faith-healing he would find our bastard substitute for the stately and gracious worship of the Æsculapian temple.[12]

Empedocles (c.495–c.435 B.C.): Greek philosopher, poet, and statesman, who first taught that all material substances are compounded of the four elements fire, air, earth, and water.

Democritus (c.460–c.370 B.C.): Greek philosopher known as "the Laughing Philosopher" because of his optimism. He was the most notable ancient exponent of the atomic theory of matter.

4. *Diogenes Laërtius* (3rd cent. A.D.): Greek writer who wrote the lives, opinions, and sayings of famous philosophers in ten volumes, which are still extant. Although often inaccurate and uncritical, they form an important contribution toward the history of philosophy.

5. Charles Victor *Daremberg* (1817–1872): French historian of medicine. Author of *État de la médecine entre Homère & Hippocrate* (1869) and *Histoire des sciences médicales* (1870).

6. A private school in Taureas, where boys were trained in physical exercises.

7. Louis Dyer, *Studies of the Gods in Greece at Certain Sanctuaries Recently Excavated* (London: Macmillan, 1891), p. 238.

8. Æsculapius (also Asclepius): Greek god of medicine. He is usually represented as a bearded old man, and his common attribute is a staff with a serpent coiled around it.

9. A town in Argolis, the chief seat of worship of Æsculapius.

10. *Miccus* (5th cent. B.C.): Teacher of the palaestra (*Lysis,* 204a).

11. *Christian Science:* A sect founded by Mary Baker Eddy in 1879 in Boston after the publication of *Science and Health* (1875).

12. Osler's original note reads: "For an account of 'Æsculapius at Epidaurus and Athens,' see chap. vi of Dyer's *Gods of Greece* (Macmillan, 1891), a chapter which contains also an excellent discussion on the relation of secular to priestly medicine. In chapter III of Pater's delightful story *Marius the Epicurean,*

From the Hippocratic writings alone we have a very imperfect knowledge of the state of medicine in the most brilliant period of Grecian history; and many details relating to the character and to the life of physicians are gleaned only from secular authors. So much of the daily life of a civilized community relates to problems of health and disease that the great writers of every age of necessity throw an important side-light, not only on the opinions of the people on these questions, but often on the condition of special knowledge in various branches. Thus a considerable literature already illustrates the medical knowledge of Shakespeare, from whose doctors, apothecaries,[13] and mad-folk much may be gathered as to the state of the profession in the latter part of the sixteenth century. So also the satire of Molière[14] malicious though it be, has preserved for us phases of medical life in the seventeenth century, for which we scan in vain the strictly medical writings of that period; and writers of our times, like George Eliot, have told for future generations in a character such as Lydgate,[15] the little every-day details of the struggles and aspirations of the profession of the nineteenth century, of which we find no account whatever in the files of the *Lancet*.[16]

We are fortunate in having had preserved the writings of the two most famous of the Greek philosophers—the great idealist, Plato, whose "contemplation of all time and all existence"[17] was more searching than that of his predecessors, fuller than that of any of his disciples, and the great realist, Aristotle, to whose memory every department of knowledge still pays homage, and who has swayed the master-minds of twenty-two centuries. From the writings of both much may be gathered about Greek physic and physicians; but I propose in this essay to restrict myself to what I have culled from the *Dialogues of Plato*. I shall first speak of his physiological and pathological speculations; then I shall refer to the many interesting allusions to, and analogies drawn from, medicine and physicians; and, lastly, I shall try to estimate from the *Dialogues* the social standing of the Greek doctor, and shall speak on other points which bear upon the

---

is a description of one of the Roman Æsculapia, and an account of the method of procedure in the 'cure,' the ridiculous aspects of which are so graphically described in the 'Plutus' of Aristophanes."

13. *apothecaries:* Pharmacists.

14. *Molière* (1622–1673): French writer of comedies. In *L'Amour médecin* (1665) Molière caricatures doctors who can do nothing to cure the illness.

15. *Lydgate:* Hero of George Eliot's novel *Middlemarch* (1871–1872).

16. Influential journal of British and foreign medicine, which has been published in London since 1823.

17. Jowett's introduction to *Timæus:* "To the 'spectator of all time and all existence' the universe remains at rest," vol. 3, p. 676. The general idea is found in *Timæus,* 37–38.

general condition of the profession. The quotations are made in every instance from Professor Jowett's translation, the third edition, 1892.[18]

I

To our enlightened minds the anatomy and physiology of Plato are crude and imperfect; as much or even more so than those of Hippocrates. In the *Timæus* he conceived the elements to be made up of bodies in the form of triangles, the different varieties and combinations of which accounted for the existence of the four elementary bodies of Empedocles[19] — fire, earth, water, and air. The differences in the elementary bodies are due to differences in the size and arrangement of the elementary triangles, which, like the atoms of the atomist, are too small to be visible. Marrow had the most perfect of the elementary triangles, and from it bone, flesh, and the other structures of the body were made. "God took such of the primary triangles as were straight and smooth, and were adapted by their perfection to produce fire and water, and air and earth; these, I say, he separated from their kinds, and mingling them in due proportions with one another, made the marrow out of them to be a universal seed of the whole race of mankind; and in this seed he then planted and enclosed the souls, and in the original distribution gave to the marrow as many and various forms as the different kinds of souls were hereafter to receive. That which, like a field, was to receive the divine seed, he made round every way, and called that portion of the marrow brain, intending that, when an animal was perfected, the vessel containing this substance should be the head; but that which was intended to contain the remaining and mortal part of the soul he distributed into figures at once round and elongated, and he called them all by the name 'marrow'; and to these, as to anchors, fastening the bonds of the whole soul, he proceeded to fashion around them the entire framework of our body, constructing for the marrow, first of all, a complete covering of bone."[20]

The account of the structure of bone and flesh, and of functions of respiration, digestion, and circulation is unintelligible to our modern notions. Plato knew that the blood was in constant motion; in speaking of inspiration and expiration, and the network of fire which interpenetrates the body, he says: "For when the respiration is going in and out, and the fire, which is fast bound within,

18. *The Dialogues of Plato,* trans. Benjamin Jowett, 1st ed., 1871; 3rd ed., 1892.

Benjamin *Jowett* (1817–1893): Regius professor of Greek at Oxford University, but best known as the master of Balliol College, which he made into one of the most respected colleges in the university.

19. See p. 127, n. 3.

20. *Timæus,* 73c–d.

follows it, and ever and anon moving to and fro, enters the belly and reaches the meat and drink, it dissolves them, and dividing them into small portions, and guiding them through the passages where it goes, pumps them as from a fountain into the channels of the veins, *and makes the stream of the veins flow through the body as through a conduit.*"[21] A complete circulation was unknown; but Plato understood fully that the blood was the source of nourishment,—"the liquid itself we call blood, which nourishes the flesh and the whole body, whence all parts are watered and empty spaces filled."[22] In the young, the triangles, or in modern parlance we would say the atoms, are new, and are compared to the keel of a vessel just off the stocks.[23] They are locked firmly together, but form a soft and delicate mass freshly made of marrow and nourished on milk. The process of digestion is described as a struggle between the triangles out of which the meats and drinks are composed, and those of the bodily frame; and as the former are older and weaker the newer triangles of the body cut them up, and in this way the animal grows great, being nourished by a multitude of similar particles. The triangles are in constant fluctuation and change, and in the "Symposium" Socrates makes Diotima[24] say, "A man is called the same, and yet in the short interval which elapses between youth and age, and in which every animal is said to have life and identity, he is undergoing a perpetual process of loss and reparation—hair, flesh, bones, and the whole body are always changing."[25]

131

PHYSICIANS IN

PLATO

The description of senility, euthanasia, and death is worth quoting: "But when the roots of the triangles are loosened by having undergone many conflicts with many things in the course of time, they are no longer able to cut or assimilate the food which enters, but are themselves easily divided by the bodies which come in from without. In this way every animal is overcome and decays, and this affection is called old age. And at last, when the bonds by which the triangles of the marrow are united no longer hold, and are parted by the strain of existence, they in turn loosen the bonds of the soul, and she,[26] obtaining a natural release, flies away with joy. For that which takes place according to nature is pleasant, but that which is contrary to nature is painful. And thus death, if caused by disease or produced by wounds, is painful and violent; but that sort

21. *Timæus,* 78e–79a.

22. Ibid., 80e–81a.

23. Ibid., 81b.

24. *Diotima:* Wise woman of Mantinea, who spoke to Socrates first of love and then of his works (*Symposium,* 201d–212a).

25. *Symposium,* 207d.

26. *She:* The soul.

of death which comes with old age and fulfils the debt of nature is the easiest of deaths, and is accompanied with pleasure rather than with pain."[27]

The mode of origin and the nature of disease, as described in the *Timæus*, are in keeping with this primitive and imperfect science. The diseases of the body arise when any one of the four elements is out of place, or when the blood, sinews and flesh are produced in a wrong order. Much influence is attributed to the various kinds of bile. The worst of all diseases, he thinks, are those of the spinal marrow, in which the whole course of the body is reversed. Other diseases are produced by disorders of respiration; as by phlegm "when detained within by reason of the air bubbles."[28] This, if mingled with black bile and dispersed about the courses of the head produces epilepsy, attacks of which during sleep, he says, are not so severe, but when it assails those who are awake it is hard to be got rid of, and "being an affection of a sacred part, is most justly called sacred"[29] *morbus sacer*.[30] Of other disorders, excess of fire causes a continuous fever; of air, quotidian fever; of water, which is a more sluggish element than either fire or air, tertian fever; of earth, the most sluggish element of the four, is only purged away in a four-fold period, that is in a quartan fever.[31]

The psychology of Plato, in contrast to his anatomy and physiology, has a strangely modern savour, and the three-fold divisions of the mind into reason, spirit and appetite, represents very much the mental types recognized by students of the present day. The rational, immortal principle of the soul "the golden cord of reason"[32] dwells in the brain "and inasmuch as we are a plant not of earthly but of heavenly growth, raises us from earth to our kindred who are in heaven."[33] The mortal soul consists of two parts; the one with which man "loves and hungers and thirsts, and feels the fluttering of any other desire,"[34] is placed between the midriff and the boundary of the navel; the other, passion or spirit, is situated in the breast between the midriff and the neck, "in order that it might be under the rule of reason and might join with it in controlling and restraining the desires when they are no longer willing of their own accord to obey the word of command issuing from the citadel."[35]

27. *Timæus*, 81c–e.

28. Ibid., 85a.

29. *Timæus*, 85b.

30. *morbus sacer:* (Latin) sacred disease.

31. *quotidian fever:* A fever characterized by daily paroxysms; *tertian fever:* A fever characterized by paroxysms that recur every third day; *quartan fever:* A fever characterized by paroxysms that recur every fourth day.

32. *Laws*, book 1, 645a.

33. *Timæus*, 90a.

34. *Republic*, book 4, 439d.

35. *Timæus*, 70a.

No more graphic picture of the struggle between the rational and appetitive parts of the soul has ever been given than in the comparison of man in the *Phædrus* to a charioteer driving a pair of winged horses, one of which is noble and of noble breed; the other ignoble and of ignoble breed, so that "the driving of them of necessity gives a great deal of trouble to him."[36]

The comparison of the mind of man in the *Theætetus* to a block of wax, "which is of different sizes in different men; harder, moister, and having more or less of purity in one than another, and in some of an intermediate quality,"[37] is one of the happiest of Plato's conceptions. This wax tablet is a gift of Memory, the mother of the Muses;[38] "and when we wish to remember anything which we have seen, or heard or thought in our own minds, we hold the wax to the perceptions and thoughts, and in that material receive the impression of them as from the seal of a ring; and that we remember and know what is imprinted as long as the image lasts; but when the image is effaced, or cannot be taken, then we forget and do not know."[39]

Another especially fortunate comparison is that of the mind to an aviary which is gradually occupied by different kinds of birds, which correspond to the varieties of knowledge. When we were children the aviary was empty, and as we grow up we go about "catching" the various kinds of knowledge.[40]

Plato recognized, in the *Timæus*, two kinds of mental disease, to wit, madness and ignorance. He has the notion advocated by advanced psychologists today, that much of the prevalent vice is due to an ill disposition of the body, and is involuntary; "for no man is voluntarily bad; but the bad become bad by reason of ill disposition of the body and bad education, things which are hateful to every man and happen to him against his will."[41] A fuller discussion of the theorem that madness and the want of sense are the same is found in the *Alcibiades* (II.); which is not, however, one of the genuine *Dialogues*. The different kinds of want of sense are very graphically described:

Socrates. In like manner men differ in regard to want of sense. Those who are most out of their wits we call "madmen," while we term those who are less far gone "stupid," or "idiotic," or if we prefer gentle language, describe them as "romantic" or "simple-minded," or again as "innocent," or "inex-

36. *Phædrus*, 246b.
37. *Theætetus*, 191c.
38. (Greek myth.) Mnemosyne is the goddess of memory and mother (by Zeus) of the Muses, nine sister goddesses who preside over various arts.
39. *Theætetus*, 191d.
40. Ibid., 197d–e.
41. *Timæus*, 86e.

perienced," or "foolish." You may even find other names if you seek for them, but by all of them lack of sense is intended. They only differ as one art appears to us to differ from another, or one disease from another.[42]

There is a shrewd remark in the *Republic* "that the most gifted minds, when they are ill-educated, become pre-eminently bad. Do not great crimes and the spirit of pure evil spring out of a fulness of nature ruined by education rather than from any inferiority, whereas weak natures are scarcely capable of any very great good or very great evil."[43]

In the *Phædrus* there is recognized a form of madness "which is a divine gift and a source of the chiefest blessings granted to man."[44] Of this there are four kinds—prophecy, inspiration, poetry and love. That indefinable something which makes the poet as contrasted with the rhymester and which is above and beyond all art, is well characterized in the following sentence: "But he who, having no touch of the Muse's madness in his soul, comes to the door and thinks that he will get into the temple by the help of art—he, I say, and his poetry are not admitted. The sane man disappears and is nowhere when he enters into rivalry with a madman."[45] Certain crimes, too, are definitely recognized as manifestations of insanity; in the *Laws* the incurable criminal is thus addressed: "Oh, sir, the impulse which moves you to rob temples is not an ordinary human malady, nor yet a visitation of heaven, but a madness which is begotten in man from ancient and unexpiated crimes of his race."[46] In the *Laws*, too, it is stated that there are many sorts of madness, some arising out of disease, and others originating in an evil and passionate temperament, and increased by bad education. Respecting the care of the insane, it is stated that a madman shall not be at large in the city, but his relations shall keep him at home in any way they can, or if not, certain fines are mentioned.[47]

The greatest aid in the prevention of disease is to preserve the due proportion of mind and body, "for there is no proportion or disproportion more productive of health and disease, and virtue and vice, than that between soul and body."[48] In the double nature of the living being if there is in this compound an impassioned soul more powerful than the body, "that soul, I say, convulses and fills with disorders the whole inner nature of man; and when eager in the pur-

42. 2 *Alcibiades*, 140c–d.
43. *Republic*, book 6, 491e.
44. *Phædrus*, 244a.
45. Ibid., 245a.
46. *Laws*, book 9, 854b.
47. Ibid., book 11, 934d.
48. *Timæus*, 87d.

suit of some sort of learning or study, causes wasting; or again, when teaching or disputing in private or in public, and considerations and controversies arise, inflames and dissolves the composite form of man and introduces rheums; and the nature of this phenomenon is not understood by most professors of medicine, who ascribe it to the opposite of the real cause."[49] . . . Body and mind should both be equally exercised to protect against this disproportion, and "we should not move the body without the soul or the soul without the body. In this way they will be on their guard against each other, and be healthy and well balanced." He urges the mathematician to practise gymnastic, and the gymnast to cultivate music and philosophy.[50]

The modes of treatment advised are simple, and it is evident that Plato had not much faith in medicines. Professor Jowett's commentary is here worth quoting: "Plato is still the enemy of the purgative treatment of physicians, which, except in extreme cases, no man of sense will ever adopt. For, as he adds, with an insight into the truth, 'every disease is akin to the nature of the living being and is only irritated by stimulants.'[51] He is of opinion that nature should be left to herself, and is inclined to think that physicians are in vain (cf. Laws, VI. 761 C., where he says that warm baths would be more beneficial to the limbs of the aged rustic than the prescriptions of a not overwise doctor). If he seems to be extreme in his condemnation of medicine and to rely too much on diet and exercise, he might appeal to nearly all the best physicians of our own age in support of his opinions, who often speak to their patients of the worthlessness of drugs. For we ourselves are sceptical about medicine, and very unwilling to submit to the purgative treatment of physicians. May we not claim for Plato an anticipation of modern ideas as about some questions of astronomy and physics, so also about medicine? As in the *Charmides* (156, 7) he tells us that the body cannot be cured without the soul, so in the *Timæus* he strongly asserts the sympathy of soul and body; any defect of either is the occasion of the greatest discord and disproportion in the other.[52] Here too may be a presentiment that in the medicine of the future the interdependence of mind and body will be more fully recognized, and that the influence of the one over the other may be exerted in a manner which is not now thought possible."[53]

The effect of the purgative method to which Plato was so opposed is probably referred to in the following passage. "When a man goes of his own accord to a doctor's shop and takes medicine, is he not quite aware that soon and for

49. Ibid., 88e.
50. Ibid., 88b–c.
51. Introduction to *Timæus*, making reference to *Timæus*, 89b.
52. Ibid., 87d.
53. Jowett's introduction to *Timæus*, vol. 3, p. 688.

many days afterwards, he will be in a state of body which he would rather die than accept as a permanent condition of his life?"[54]

It is somewhat remarkable that nowhere in the *Dialogues* is any reference made to the method of healing at the Æsculapian temples. The comments upon physic and physicians are made without allusion to these institutions. Hippocrates and other practitioners at Athens were probably secular Asclepiads,[55] but as Dyer remarks, "in spite of the severance the doctors kept in touch with the worship of Æsculapius, and the priests in his temples did not scorn such secular knowledge as they could gain from lay practitioners."[56]

II

So much for the general conception of the structure and functions of the body, in order and disorder, as conceived by Plato. Were nothing more to be gleaned, the thoughts on these questions of one of the greatest minds of what was intellectually the most brilliant period of the race, would be of interest, but scattered throughout his writings are innumerably little *obiter dicta*,[57] which indicate a profound knowledge of that side of human nature which turns uppermost when the machinery is out of gear. There are, in addition, many charming analogies drawn from medicine, and many acute suggestions, some of which have a modern flavour. The noble pilot and the wise physician[58] who, as Nestor[59] remarks, "is worth many another man,"[60] furnish some of the most striking illustrations of the *Dialogues*.

One of the most admirable definitions of the Art of Medicine I selected as a rubric with which to grace my text-book, "And I said of medicine, that this is an Art which considers the constitution of the patient, and has principles of action and reasons in each case."[61] Or, again, the comprehensive view taken in the statement, "There is one science of medicine which is concerned with the inspection of health equally in all times, present, past and future."[62]

---

54. *Laws,* book 1, 646c.

55. Lay physicians.

56. Louis Dyer, *Studies of the Gods in Greece,* p. 230.

57. *obiter dicta:* (Latin) things said incidentally.

58. *Statesman,* 297e. Originally in Homer's *Iliad.*

59. *Nestor:* Homeric hero, king of Pylos, famous for his wisdom and old age, who was one of the few Greek leaders to reach home safely after the fall of Troy.

60. Homer, *Iliad,* book 11, line 514.

61. *Gorgias,* 501a. Not the exact quotation, but the same idea. Osler may be following another translation or making his own from the Greek.

62. *Laches,* 198d.

Plato gives a delicious account of the origin of the modern medicine, as contrasted with the art of the guild of Asclepius.[63]

Well, I said, and to require the help of medicine, not when a wound has to be cured, or on occasion of an epidemic, but just because by indolence and a habit of life such as we have been describing, men fill themselves with waters and winds, as if their bodies were a marsh, compelling the ingenious sons of Asclepius to find more names for diseases, such as flatulence and catarrh; is not this, too, a disgrace?

Yes, he said, they do certainly give very strange and new-fangled names to diseases.

Yes, I said, and I do not believe there were any such diseases in the days of Asclepius; and this I infer from the circumstance that the hero Eurypylus,[64] after he has been wounded in Homer, drinks a posset of Pramnian wine[65] well besprinkled with barley-meal and grated cheese, which are certainly inflammatory, and yet the sons of Asclepius who were at the Trojan war do not blame the damsel who gives him the drink, or rebuke Patroclus,[66] who is treating his case.

Well, he said, that was surely an extraordinary drink to be given to a person in his condition.

Not so extraordinary, I replied, if you bear in mind that in former days, as is commonly said, before the time of Herodicus, the guild of Asclepius did not practise our present system of medicine, which may be said to educate diseases. But Herodicus,[67] being a trainer, and himself of a sickly constitution, by a combination of training and doctoring found out a way of torturing first and chiefly himself, and secondly the rest of the world.

How was that? he said.

By the invention of lingering death; for he had a mortal disease which he perpetually tended, and as recovery was out of the question, he passed his entire life as a valetudinarian;[68] he could do nothing but attend upon

---

63. *Republic,* book 3, 405c–406b.

64. *Eurypylus:* Trojan leader in the Trojan War. Plato quotes this story incorrectly from the *Iliad,* book 11, lines 618–654, where the cup is given to Machaon and Nestor, not Eurypylus.

65. Wine from the neighborhood of Smyrna, used as a posset for the injured Eurypylus. Refer to *Republic,* book 3, 405e.

66. *Patroclus:* Greek hero who accompanied Achilles to the Trojan War; according to Plato, he was Achilles' devoted lover. Achilles died to avenge Patroclus (*Symposium,* 179e/208d).

67. *Herodicus* (5th cent. B.C.): Athenian physician and sophist and teacher of Hippocrates. "His teacher, Herodicus of Selymbria, formed his art by accustoming him to rely upon diet and exercise rather than upon drugs." Will Durant, *The Life of Greece* (New York: Simon & Schuster, 1939), p. 343.

68. *valetudinarian:* An invalid.

himself, and he was in constant torment whenever he departed in anything from his usual regimen, and so dying hard, by the help of science he
struggled on to old age.

A rare reward of his skill!

He goes on to say that Asclepius did not instruct his descendants in valetudinarian arts[69] because he knew that in well-ordered states individuals with occupations had no time to be ill. If a carpenter falls sick, he asks the doctor for a
"rough and ready cure—an emetic, or a purge, or a cautery, or the knife—these
are his remedies."[70] Should any one prescribe for him a course of dietetics and
tell him to swathe and swaddle his head, and all that sort of thing, he says, "he
sees no good in a life spent in nursing his disease to the neglect of his customary employment; and therefore bidding good-bye to this sort of physician, he
resumes his ordinary habits, and either gets well and lives and does his business,
or, if his constitution fails, he dies and has no more trouble."[71]

He is more in earnest in another place (*Gorgias*) in an account of the relations of the arts of medicine and gymnastics: "The soul and the body being two,
have two arts corresponding to them: there is the art of politics attending on the
soul; and another art attending on the body, of which I know no specific name,
but which may be described as having two divisions, one of them gymnastic, and
the other medicine. And in politics there is a legislative part, which answers to
gymnastic, as justice does to medicine; and the two parts run into one another,
justice having to do with the same subject as legislation, and medicine with the
same subject as gymnastic, but with a difference . . . Cookery simulates the disguise of medicine, and pretends to know what food is the best for the body; and
if the physician and the cook had to enter into a competition in which children
were the judges, or men who had no more sense than children, as to which of
them best understands the goodness or badness of food, the physician would be
starved to death."[72]

And later in the same dialogue Socrates claims to be the only true politician of his time who speaks, not with any view of pleasing, but for the good of
the State, and is unwilling to practise the graces of rhetoric—and so would make
a bad figure in a court of justice. He says: "I shall be tried just as a physician
would be tried in a court of little boys at the indictment of the cook. What would

69. Arts to treat people in weak health, especially those who are constantly concerned with their own
ailments; hypochondriacs.
70. *Republic*, book 3, 406d.
71. Ibid., 406d–e.
72. *Gorgias*, 464b–e.

he reply under such circumstances, if some one were to accuse him, saying, 'O my boys, many evil things has this man done to you; he is the death of you, especially of the younger ones among you, cutting and burning and starving and suffocating you, until you know not what to do; he gives you the bitterest potions, and compels you to hunger and fast? How unlike the variety of meats and sweets on which I feasted for you.' What do you suppose that the physician would be able to reply when he found himself in such a predicament? If he told the truth he could only say: 'All these evil things, my boys I did for your health,' and then would there not just be a clamour among a jury like that? How they would cry out!"[73]

The principle of continuity, of uniformity, so striking in ancient physics was transferred to the body, which, like the world, was conceived as a whole. Several striking passages illustrative of this are to be found. Thus to the question of Socrates, "Do you think that you can know the nature of the soul intelligently without knowing the nature of the whole?" Phædrus replies, "Hippocrates, the Asclepiad, says that the nature even of the body can only be understood as a whole."[74] The importance of treating the whole and not the part is insisted upon. In the case of a patient who comes to them with bad eyes the saying is "that they cannot cure his eyes by themselves, but that if his eyes are to be cured his head must be treated": and then again they say "that to think of curing the head alone and not the rest of the body also is the height of folly."[75]

Charmides[76] had been complaining of a headache, and Critias[77] had asked Socrates to make believe that he could cure him of it. He said that he had a charm, which he had learnt, when serving with the army, of one of the physicians of the Thracian king, Zamolxis.[78] This physician had told Socrates that the cure of the part should not be attempted without treatment of the whole, and also that no attempt should be made to cure the body without the soul, "and, therefore, if the head and body are to be well you must begin by curing the soul; that is the first thing . . . And he who taught me the cure and the charm added a special direction, 'Let no one,' he said, 'persuade you to cure the head until he has first given you his soul to be cured. For this,' he said, 'is the great error of our day

73. Ibid., 521e–522a.

74. *Phædrus*, 270c. Not the exact quotation, but the same idea. Osler may be following another translation or making his own from the Greek.

75. *Charmides*, 156b–c.

76. *Charmides* (d.404 B.C.): Beautiful young Athenian who was renowned for his moderation.

77. *Critias* (c.460–403 B.C.): Athenian orator and politician, cousin of Charmides. Plato, who was related to him, made him one of the interlocutors in his *Timæus* and *Critias*.

78. *Zamolxis:* A legendary Thracian king (*Charmides*, 156d).

in the treatment of the human body, that physicians separate the soul from the body." The charms to which he referred were fair words by which temperance was implanted in the soul.[79]

Though a contemporary, Hippocrates is only once again referred to in the *Dialogues*—where the young Hippocrates, son of Apollodorus, who has come to Protagoras,[80] "that almighty wise man,"[81] as Socrates terms him in another place, to learn the science and knowledge of human life, is asked by Socrates, "If you were going to Hippocrates of Cos, the Asclepiad, and were about to give him your money, and some one had said to you, 'You are paying money to your namesake, Hippocrates, O Hippocrates; tell me, what is he that you give him money?' how would you have answered?" "I should say," he replied, "that I gave money to him as a physician." "And what will he make of you?" "A physician," he said[82]—a paragraph which would indicate that Hippocrates was in the habit of taking pupils and teaching them the art of medicine; and in the *Euthydemus*, with reference to the education of physicians, Socrates says, "that he would send such to those who profess the art, and to those who demand payment for teaching the art, and profess to teach it to any one who will come and learn."[83]

We get a glimpse of the method of diagnosis, derived doubtless from personal observation, possibly of the great Hippocrates himself, whose critical knowledge of pulmonary complaints we daily recognize in the use of his name in association with the clubbed fingers of phthisis, and with the succussion splash of pneumo-thorax.[84] "Suppose some one, who is inquiring into the health or some other bodily quality of another: he looks at his face and at the tips of his fingers, and then he says, 'Uncover your chest and back to me that I may have a better view.'" And then Socrates says to Protagoras, "Uncover your mind to me; reveal your opinion, etc."[85]

79. *Charmides,* 157a–b. Wording is slightly different, but the meaning is the same. Osler may be following another translation or making his own from the Greek.

80. *Protagoras* (c.483–c.414 B.C.): Greek philosopher, called Protagoras of Abdera. He maintained that his famous apophthegm, "man is the measure of all things" would belong to philosophy eternally and would never lose its significance. He was the first to assume the title of sophist, and the first to teach for pay. Plato's *Protagoras* gives us some information about his way of teaching.

81. Socrates once said, "the wisest of all living men, if you are willing to accord that title to Protagoras." See *Protagoras,* 309d.

82. *Protagoras,* 311b–c.

83. This quote is not from *Euthydemus,* but *Meno,* 90d. Socrates does refer to the education of physicians in the *Euthydemus,* 304c and 279e–280a. Probably Osler got this quote from his notebooks and did not go back to verify the original text.

84. Hippocratic fingers and Hippocratic succussion splash.

85. *Protagoras,* 352a–b.

One of the most celebrated medical passages is that in which Socrates professes the art of a midwife practising on the souls of men when they are in labour, and diagnosing their condition, whether pregnant with the truth or with some "darling folly."[86] The entire section, though long, must be quoted. Socrates is in one of his "little difficulties"[87] and wishes to know of the young Theætetus,[88] who has been presented to him as a paragon of learning, and whose progress in the path of knowledge has been sure and smooth—"flowing on silently like a river of oil"[89]—what is knowledge? Theætetus is soon entangled and cannot shake off a feeling of anxiety.

> *Theæt.* I can assure you, Socrates, that I have tried very often, when the report of questions asked by you was brought to me; but I can neither persuade myself that I have any answer to give, nor hear of any one who answers as you would have him; and I cannot shake off a feeling of anxiety.
>
> *Soc.* These are the pangs of labour, my dear Theætetus; you have something within you which you are bringing to the birth.
>
> *Theæt.* I do not know, Socrates; I only say what I feel.
>
> *Soc.* And did you never hear, simpleton, that I am the son of a midwife, brave and burly, whose name was Phænarete?[90]
>
> *Theæt.* Yes, I have.
>
> *Soc.* And that I myself practise midwifery?
>
> *Theæt.* No, never.
>
> *Soc.* Let me tell you that I do though, my friend; but you must not reveal the secret, as the world in general have not found me out; and therefore they only say of me, that I am the strangest of mortals, and drive men to their wits' end. Did you ever hear that too?
>
> *Theæt.* Yes.
>
> *Soc.* Shall I tell you the reason?
>
> *Theæt.* By all means.
>
> *Soc.* Bear in mind the whole business of the midwives, and then you will see my meaning better. No woman, as you are probably aware, who is still able to conceive and bear, attends other women, but only those who are past bearing.

86. *Theætetus*, 151c.

87. The term "difficulty" is an example of Socrates' characteristic irony. He would very often pretend to have trouble understanding a subject and ask some young man for help as a way of starting a conversation on some topic on which he in fact thought the youth needed instruction.

88. *Theætetus* (d.369 B.C.): Athenian mathematician and disciple of Socrates.

89. *Theætetus*, 144b.

90. *Phænarete* (5th cent. B.C.): Mother of Socrates, a midwife.

Theæt. Yes, I know.

Soc. The reason of this is said to be that Artemis—the goddess of child-birth—is not a mother, and she honours those who are like herself; but she could not allow the barren to be midwives, because human nature cannot know the mystery of an art without experience; and therefore she assigned this office to those who are too old to bear.

Theæt. I dare say.

Soc. And I dare say, too, or rather I am absolutely certain, that the midwives know better than others who is pregnant and who is not?

Theæt. Very true.

Soc. And by the use of potions and incantations they are able to arouse the pangs and to soothe them at will; they can make those bear who have a difficulty in bearing, and if they think fit, they can smother the embryo in the womb.

Theæt. They can.

Soc. Did you ever remark that they are also most cunning matchmakers, and have a thorough knowledge of what unions are likely to produce a brave brood?

Theæt. No, never.

Soc. Then let me tell you that this is their greatest pride, more than cutting the umbilical cord. And if you reflect, you will see that the same art which cultivates and gathers in the fruits of the earth, will be most likely to know in what soils the several plants or seeds should be deposited.

Theæt. Yes, the same art.

Soc. And do you suppose that with women the case is otherwise?

Theæt. I should think not.

Soc. Certainly not; but midwives are respectable women and have a character to lose, and they avoid this department of their profession, because they are afraid of being called procuresses, which is a name given to those who join together man and woman in an unlawful and unscientific way; and yet the true midwife is also the true and only matchmaker.

Theæt. Clearly.

Soc. Such are the midwives, whose task is a very important one, but not so important as mine; for women do not bring into the world at one time real children, and at another time counterfeits which are with difficulty distinguished from them; if they did, then the discernment of the true and false birth would be the crowning achievement of the art of midwifery— you would think so?

Theæt. Indeed I should.

Soc. Well, my art of midwifery is in most respects like theirs; but differs in that I attend men and not women, and I look after their souls when they are in labour, and not after their bodies; and the triumph of my art is in thoroughly examining whether the thought which the mind of the young man is bringing to the birth, is a false idol or a noble and true birth. And like the midwives, I am barren, and the reproach which is often made against me, that I ask questions of others and have not the wit to answer them myself, is very just; the reason is, that the god compels me to be a midwife, but forbids me to bring forth. And therefore I am not myself at all wise, nor have I anything to show which is the invention or birth of my own soul, but those who converse with me profit. Some of them appear dull enough at first, but afterwards, as our acquaintance ripens, if the god is gracious to them, they all make astonishing progress; and this in the opinion of others as well as their own. It is quite clear that they had never learned anything from me; the many fine discoveries to which they cling are of their own making. But to me and the god they owe their delivery. And the proof of my words is, that many of them in their ignorance, either in their self-conceit despising me, or falling under the influence of others, have gone away too soon; and have not only lost the children of whom I had previously delivered them by an ill bringing up, but have stifled whatever else they had in them by evil communications, being fonder of lies and shams than of the truth; and they have at last ended by seeing themselves, as others see them, to be great fools. Aristeides,[91] the son of Lysimachus, is one of them, and there are many others. The truants often return to me, and beg that I would consort with them again — they are ready to go to me on their knees — and then, if my familiar allows, which is not always the case, I receive them and they begin to grow again. Dire are the pangs which my art is able to arouse and to allay in those who consort with me, just like the pangs of women in childbirth; night and day they are full of perplexity and travail which is even worse than that of the women. So much for them. And there are others, Theætetus, who come to me apparently having nothing in them; and as I know that they have no need of my art, I coax them into marrying some one, and by the grace of God I can generally tell who is likely to do them good. Many of them I have given away to Prodicus,[92] and many to other inspired sages. I tell you this long story, friend Theætetus, because

---

91. *Aristeides* (also *Aristides*) (c.530–c.468 B.C.): Athenian statesman and general, surnamed "the Just." For further information, see "Chauvinism in Medicine," p. 241.

92. *Prodicus* of Ceos (5th cent. B.C.): Greek sophist and itinerant teacher known for his distinctions of words.

I suspect, as indeed you seem to think yourself, that you are in labour—great with some conception. Come then to me, who am a midwife's son and myself a midwife, and try to answer the questions which I will ask you. And if I abstract and expose your first-born, because I discover upon inspection that the conception which you have formed is a vain shadow, do not quarrel with me on that account, as the manner of women is when their first children are taken from them. For I have actually known some who were ready to bite me when I deprived them of a darling folly; they did not perceive that I acted from good will, not knowing that no god is the enemy of man—that was not within the range of their ideas; neither am I their enemy in all this, but it would be wrong in me to admit falsehood, or to stifle the truth. Once more, then, Theætetus, I repeat my old question, "What is knowledge?" and do not say that you cannot tell; but quit yourself like a man, and by the help of God you will be able to tell.[93]

Socrates proceeds to determine whether the intellectual babe brought forth by Theætetus is a wind-egg [94] or a real and genuine birth. "This then is the child, however he may turn out, which you and I have with difficulty brought into the world, and now that he is born we must run round the hearth with him and see whether he is worth rearing or only a wind-egg and a sham. Is he to be reared in any case and not exposed? or will you bear to see him rejected and not get into a passion if I take away your first-born?"[95] The conclusion is "that you have brought forth wind, and that the offspring of your brain are not worth bringing up."[96] And the dialogue ends as it began with a reference to the midwife: "The office of a midwife I, like my mother, have received from God; she delivered women, and I deliver men; but they must be young and noble and fair."[97]

III

From the writings of Plato we may gather many details about the status of physicians in his time. It is very evident that the profession was far advanced and had been progressively developing for a long period before Hippocrates, whom we erroneously, yet with a certain propriety, call the *Father of Medicine.* The little

93. *Theætetus*, 148e–151d.

94. *wind-egg:* Literally, an unfertilized egg that cannot hatch; here, figuratively, an imperfect or unproductive idea.

95. Ibid., 160e–161a.

96. Ibid., 210b.

97. Ibid., 210c.

by-play between Socrates and Euthydemus[98] suggests an advanced condition of medical literature: "Of course, you who have so many books are going in for being a doctor," says Socrates, and then he adds, "there are so many books on medicine, you know."[99] As Dyer remarks, whatever the quality of these books may have been, their number must have been great to give point to this chaff.[100]

It may be clearly gathered from the writings of Plato that two sorts of physicians (apart altogether from quacks and the Æsculapian guild) existed in Athens, the private practitioner, and the State-physician. The latter, though the smaller numerically, representing apparently the most distinguished class. From a reference in one of the dialogues (*Gorgias*) they evidently were elected by public assembly,—"when the assembly meets to elect a physician."[101] The office was apparently yearly, for in the *Statesman* is the remark, "when the year of office has expired, the pilot or physician has to come before a court of review"[102] to answer any charges that may be made against him. In the same dialogue occurs the remark, "and if anyone who is in a private station has the art to advise one of the public physicians, must he not be called a physician?"[103] Apparently a physician must have been in practice for some time and attained great eminence before he was deemed worthy of the post of State-physician. "If you and I were physicians, and were advising one another that we were competent to practise as state-physicians, should I not ask you, and would you not ask me, Well, but how about Socrates himself, has he good health? And was any one else ever known to be cured by him whether slave or freeman?"[104]

A reference to the two sorts of doctors is also found in the *Republic:* "Now you know that when patients do not require medicine, but have only to be put under a regimen, the inferior sort of practitioner is deemed to be good enough; but when medicine has to be given, then the doctor should be more of a man."[105]

The office of State-physician was in existence fully two generations before this time, for Democedes[106] held this post at Athens in the second half of the sixth century at a salary of £406 and, very much as a modern professor might be, he was seduced away by the offer of a great increase in salary by Polycrates,[107] the

PHYSICIANS IN

PLATO

98. *Euthydemus:* See p. 140, n. 83.

99. Louis Dyer, *Studies of the Gods in Greece,* pp. 224–25.

100. Ibid., p. 225.

101. *Gorgias,* 455b.

102. *Statesman,* 299a.

103. Ibid., 259a.

104. *Gorgias,* 514d.

105. *Republic,* book 5, 459c.

106. *Democedes* (c.550–504 B.C.): The most skilled physician of his day.

107. *Polycrates* (6th cent. B.C.): Tyrant of Samos from c.540 to 522 B.C. He is said to have been "the most daring, successful and treacherous of the Greek tyrants."

tyrant of Samos. It is evident, too, from the *Laws,* that the doctors had assistants, often among the slaves.

> For of doctors, as I may remind you, some have a gentler, others a ruder method of cure; and as children ask the doctor to be gentle with them, so we will ask the legislator to cure our disorders with the gentlest remedies. What I mean to say is, that besides doctors there are doctors' servants, who are also styled doctors.
>
> *Cle.* Very true.
>
> *Œth.* And whether they are slaves or freemen makes no difference; they acquire their knowledge of medicine by obeying and observing their masters; empirically and not according to the natural way of learning, as the manner of freemen is, who have learned scientifically themselves the art which they impart scientifically to their pupils. You are aware that there are these two classes of doctors?
>
> *Cle.* To be sure.
>
> *Œth.* And did you ever observe that there are two classes of patients in states, slaves and freemen; and the slave doctors run about and cure the slaves, or wait for them in the dispensaries—practitioners of this sort never talk to their patients individually, or let them talk about their own individual complaints? The slave-doctor prescribes what mere experience suggests, as if he had exact knowledge; and when he has given his orders, like a tyrant, he rushes off with equal assurance to some other servant who is ill; and so he relieves the master of the house of the care of his invalid slaves. But the other doctor, who is a freeman, attends and practises upon freemen; and he carries his inquiries far back, and goes into the nature of the disorder; he enters into discourse with the patient and with his friends, and is at once getting information from the sick man, and also instructing him as far as he is able, and he will not prescribe for him until he has first convinced him; at last, when he has brought the patient more and more under his persuasive influences and set him on the road to health, he attempts to effect a cure. Now which is the better way of proceeding in a physician and in a trainer? Is he the better who accomplishes his ends in a double way, or he who works in one way, and that the ruder and inferior? [108]

This idea of first convincing a patient by argument is also mentioned in the *Gorgias,* and would appear indeed to have furnished occupation for some of the numerous sophists of that period. Gorgias,[109] lauding the virtues of rhetoric and

108. *Laws,* book 4, 720a–e.
109. *Gorgias* (c.480–c.380 B.C.): Greek sophist. "He was one of the first to analyse the emotional effect on

146

PHYSICIANS IN

PLATO

claiming that she holds under her sway all the inferior arts, says: "Let me offer you a striking example of this. On several occasions I have been with my brother Herodicus,[110] or some other physician, to see one of his patients, who would not allow the physician to give him medicine or apply the knife or hot iron to him; and I have persuaded him to do for me what he would not do for the physician just by the use of rhetoric. And I say that if a rhetorician and a physician were to go to any city, and had there to argue in the Ecclesia[111] or any other assembly as to which of them should be elected state-physician, the physician would have no chance; but he who could speak would be chosen if he wished."[112] In another place (*Laws*) Plato satirizes this custom: "For of this you may be very sure, that if one of those empirical physicians, who practise medicine without science, were to come upon the gentleman physician talking to his gentleman patient, and using the language almost of philosophy—beginning at the beginning of the disease, and discoursing about the whole nature of the body, he would burst into a hearty laugh—he would say what most of those who are called doctors always have at their tongue's end:[113] foolish fellow, he would say, you are not healing the sick man, but you are educating him; and he does not want to be made a doctor, but to get well."[114]

Of the personal qualifications of the physician not much is said; but in the *Republic* (III. 408) there is an original, and to us not very agreeable, idea: "Now the most skilful physicians are those who, from their youth upwards, have combined with a knowledge of their art, the greatest experience of disease; they had better not be in robust health, and should have had all manner of diseases in their own person. For the body, as I conceive, is not the instrument with which they cure the body; in that case we could not allow them ever to be or to have been sickly; but they cure the body with the mind, and the mind which has become and is sick can cure nothing."[115]

Some idea of the estimate which Plato put on the physician may be gathered from the mystical account in the *Phædrus* of the nature of the soul and of life in the upper world. We are but animated failures—the residua of the souls above, which have attained a vision of truth, but have fallen "hence beneath the double

the audience of different rhetorical techniques—hence the view, criticized by Plato (*Gorgias*), that a good speaker must be able to make the worse case seem to be the better" (*Who Was Who in the Greek World*).

110. *Herodicus:* See p. 137, n. 67.

111. *the Ecclesia:* Popular assembly, especially the general assembly of the voting Athenian citizens. There the people had full sovereignty, and any citizen twenty years of age or older could vote.

112. *Gorgias,* 456b–c.

113. *have at their tongue's end:* Are ready to say whatever they have in mind.

114. *Laws,* book 9, 857c–d.

115. *Republic,* book 3, 408d-e.

load of forgetfulness and vice."[116] There are nine grades of human existence into which these souls may pass, from that of a philosopher or artist to that of a tyrant. The physician or lover of gymnastic toils comes in the fourth class.[117]

But if Plato assigns the physician a place in the middle tier in his mystery, he welcomes him socially into the most select and aristocratic circle of Athens. In that most festive of all festal occasions, at the house of Agathon,[118] described in the *Symposium*, Eryximachus,[119] a physician and the son of one, is a chief speaker, and in his praise of love says, "from medicine I will begin that I may do honour to my art."[120] We find him, too, on the side of temperance and sobriety: "The weak heads like myself, Aristodemus,[121] Phædrus,[122] and others who never can drink, are fortunate in finding that the stronger ones are not in a drinking mood. (I do not include Socrates, who is able either to drink or to abstain, and will not mind, whichever we do.) Well, as none of the company seem disposed to drink much, I may be forgiven for saying, as a physician, that drinking deep is a bad practice, which I never follow, if I can help, and certainly do not recommend to another, least of all to any one who still feels the effect of yesterday's carouse."[123] The prescriptions for hiccough, given by Eryximachus, give verisimilitude to the dialogue. When the turn of Aristophanes[124] came he had eaten too much and had the hiccough, and he said to Eryximachus, "You ought either to stop my hiccough or speak in my turn."[125] Eryximachus recommended him to hold his breath, or if that failed to gargle with a little water, and if the hiccough still continued, to tickle his nose with something and sneeze, adding, "if you sneeze once or twice even the most violent hiccough is sure to go."[126]

Upon the medical symptoms narrated in that memorable scene, unparalleled in literature, after Socrates had drunk the poison in prison, it is unnecessary to dwell; but I may refer to one aspect as indicating the reverence felt for the representative of the great Healer.[127] Denied his wish (by the warning of the jailor,

116. *Phædrus*, 248c: And through some ill-hap sinks beneath the double load."

117. Ibid., 248d.

118. *Agathon* (c.450–c.400 B.C.): Athenian tragic poet and friend of Plato. The scene is the banquet held at the Lenaea to celebrate his first dramatic victory.

119. *Eryximachus* (4th cent. B.C.): Greek physician.

120. *Symposium*, 186b.

121. *Aristodemus* (Plato's contemporary): An Athenian and an early and devoted follower of Socrates.

122. *Phædrus* (c.450–c.400 B.C.): Athenian philosopher and friend of Socrates.

123. *Symposium*, 176c–d.

124. *Aristophanes* (c.445–c.385 B.C.): Athenian poet and writer of comedy. He wrote a satirical play on Socrates called *The Clouds* and one against Euripides called *The Frogs*.

125. *Symposium*, 185d.

126. *Symposium*, 185e.

127. Æsculapius: See p. 128, n. 8.

who says that there is only sufficient poison) to offer a libation [128] to a god, Socrates' dying words were, "Crito, we owe a cock to Æsculapius." [129] "The meaning of this solemnly smiling farewell of Socrates would seem to be," according to Dyer, "that to Æsculapius, a god who always is prescribing potions and whose power is manifest in their effects, was due that most welcome and sovereign remedy which cured all the pains and ended all the woes of Socrates—the hemlock,[130] which cured him of life which is death, and gave him the glorious realities of hereafter. For this great boon of awakening into real life Socrates owed Æsculapius a thankoffering. This offering of a cock to Æsculapius was plainly intended for him as the awakener of the dead to life everlasting." [131]

And permit me to conclude this already too long account with the eulogium of Professor Jowett [132]—words worthy of the master, worthy of his great interpreter to this generation:

> More than two thousand two hundred years have passed away since he returned to the place of Apollo and the Muses. Yet the echo of his words continues to be heard among men, because of all philosophers he has the most melodious voice. He is the inspired prophet or teacher who can never die, the only one in whom the outward form adequately represents the fair soul within; in whom the thoughts of all who went before him are reflected and of all who come after him are partly anticipated. Other teachers of philosophy are dried up and withered—after a few centuries they have become dust; but he is fresh and blooming, and is always begetting new ideas in the minds of men. They are one-sided and abstract; but he has many sides of wisdom. Nor is he always consistent with himself, because he is always moving onward, and knows that there are many more things in philosophy than can be expressed in words, and that truth is greater than consistency. He who approaches him in the most reverent spirit shall reap most of the fruits of his wisdom; he who reads him by the light of ancient commentators will have the least understanding of him.
>
> "We may see him with the eye of the mind in the groves of the Acad-

128. *libation:* Liquid poured out before drinking as an offering to a god.

129. *Phædo,* 118a. Jowett's translation reads: "Crito, I owe a cock to Aesculapius," but "we owe," as Osler writes, is the accurate translation of the original Greek. Jowett must have taken "we" as authorial, but Socrates is including his friends, not merely speaking of himself.

130. *hemlock:* A poisonous herb, used medicinally as a powerful sedative. Socrates had been sentenced to death for allegedly subverting young Athenians' morals and religious beliefs, and hemlock was the poison he was made to drink to carry out the sentence.

131. Louis Dyer, *Studies of the Gods in Greece,* p. 239.

132. Benjamin *Jowett:* See p. 129, n. 17.

emy,[133] or on the banks of the Ilissus,[134] or in the streets of Athens, alone or walking with Socrates, full of these thoughts which have since become the common possession of mankind. Or we may compare him to a statue hid away in some temple of Zeus or Apollo, no longer existing on earth, a statue which has a look as of the God himself. Or we may once more imagine him following in another state of being the great company of heaven which he beheld of old in a vision (*Phædrus*, 248). So, 'partly trifling but with a degree of seriousness' (*Symposium*, 197, E), we linger around the memory of a world which has passed away (*Phædrus*, 250, C)."[135]

133. Gymnasium near Athens where Plato taught. The name was derived from a mythical hero Academus.

134. A small river in Attica, Greece, which flowed just south of Athens.

135. Jowett's translation of *Plato*, vol. 4, p. 188.

8

THE LEAVEN OF SCIENCE

Knowledge comes, but wisdom lingers.
ALFRED TENNYSON, *Locksley Hall*

Who loves not knowledge? Who shall rail
    Against her beauty? May she mix
    With men and prosper! Who shall fix
Her pillars? Let her work prevail.
ALFRED TENNYSON, "In Memoriam A.H.H."

OSLER EXPRESSES REGRET that the current emphasis on the individual has lessened the sense of continuity with the past. This address was given at the dedication of the Wistar Institute of Anatomy and Biology at the University of Pennsylvania in 1894.

Caspar Wistar the second of four exceptional professors of anatomy at the University of Pennsylvania. The school had achieved an excellence in anatomy unmatched elsewhere, except perhaps at the University of Edinburgh, Scotland, where several of the early Pennsylvania faculty members had studied with John Hunter. The first anatomy professor was William Shippen, who founded the medical school after studying with Hunter. Wistar followed him, wrote the first anatomy textbook, and established a museum for anatomical specimens. He was a brilliant, innovative teacher, remembered for his vibrant, sociable personality. The third professor, William Horner, had made the first contributions to human anatomy in the United States. Then came Joseph Leidy, a great comparative anatomist, whom Osler compares to Darwin.

Osler discusses how much modern thinking has been changed by anatomy and biology. Early in the century, it was believed that everything about anatomy was known. Then Hunter opened anatomy to include the relationship of structure to function. As an example, Osler discusses the growing knowledge concerning the functions of various parts of the brain and the impact that this has had on diagnosis and treatment. Biology, with its wider scope, provides a framework for looking at life as a whole, and trains the mind in accurate observation and reasoning. With *On the Origin of Species*, biology has affected all aspects of human thought.

Osler extols the benefits of science to a physician as enlarged vision, exactness, skepticism, an independent mind, and avoidance of self-deception. He stresses the need for universities to be places where thinkers can explore science deeply. He adds that medical education must include art and charity as well as science.

THE LEAVEN OF
SCIENCE

I

IN THE CONTINUAL REMEMBRANCE of a glorious past individuals and nations
find their noblest inspiration, and if to-day this inspiration, so valuable for
its own sake, so important in its associations, is weakened, is it not because
in the strong dominance of the individual, so characteristic of a democracy,
we have lost the sense of continuity? As we read in Roman history of the ceremonies commemorative of the departed, and of the scrupulous care with which,
even at such private festivals as the Ambarvalia,[1] the dead were invoked and remembered, we appreciate, though feebly, the part which this sense of continuity
played in the lives of their successors—an ennobling, influence, through which
the cold routine of the present received a glow of energy from "the touch divine
of noble natures gone."[2] In our modern lives no equivalent to this feeling exists,
and the sweet and gracious sense of an ever-present immortality, recognized so
keenly and so closely in the religion of Numa,[3] has lost all value to us. We are

An address delivered at the opening of the Wistar Institute of Anatomy and Biology, May 21, 1894.
Leaven refers to an agent, usually yeast, that causes bread dough to rise; here meaning an agent or element
that acts in or upon something to produce a gradual change or modification. "The kingdom of heaven is
like unto leaven, which a woman took, and hid in three measures of meal, till the whole was leavened"
Matthew 13:33. Osler is thinking of leaven as an enlivening influence.
1. A solemn annual purification of the fields by ancient Roman farmers, involving the sacrifice of animals.
This festival, held in May, was celebrated in honor of Ceres, goddess of agriculture, for fruitful harvests.
2. James Russell Lowell, "Memoriæ Positum," part 1, stanza 2, lines 9–10.
3. *Numa* Pompilius (715–673 B.C.) is a legendary king of Rome, successor of Romulus, who founded the
city in 753 B.C. This period was considered a golden age in which many religious institutions began. Numa
established the priestly offices of the Roman state.

even impatient of those who would recall the past, and who would insist upon the importance of its recognition as a factor in our lives, impatient as we are of everything save the present with its prospects, the future with its possibilities. Year by year the memory of the men who made this institution fades from out the circle of the hills, and the shadow of oblivion falls deeper and deeper over their forms, until a portrait, or perhaps a name alone, remains to link the dead with the quick.[4] To be forgotten seems inevitable, but not without a sense of melancholy do we recognize that the daily life of three thousand students and teachers is passed heedless of the fame, careless of the renown of these men; and in the second state sublime it must sadden the "circle of the wise,"[5] as they cast their eyes below, to look down on festivals in which they play no part, on gatherings in which their names are neither invoked nor blessed. But ours the loss, since to us, distant in humanity, the need is ever present to cherish the memories of the men who in days of trial and hardship laid on broad lines the foundations of the old colonial colleges.

To-day, through the liberality of General Wistar,[6] we dedicate a fitting monument to one of the mighty dead of the University[7]—Caspar Wistar.[8] The tribute of deeds has already been paid to him in this splendid structure, to all in the stately group of academic buildings which you now see adorning the campus—the tribute of words remains, to be able to offer which I regard a very special honour.

But as this is an Institute of Anatomy, our tribute to-day may be justly restricted, in its details at least, to a eulogy upon the men who have taught the subject in this University. About the professorship of anatomy cluster memories which give it precedence of all others, and in the septemviri of the old school[9] the

4. *the quick:* Living people. This is a reminiscence of the phrase "the quick and the dead," which occurs in the *Book of Common Prayer* in both the Apostles' Creed and the Nicene Creed.

5. Probably a reference to *Paradiso,* the third and concluding part of *La Divina Commedia* (1307–1321) by Dante, depicting heaven.

6. Isaac Jones *Wistar* (1827–1905): Penologist and great-nephew of Caspar Wistar. Isaac founded the Wistar Institute of Anatomy and Biology in honor of his great-uncle. Author of *Autobiography* (1914), with portraits, maps, and an appendix on the Wistar Institute.

7. Seven early professors of the University of Pennsylvania Medical School who were mostly anatomists: Wistar, Leidy, Dorsey, Physick, Horner, Gibson, and Shippen.

8. Caspar *Wistar* (1761–1818): Physician and anatomist. In 1808 Wistar succeeded William Shippen as full professor of anatomy at the University of Pennsylvania, serving until his death. His family later presented his large anatomical collection to the University to start a museum. He wrote *A System of Anatomy for the Use of Students of Medicine* (1811–1814), and was president of the American Philosophical Society (1815–1818) and of the Society for the Abolition of Slavery (1813). For further information, see pp. 158–159.

9. *the septemviri:* (Latin) a body of seven early professors associated in the medical school

chairs were arranged, with that of anatomy in the centre, with those of physiology, chemistry, and materia medica on the left, and with those of practice, surgery, and obstetrics on the right. With the revival of learning anatomy brought life and liberty to the healing art, and throughout the sixteenth, seventeenth, and eighteenth centuries the great names of the profession, with but one or two exceptions, are those of the great anatomists. The University of Pennsylvania has had an extraordinary experience in the occupancy of this important chair. In the century and a quarter which ended with the death of Leidy,[10] six names appear on the faculty roll as professors of this branch. Dorsey,[11] however, only delivered the introductory lecture to the course, and was seized the same evening with his fatal illness; and in the next year Physick[12] was transferred from the chair of surgery, with Horner[13] as his adjunct. In reality, therefore, only four men have taught anatomy in this school since its foundation. Physick's name must ever be associated with the chair of surgery. We do not know the faculty exigencies which led to the transfer, but we can readily surmise that the youthfulness of Horner, who was only twenty-six, and the opportunity of filching for surgery so strong a man as Gibson[14] from the Faculty of the University of Maryland, then a stout rival, must have been among the most weighty considerations.

If in the average length of the period of each incumbency the chair of anatomy in the University is remarkable, much more so is it for the quality of the men who followed each other at such long intervals. It is easy to praise the Athenians among the Athenians,[15] but where is the school in this country which can show such a succession of names in this branch: Shippen,[16] the first

10. Joseph *Leidy* (1823–1891): Anatomist, botanist, paleontologist, zoologist, and mineralogist. He succeeded to the chair of anatomy at the University of Pennsylvania upon Horner's death in 1853. He was one of the foremost American anatomists of his time, author of 553 volumes, papers, and communications at the time of his death.

11. John Syng *Dorsey* (1802–1818): Surgeon and professor of materia medica at the University of Pennsylvania.

12. Philip Syng *Physick* (1768–1837): Surgeon and professor of surgery at the University of Pennsylvania. He contributed many inventions and improvements in surgical procedures and instruments.

13. William Edmonds *Horner* (1793–1853): Anatomist and professor at the University of Pennsylvania. Author of *Treatise on Pathological Anatomy* (1829), the first book of its kind in the United States. For further information, see pp. 160–161.

14. William *Gibson* (1788–1868): Surgeon and professor of surgery at the University of Pennsylvania after teaching at the University of Maryland. He did much to advance knowledge about surgery, and he was known for performing a Caesarean section twice on the same patient. The woman lived for fifty years after the first operation.

15. It is easy (pleasant and comfortable) to praise people among their own countrymen or kinsmen.

16. William *Shippen* (1736–1808): Pioneer teacher of anatomy. He studied midwifery under William Hunter and Colin McKenzie in Scotland and also became friends with John Fothergill (1712–1780), the

teacher of anatomy; Wistar, the author of the first text-book of anatomy; Horner, the first contributor to human anatomy in this country; and Leidy, one of the greatest comparative anatomists of his generation? Of European schools, Edinburgh alone presents a parallel picture, as during the same period only four men have held the chair. The longevity and tenacity of the three Monros[17] have become proverbial; in succession they held the chair of anatomy for 126 years. Shortly before the foundation of this school Monro *secundus* had succeeded his father, and taught uninterruptedly for fifty years. His son, Monro *tertius*, held the chair for nearly the same length of time, and the remainder of the period has been covered by the occupancy of John Goodsir,[18] and his successor, Sir William Turner,[19] the present incumbent.

To one feature in the history of anatomy in this school I must refer in passing. Shippen[20] was a warm personal friend and house-pupil of John Hunter.[21] Physick[22] not only had the same advantages, but became in addition his house-surgeon at St. George's Hospital. Both had enjoyed the intimate companionship of the most remarkable observer of nature since Aristotle, of a man with wider and more scientific conceptions and sympathies than had ever before been united in a member of our profession, and whose fundamental notions of disease are only now becoming prevalent. Can we doubt that from this source was derived the powerful inspiration which sustained these young men. One of them, on his

---

famous Quaker physician. In 1762 he established courses in midwifery and anatomy in Philadelphia, and he was appointed professor of anatomy, surgery, and midwifery in 1791 when the College of Philadelphia and the University of the State of Pennsylvania agreed to come together as one body under the name of the University of Pennsylvania.

17. Alexander *Monro*, primus (1697–1767): Professor of anatomy at the University of Edinburgh in 1720. Author of *Osteology, A Treatise on the Anatomy of the Human Bones* (1726), which was used as a popular textbook.

Alexander *Monro*, secundus (1733–1817): Professor of anatomy at the University of Edinburgh, succeeding to his father's chair of anatomy (1759–1808). Author of *Treatises on the Brain, the Eye, and the Ear* (1797).

Alexander *Monro*, tertius (1773–1859): Professor of anatomy at the University of Edinburgh. He first held a joint professorship with his father and then from 1817 to 1846 he was sole professor after his father died. Author of *Observations on Crural Hernia* (1803).

18. John *Goodsir* (1814–1867): Professor of anatomy at the University of Edinburgh, who succeeded Monro tertius in the chair in 1846. Author of *Anatomical and Pathological Observations* (1845).

19. William *Turner* (1832–1916): Scottish anatomist who later became president of the University of Edinburgh. Author of *An Introduction to Human Anatomy* (1875) and numerous papers on anthropological and comparative anatomy.

20. *Shippen:* See p. 155, n. 16 and p. 157, n. 27.

21. John *Hunter* (1728–1793): Scottish anatomist and surgeon. For further information, see "The Old Humanities and the New Science," p. 93, n. 214.

22. *Physick:* See p. 155, n. 12.

return from England, at once began the first anatomical classes which were held in the colonies; the other entered upon that career so notable and so honourable, which led to the just title of the Father of American Surgery. It is pleasant to think that direct from John Hunter came the influence which made anatomy so strong in this school, and that zeal in the acquisition of specimens which ultimately led to the splendid collections of the Wistar-Horner Museum.

William Shippen the younger shares with John Morgan[23] the honour of establishing medical instruction in this city. When students in England they had discussed plans, but it was Morgan who seems to have had the ear of the trustees, and who broached a definite scheme in his celebrated "Discourse,"[24] delivered in May 1765. It was not until the autumn of the year that Shippen signified to the board his willingness to accept a professorship of anatomy and surgery. He had enjoyed, as I have mentioned, the friendship of John Hunter, and had studied also with his celebrated brother, William.[25] Associated with him as fellow-pupil was William Hewson,[26] who subsequently became so famous as an anatomist and physiologist, and as the discoverer of the leucocytes of the blood, and whose descendants have been so prominent in the profession of this city. No wonder, then, with such an education, that Shippen, on his return in 1762, in his twenty-sixth year, should have begun a course of lectures in anatomy, the introductory to which was delivered in the State House on November 16.[27] To him belongs the great merit of having made a beginning, and of having brought from the Hunters methods and traditions which long held sway in this school. Wistar in his eulogium pays a warm tribute to his skill as a lecturer and as a demonstrator, and

23. John *Morgan* (1735–1789): American surgeon and anatomist, who founded the University of Pennsylvania medical school and taught the theory and practice of physics. He went overseas in 1760, going first to London to study with the Hunters, then to Edinburgh, Paris, and Rome, and finally back to London. When he returned to Philadelphia in 1765, he made a proposal to establish a medical school affiliated with the college, which was later approved.

24. *A Discourse upon the Institution of Medical Schools in America* was delivered at the annual Commencement of the College of Philadelphia (now the University of Pennsylvania) Medical School in May 1765.

25. William *Hunter* (1718–1783): Scottish physiologist and anatomist. He became professor of anatomy at the Royal Academy in 1768.

26. William *Hewson* (1739–1774): English anatomist and physiologist who attended and assisted at William Hunter's anatomy school in London and later established his own school in 1772. He published many papers in the field of hematology. He described blood coagulation and isolated fibrinogen, a key protein in the coagulation process.

27. Shippen began to teach on November 16, 1762, in temporary quarters in the State House. Although Fothergill's pictures and casts were used, Shippen's teaching relied most heavily on the dissection of human bodies, a method originated by Hunter. This practice aroused much controversy and attacks from angry crowds.

to the faithfulness with which he taught the subject for more than forty years. Apart from his connection with this institution he served as Director-General of the Military Hospitals from 1777 to 1781, and was the second president of the College of Physicians.

In the history of the profession of this country Caspar Wistar holds an unique position. He is its Avicenna,[28] its Mead,[29] its Fothergill,[30] the very embodiment of the physician who, to paraphrase the words of Armstrong,[31] used by Wistar in his Edinburgh Graduation Thesis,[32] "Sought the cheerful haunts of men, and mingled with the bustling crowd."[33] He taught anatomy in this school as adjunct and professor for twenty-six years. From the records of his contemporaries we learn that he was a brilliant teacher, "the idol of his class,"[34] as one of his eulogists says. As an anatomist he will be remembered as the author of the first American Text-Book on Anatomy,[35] a work which was exceedingly popular, and ran through several editions. His interest in the subject was not, however, of the "knife and fork"[36] kind, for he was an early student of mammalian palæontology, in the development of which one of his successors[37] was to be a chief promotor. But Wistar's claim to remembrance rests less upon his writings than upon the impress which remains to this day of his methods of teaching anatomy.

28. *Avicenna* (also known as Ibn-Sina) (980–1037): Arab physician and philosopher. He wrote on many subjects, including medicine, theology, and mathematics. His philosophy (Avicennism) is based on Aristotle with Neoplatonic additions. His chief medical work is his *Canon of Medicine,* based on Greek writings. He also wrote *Kitab Ash-shifa* (the Book of Healing).

29. Richard *Mead* (1673–1754): English physician known for his learning and his hospitality. He made a great contribution to the study of preventative medicine. Author of *Mechanical Account of Poisons* (1702), a book on his observations of the action of snake venom.

30. John *Fothergill* (1712–1780): English physician. He encouraged his friend, William Shippen, to establish courses in midwifery and anatomy in Philadelphia, and sent him anatomical drawings and casts.

31. John *Armstrong* (1709–1779): Scottish physician, poet, and essayist. Author of *Edinburgh Medical Essays* (1734).

32. Wistar received the degree of M.D. from Edinburgh University in 1786. His graduation thesis, *De Animo Demisso* (1786), was dedicated to Benjamin Franklin and Dr. William Cullen (1710–1790), professor of the theory of physic at Edinburgh.

33. This may be a casual, inexact reference to Cowper or Milton, or perhaps simply a statement of Wistar's attitude. Cf. "The cheerful haunts of man; to wield the axe," William Cowper, "The Task," book 5, line 42 and "The cheerful ways of men," John Milton, *Paradise Lost,* book 3, line 46.

34. None of the three eulogists we found used precisely this expression. Charles Caldwell (1772–1853), however, in "An Eulogium on Caspar Wistar" discusses his excellence as a teacher at great length.

35. *A System of Anatomy for the Use of Students of Medicine* (1811–1814).

36. *knife and fork:* (Practical kind.) Osler refers to the fact that Wistar was not primarily interested in anatomical study dependent on operations on specimens.

37. Joseph Leidy (1823–1891), who was distinguished not only as an anatomist, but also as a paleontologist. For further information, see pp. 160–162.

Speaking of these, Horner, who was his adjunct and intimate associate, in a letter dated February 1, 1818, says, "In reviewing the several particulars of his course of instruction, it is difficult to say in what part his chief merit consisted; he undertook everything with so much zeal, and such a conscientious desire to benefit those who came to be instructed by him, that he seldom failed of giving the most complete satisfaction. There were, however, some parts of his course peculiar to himself. These were the addition of models on a very large scale to illustrate small parts of the human structure; and the division of the general class into a number of sub-classes, each of which he supplied with a box of bones, in order that they might become thoroughly acquainted with the human skeleton, a subject which is acknowledged by all to be at the very foundation of anatomical knowledge. The idea of the former mode of instruction was acted on for the first time about fifteen years ago." We have no knowledge of a collection of specimens by Shippen, though it is hard to believe that he could have dwelt in John Hunter's house and remained free from the insatiable hunger for specimens which characterized his master. But the establishment of a museum as an important adjunct to the medical school was due to Wistar, whose collections formed the nucleus of the splendid array which you will inspect to-day. The trustees, in accepting the gift on the death of Dr. Wistar, agreed that it should be styled the Wistar Museum, and now, after the lapse of seventy-six years, the collection has found an appropriate home in an Institute of Anatomy which bears his honoured name.

But Wistar has established a wider claim to remembrance. Genial and hospitable, he reigned supreme in society by virtue of exceptional qualities of heart and head, and became, in the language of Charles Caldwell,[38] "the *sensorium commune* of a large circle of friends."[39] About no other name in our ranks cluster such memories of good fellowship and good cheer, and it stands to-day in this city a synonym for *esprit* and social intercourse. Year by year his face, printed on the invitations to the "Wistar Parties"[40] (still an important function of winter life in Philadelphia) perpetuates the message of his life, "Go seek the cheerful haunts of men."[41]

How different was the young prosector and adjunct who next taught the subject! Horner was naturally reserved and diffident, and throughout his

38. Charles *Caldwell* (1772–1853): American surgeon. His *Autobiography* (1855) describes American medicine of his day. He experimented with X-rays in diagnosis.
39. *sensorium commune:* In anatomy the phrase means "the supposed seat of sensation in the brain, usually taken as the cortex or gray matter," but Caldwell uses it playfully to mean "brain" or "mind."
40. Once a week Wistar held open houses for the members of the American Philosophical Society, visiting scientists, students, and citizens. After his death a group was organized to perpetuate these gatherings.
41. See p. 158, n. 33.

life those obstinate questionings which in doubt and suffering have so often wrung the heart of man were ever present. Fightings within and fears without [42] harassed his gentle and sensitive soul, on which mortality weighed heavily, and to which the four last things [43] were more real than the materials in which he worked. He has left us a *journal intime*,[44] in which he found, as did Amiel,[45] of whom he was a sort of medical prototype, "a safe shelter wherein his questionings of fate and the future, the voice of grief, of self-examination and confession, the soul's cry for inward peace, might make themselves freely heard." [46] Listen to him: "I have risen early in the morning, ere yet the watchman had cried the last hour of his vigil, and in undisturbed solitude giving my whole heart and understanding to my Maker, prayed fervently that I might be enlightened on this momentous subject, that I might be freed from the errors of an excited imagination, from the allurements of personal friendship, from the prejudices of education, and that I might, under the influence of Divine grace, be permitted to settle this question in its true merits." [47] How familiar is the cry, the great and exceeding bitter cry of the strong soul in the toils and doubtful of the victory! Horner, however, was one of those on whom both blessings rested. Facing the spectres of the mind, he laid them, and reached the desired haven. In spite of feeble bodily health and fits of depression, he carried on his anatomical studies with zeal, and as an original worker and author brought much reputation to the University. Particularly he enriched the museum with many valuable preparations, and his name will ever be associated with that of Wistar in the anatomical collection which bears their names.

But what shall I say of Leidy,[48] the man in whom the leaven of science

42. Hymn 606:3. The exact quotation is: "Fightings and fears within, without, O Lamb of God, I come." Osler's version of the line is from Charlotte Elliott's *Invalid's Hymm Book* (2nd ed., 1841). Cf. 2 Corinthians 7:5.

43. Death, judgement, heaven, and hell. Thomas Browne, *Religio Medici*, part 1, sect. 45. The full quotation is: "I have therefore enlarged that common *Memento mori* into a more Christian memorandum: *Memento quatuor novissima*—those four inevitable points of us all, death, judgement, heaven, and hell." *Memento quatuor novissima* here means "remember the four last things." While Osler probably got the notion from Thomas Browne, the Latin phrase can be found much earlier.

44. Horner maintained a journal intermittently throughout his life. Parts of it are now in the Archives of the University of Pennsylvania, but Osler seems to have had access to extensive portions that cannot now be found. Osler calls this diary a "journal intime" because it is similar to Amiel's.

45. Henri Frederic *Amiel* (1821–1881): Swiss poet and philosophical critic and essayist. Author of *Journal Intime* (1883–1884), an introspective, intimate diary, which was the work chiefly responsible for his fame.

46. Humphrey Ward, "Introduction," *Amiel's Journal*, 2nd ed., trans. Humphrey Ward (1883–1884; New York: Macmillan, 1906), p. xiv.

47. From Horner's journal.

48. *Leidy:* See p. 155, n. 10.

wrought with labour and travail for so many years? The written record[49] survives, scarcely equalled in variety and extent by any naturalist, but how meagre is the picture of the man as known to his friends. The traits which made his life of such value—the patient spirit, the kindly disposition, the sustained zeal—we shall not see again incarnate. The memory of them alone remains. As the echoes of the eulogies upon his life have scarcely died away, I need not recount to this audience his ways and work, but upon one aspect of his character I may dwell for a moment, as illustrating an influence of science which has attracted much attention and aroused discussion. So far as the facts of sense were concerned, there was not a trace of Pyrrhonism[50] in his composition, but in all that relates to the ultra-rational no more consistent disciple of the great sceptic ever lived.[51] There was in him, too, that delightful "ataraxia,"[52] that imperturbability which is the distinguishing feature of the Pyrrhonist, in the truest sense of the word. A striking parallel exists between Leidy and Darwin[53] in this respect, and it is an interesting fact that the two men of this century who have lived in closest intercourse with nature should have found full satisfaction in their studies and in their domestic affections. In the autobiographical section of the life of Charles Darwin, edited by his son Francis,[54] in which are laid bare with such charming frankness the inner thoughts of the great naturalist, we find that he, too, had reached in suprasensuous affairs that state of mental imperturbability in which, to borrow the quaint expression of Sir Thomas Browne, they stretched not his *pia mater*.[55] But while acknowledging that in science scepticism is advisable, Darwin says that he was not himself very sceptical. Of these two men, alike in this point, and with minds distinctly of the Aristotelian type, Darwin yet retained amid an overwhelming accumulation of facts—and here was his great superi-

49. Some of his important publications are *Elementary Treatise on Human Anatomy* (1861), "On the Fossil Horse of America" (1847), "On the Extinct Mammalia of Dakota and Nebraska" (1869), and *Fresh Water Rhizopods of North America* (1879).

50. Extreme or absolute skepticism or philosophic doubt, named from Pyrrho, whose school maintained that nothing but sensation was capable of proof.

51. *Pyrrho* (c.365–c.275 B.C.): Greek philosopher who founded a skeptic school in Elis. Leidy had a healthy skepticism about research but it did not infect the rest of his life with the self-doubt that troubled Horner.

52. *ataraxia*: A state of tranquillity, calmness of the mind.

53. Charles Robert *Darwin* (1809–1882): English naturalist. He published *Zoology of the Voyage of the Beagle* (1840–1842) and *On the Origin of Species by Means of Natural Selection* (1859), an epoch-making book on the theory of evolution, which aroused a storm of controversy.

54. *Francis Darwin* (1848–1925): English botanist, son of Charles, and his father's editor and biographer. Author of *Life and Letters of Charles Darwin* (1887).

55. Thomas Browne, *Religio Medici*, part I, sect. 9. The *pia mater*, in this context means the delicate fibrous and highly vascular membrane forming the innermost of the three coverings of the brain and spinal cord. So, to "not stretch his pia mater" means not to overexert his mental faculties.

ority—an extraordinary power of generalizing principles from them. Deficient as was this quality in Leidy, he did not, on the other hand, experience "the curious and lamentable loss of the higher æsthetic taste"[56] which Darwin mourned, and which may have been due in part to protracted ill health, and to an absolute necessity of devoting all his powers to collecting facts in support of his great theory.

When I think of Leidy's simple life, of his devotion to the study of nature, of the closeness of his communion with her for so many years, there recur to my mind time and again the lines,—

> He is made one with nature: there is heard
> His voice in all her music, from the moan
> Of thunder, to the song of night's sweet bird;
> He is a presence to be felt and known
> In darkness and in light, from herb and stone,
> Spreading itself where'er that Power may move
> Which has withdrawn his being to its own.[57]

II

Turning from the men to the subject in which they worked, from the past to the present, let us take a hasty glance at some of the developments of human anatomy and biology. Truth has been well called the daughter of Time,[58] and even in anatomy, which is a science in a state of fact, the point of view changes with successive generations. The following story, told by Sir Robert Christison,[59] of Barclay,[60] one of the leading anatomists of the early part of this century, illustrates the old attitude of mind still met with among "bread and butter"[61] teachers of the subject. Barclay spoke to his class as follows: "Gentlemen, while carrying on your work in the dissecting-room, beware of making anatomical discoveries; and above all beware of rushing with them into print. Our precursors have left us

56. Charles Robert Darwin, *The Life and Letters of Charles Darwin,* ed. Francis Darwin (1887; New York: Basic Books, 1959), p. 81.

57. Percy Bysshe Shelley, "Adonais," stanza 42, lines 370–376.

58. English proverb, which derives from Latin: "Veritas temporis filia dicitur."

59. Robert *Christison* (1797–1882): Scottish toxicologist and physician. Professor at the University of Edinburgh who specialized in pathology of kidneys.

60. John *Barclay* (1758–1826): Scottish anatomist. He was an eminent "extra-academical" (private) lecturer at the University of Edinburgh, whose name is associated with an attempt to introduce a simple anatomical nomenclature.

61. *bread and butter:* Ordinary, everyday; also practical, realistic.

little to discover. You may, perhaps, fall in with a supernumerary muscle or tendon, a slight deviation or extra branchlet of an artery, or, perhaps, a minute stray twig of a nerve—that will be all. But beware! Publish the fact, and ten chances to one you will have it shown that you have been forestalled long ago. Anatomy may be likened to a harvest-field. First come the reapers, who, entering upon untrodden ground, cut down great store of corn from all sides of them. These are the early anatomists of modern Europe, such as Vesalius, Fallopius, Malpighi, and Harvey.[62] Then come the gleaners, who gather up ears enough from the bare ridges to make a few loaves of bread. Such were the anatomists of last century—Valsalva, Cotunnius, Haller, Winslow, Vicq d'Azyr, Camper, Hunter, and the two Monros.[63] Last of all come the geese, who still contrive to pick up a few grains scattered here and there among the stubble, and waddle home in the evening, poor things, cackling with joy because of their success. Gentlemen, we are the geese."[64] Yes, geese they were, gleaning amid the stubble of a restricted field, when the broad acres of biology were open before them. Those were the days when anatomy meant a knowledge of the human frame alone; and yet the way had been opened to the larger view by the work of John Hunter, whose comprehensive mind grasped as proper subjects of study for the anatomist all the manifestations of life in order and disorder.

The determination of structure with a view to the discovery of function has

163

THE LEAVEN OF

SCIENCE

62. All early anatomists.

Andreas *Vesalius* (1514–1564): Belgian anatomist and physician, one of the first to dissect the human body. He taught at Padua, Basel, Pisa, and Bologna. Author of *De Corporis Humani Fabrica* (1543), which exposed the errors of the Galenian school. Because of his work, anatomy became a scientific discipline.

Gabriel *Fallopius* (1523–1562): Italian anatomist who discovered the function of the oviducts (fallopian tubes). He became the first anatomist to describe with accuracy the vessels and bones of the fetus.

Marcello *Malpighi* (1628–1694): Italian physician, called the founder of microscopic anatomy.

William *Harvey* (1578–1657): See "Teacher and Student," p. 116, n. 22.

63. Antonio Maria *Valsalva* (1666–1723): Italian anatomist who studied the ear.

Domenico *Cotunnius* (Cotugno) (1736–1822): Italian anatomist who described the endolymph and sciatica of the inner ear.

Albrecht von *Haller* (1708–1777): Swiss anatomist, physiologist, botanist, physician, and poet. He was professor of anatomy, surgery, and botany at Göttingen.

Jakob Benignus *Winslow* (1669–1760): Danish naturalist who wrote *Exposition Anatomique de la Structure du Corps Humain* (1732).

Félix *Vicq d'Azyr* (1748–1794): French anatomist who studied neuroanatomy.

Pieter *Camper* (1722–1789): Dutch anatomist, who distinguished himself in surgery, obstetrics, and medical jurisprudence as well as in anatomy.

Hunter: See "The Old Humanities and the New Science," p. 93, n. 214.

the two *Monros*: See p. 156, n. 17.

64. Robert Christison, *The Life of Sir Robert Christison*, ed. by his sons (Edinburgh: William Blackwood and Sons, 1885–1886), vol. 1, pp. 71–72.

been the foundation of progress. The meaning may not always have been for "him who runs to read;"[65] often, indeed, it has been at the time far from clear; and yet a knowledge in full detail of the form and relations must precede a correct physiology. The extraordinary development of all the physical sciences, and the corresponding refinement of means of research, have contributed most largely to the enlightenment of the "geese" of Barclay's witticism. Take the progress in any one department which has a practical aspect, such as, in the anatomy and physiology of the nervous system. Read, for example, in the third edition of Wistar's *Anatomy*, edited by Horner in 1825, the description of the convolutions of the brain, on which to-day a whole army of special students are at work, medical, surgical, and anthropological, and the functions of which are the objective point of physiological and psychological research—the whole subject is thus disposed of: "The surface of the brain resembles that of the mass of the small intestine, or of a convoluted, cylindrical tube; it is, therefore, said to be convoluted. The fissures between these convolutions do not extend very deep into the substance of the brain."[66] The knowledge of function correlated with this meagre picture of structure is best expressed, perhaps, in Shakespearian diction, "that when the brains were out, the man would die."[67] The laborious, careful establishment of structure by the first two generations in this century led to those brilliant discoveries in the functions of the nervous system which have not only revolutionized medicine, but have almost enabled psychologists to dispense with metaphysics altogether. It is particularly interesting to note the widespread dependence of many departments on accurate anatomical knowledge. The new cerebral anatomy, particularly the study of the surface of the brain, so summarily dismissed in a few lines by Wistar, made plain the path for Hitzig and Fritsch,[68] the careful dissection of cases of disease of the brain prepared the way for Hughlings Jackson;[69] and gradually a new phrenology on a scientific basis has replaced

65. The meaning may not be clear to one who goes quickly past (Habakkuk 2:2). In the biblical passage, God is commanding the prophet to write his revelation so clearly that someone running by can read it at a glance. However, Osler's point is virtually the reverse, meaning that a hasty reader may mistake the sense.

66. Caspar Wistar, *A System of Anatomy for the Use of Students of Medicine*, 9th ed., ed. Williams Edmonds Horner (Philadelphia: Thomas, Cowperthwait, 1846), vol. 1, sect. 2, p. 322.

67. William Shakespeare, *Macbeth*, III, iv, 79.

68. Julius Eduard *Hitzig* (1838–1907): German psychiatrist and neurophysiologist who studied the function of the cerebral cortex.

Gustav Theodor *Fritsch* (1838–1927): German anatomist who studied the electrophysiology of the brain.

69. John Hughlings *Jackson* (1835–1911): English neurologist. He correlated certain speech defects with diseases in the left cerebral hemisphere, and found that motor spasms were due to local brain irritation (Jacksonian epilepsy).

the crude notions of Gall and Spurzheim;[70] so that with the present generation, little by little, there has been established on a solid structure of anatomy, the localization of many of the functions of the brain. Excite with a rough touch, from within or from without, a small region of that mysterious surface, and my lips may move, but not in the articulate expression of thought, and I may see, but I cannot read the page before me; touch here and sight is gone, and there again and hearing fails. One by one the centres may be touched which preside over the muscles, and they may, singly or together, lose their power. All these functions may go without the loss of consciousness. Touch with the slow finger of Time the nutrition of that thin layer, and backward by slow degrees creep the intellectual faculties, back to childish simplicity, back to infantile silliness, back to the oblivion of the womb.[71]

To this new cerebral physiology, which has thus gradually developed with increasing knowledge of structure, the study of cases of disease has contributed enormously, and to-day the diagnosis of affections of the nervous system has reached an astonishing degree of accuracy. The inter-dependence and sequence of knowledge in various branches of science is nowhere better shown than in this very subject. The facts obtained by precise anatomical investigation, from experiments on animals in the laboratory, from the study of nature's experiments upon us in disease, slowly and painfully acquired by many minds in many lands, have brought order out of the chaos of fifty years ago. In a practical age this vast change has wrought a corresponding alteration in our ideas of what may or may not be done in the condition of perverted health which we call disease, and we not only know better what to do, but also what to leave undone. The localization of centres in the surface of the brain has rendered it possible to make, with a considerable degree of certainty, the diagnosis of focal disease,[72] and Macewen and Horsley[73] have supplemented the new cerebral physiology and pathology by a new cerebro-spinal surgery, the achievements of which are scarcely credible.

70. Franz Joseph *Gall* (1758–1828): German physician and founder of phrenology. He studied the brains and skulls of men and animals and sought to establish a relationship between mental faculties and the shape of the brain and skull.

Johann Kaspar *Spurzheim* (1776–1832): German physician who collaborated with Gall in founding phrenology. He wrote on the physiology and anatomy of the brain and of the nervous system.

71. *Excite with a rough touch . . . back to the oblivion of the womb:* A collection of catch phrases. This passage refers to things that can affect brain functions.

72. *focal disease:* Centrally localized disease.

73. William *Macewen* (1848–1924): Scottish surgeon and a pioneer in bone surgery.

Victor Alexander Haden *Horsley* (1857–1916): English physiologist and surgeon. His contributions include a protective treatment against rabies, as well as studies of the functions of the thyroid gland and localization of the brain functions.

But this is not all; in addition to the determination of the centres of sight, hearing, speech, and motor activities, we are gradually reaching a knowledge of the physical basis of mental phenomena. The correlation of intelligence and brain weight, of mental endowment and increased convolution of the brain surface, was recognized even by the *gleaners* of Barclay's story;[74] but within the past twenty-five years the minute anatomy of the organ has been subjected to extensive study by methods of ever-increasing delicacy, which have laid bare its complex mechanism. The pyramidal cells of the cerebral grey matter constitute the anatomical basis of thought, and with the development, association, and complex connection of these psychical cells, as they have been termed, the psychical functions are correlated. How far these mechanical conceptions have been carried, may be gathered from the recent Croonian Lecture[75] before the Royal Society, in which Ramón y Cajal[76] based the action and the degree, and the development of intelligence upon the complexity of the cell mechanism and its associations. Even the physical basis of moody madness[77] has not evaded demonstration. Researches upon the finer structure of the cerebral cortex lead to the conclusion that imbecility, mental derangement, and the various forms of insanity are but symptoms of diseased conditions of the pyramidal cells, and not separate affections of an indefinable entity, the mind. Still further; there is a school of anthropologists which strives to associate moral derangement with physical abnormalities, particularly of the brain, and urges a belief in a criminal psychosis, in which men are "villains by necessity, fools by heavenly compulsion, knaves, thieves, and treachers by spherical predominance."[78] This remarkable revolution in our knowledge of brain functions has resulted directly from the careful and accurate study by Barclay's "geese," of the anatomy of the nervous system. Truly the gleaning of the grapes of Ephraim has been better than the vintage of Abiezer.[79]

74. See p. 163.

75. Lecture held at the Royal Society in honor of William Croone (1633–1684), English physiologist and one of the founders of the Royal Society.

76. Santiago *Ramón y Cajal* (1852–1934): Spanish histologist who worked on the nervous system and established the neuron theory.

77. *moody Madness:* madness that arises from changing moods, often ill humor or depression.

78. William Shakespeare, *King Lear,* I, ii, 132–134.

79. Judges 8:2. The exact quotation is: "And he said unto them, What have I done now in comparison of you? Is not the gleaning of the grapes of Ephraim better than the vintage of Abiezer?" This is the response of Gideon, an Abiezrite, to the men of Ephraim when they complained of not being called to fight in his attack on the oppressors of Israel. Over time, it has become a set phrase. The men of Ephraim were not called to help Gideon in his attack, but afterward they were called in to kill two of the princes of the enemy people. (The "gleanings of Ephraim" indicates the princes; the "vintage of Abiezer" is the enemy host defeated by Gideon).

The study of structure, however, as the basis of vital phenomena, the strict province of anatomy, forms but a small part of the wide subject of biology, which deals with the multiform manifestations of life, and seeks to know the laws governing the growth, development, and actions of living things. John Hunter, the master of Shippen and Physick,[80] was the first great biologist of the moderns, not alone because of his extraordinary powers of observation and the comprehensive sweep of his intellect, but chiefly because he first looked at life as a whole, and studied all of its manifestations, in order and disorder, in health and in disease. He first, in the words of Buckle,[81] "determined to contemplate nature as a vast and united whole, exhibiting, indeed, at different times, different appearances, but preserving amidst every change, a principle of uniform and uninterrupted order, admitting of no division, undergoing no disturbance, and presenting no real irregularity, albeit to the common eye irregularities abound on every side."[82] We of the medical profession may take no little pride in the thought that there have never been wanting men in our ranks who have trodden in the footsteps of this great man; not only such giants as Owen,[83] Huxley,[84] and Leidy,[85] but in a more humble way many of the most diligent students of biology have been physicians. From John Hunter to Charles Darwin enormous progress was made in every department of zoology and botany, and not only in the accumulation of facts relating to structure, but in the knowledge of function, so that the conception of the phenomena of living matter was progressively widened. Then with the *Origin of Species* came the awakening, and the theory of evolution has not only changed the entire aspect of biology, but has revolutionized every department of human thought.86

Even the theory itself has come within the law; and to those of us whose biology is ten years old, the new conceptions are, perhaps, a little bewildering. The recent literature shows, however, a remarkable fertility and strength. Around

---

Osler is referring back to the "gleaners" of Barclay's speech on p. 000; he means that the scientists who follow in the wake of greater discoveries often find even more exciting facts although they have not done the groundwork themselves.

80. John *Hunter:* See "The Old Humanities and the New Science," p. 93, n. 214.

Shippen: See p. 155, n. 16 and p. 157, n. 27.

Physick: See p. 155, n. 12.

81. Henry Thomas *Buckle* (1822–1862): English historian. Author of *History of Civilization in England* (1858–1861).

82. Henry Thomas *Buckle, History of Civilization in England,* 2nd ed. (New York: Hearst's International Library, 1913), vol. 2, part 2, p. 446.

83. Richard *Owen* (1804–1892): See "Aequanimitas," p. 25, n. 21.

84. Thomas Henry *Huxley* (1825–1895): English biologist and a foremost advocate of Darwin's theory of evolution.

85. *Leidy:* See p. 155, n. 10.

the nature of cell-organization the battle wages most fiercely, and here again the knowledge of structure is sought eagerly as the basis of explanation of the vital phenomena. So radical have been the changes in this direction that a new and complicated terminology has sprung up, and the simple, undifferentiated bit of protoplasm has now its cytosome, cytolymph, caryosome, chromosome, with their somacules and biophores. These accurate studies in the vital units have led to material modifications in the theory of descent. Weismann's views,[86] particularly on the immortality of the unicellular organisms, and of the reproductive cells of the higher forms, and on the transmission or non-transmission of acquired characters, have been based directly upon studies of cell-structure and cell-fission.

In no way has biological science so widened the thoughts of men as in its application to social problems. That throughout the ages, in the gradual evolution of life, one unceasing purpose runs; that progress comes through unceasing competition, through unceasing selection and rejection; in a word, that evolution is the one great law controlling all living things, "the one divine event to which the whole creation moves,"[87] this conception has been the great gift of biology to the nineteenth century. In his work on *Social Evolution*, Kidd[88] thus states the problem in clear terms: "Nothing tends to exhibit more strikingly the extent to which the study of our social phenomena must in future be based on the biological sciences, than the fact that the technical controversy now being waged by biologists as to the transmission or non-transmission to offspring of qualities acquired during the lifetime of the parent, is one which, if decided in the latter sense, must produce the most revolutionary effect throughout the whole domain of social and political philosophy. If the old view is correct, and the effects of use and education *are* transmitted by inheritance, then the Utopian dreams of philosophy in the past are undoubtedly possible of realization. If we tend to inherit in our own persons the result of the education and mental and moral culture of past generations, then we may venture to anticipate a future society which will not deteriorate, but which may continue to make progress, even though the struggle for existence be suspended, the population regulated exactly to the means of subsistence, and the antagonism between the individual and the social

86. August *Weismann* (1834–1914): German biologist and one of the founders of the science of genetics. He held that all inheritable characteristics are carried in the germ plasm that passes from one generation to another and that is isolated from the soma. Thus, acquired characters cannot be inherited.

87. Alfred Tennyson, "In Memoriam A.H.H.," epilogue, lines 143–144. The exact quotation is:

> And one far-off divine event,
> To which the whole creation moves.

88. Benjamin *Kidd* (1858–1916): English sociologist. Author of *Social Evolution* (1894), which was widely read in Osler's age.

organism extinguished. But if the views of the Weismann party are in the main correct; if there can be no progress except by the accumulation of congenital variations above the average to the exclusion of others below; if, without the constant stress of selection which this involves, the tendency of every higher form of life *is actually retrograde;* then is the whole human race caught in the toils of that struggle and rivalry of life which has been in progress from the beginning. Then must the rivalry of existence continue, humanized as to conditions it may be, but immutable and inevitable to the end. Then also must all the phenomena of human life, individual, political, social, and religious, be considered as aspects of this cosmic process, capable of being studied and understood by science only in their relations thereto."[89]

Biology touches the problems of life at every point, and may claim, as no other science, completeness of view and a comprehensiveness which pertains to it alone. To all whose daily work lies in her manifestations the value of a deep insight into her relations cannot be overestimated. The study of biology trains the mind in accurate methods of observation and correct methods of reasoning, and gives to a man clearer points of view, and an attitude of mind more serviceable in the working-day-world than that given by other sciences, or even by the humanities. Year by year it is to be hoped that young men will obtain in this Institute a fundamental knowledge of the laws of life.

To the physician particularly a scientific discipline is an incalculable gift, which leavens his whole life, giving exactness to habits of thought and tempering the mind with that judicious faculty of distrust which can alone, amid the uncertainties of practice, make him wise unto salvation. For perdition inevitably awaits the mind of the practitioner who has never had the full inoculation with the leaven, who has never grasped clearly the relations of science to his art, and who knows nothing, and perhaps cares less, for the limitations of either.

And I may be permitted on higher grounds to congratulate the University of Pennsylvania on the acquisition of this Institute. There is great need in the colleges of this country of men who are thinkers as well as workers—men with ideas, men who have drunk deep of the Astral wine,[90] and whose energies are not sapped in the tread-mill of the class-room. In these laboratories will be given opportunities for this higher sort of university work. The conditions about us are changing rapidly: in the older states utility is no longer regarded as the test of fitness, and the value of the intellectual life has risen enormously in every department. Germany must be our model in this respect. She is great because she

89. Benjamin Kidd, *Social Evolution* (London: Macmillan, 1894), pp. 203–204.

90. Drinking deeply of something for inspiration or knowledge is a common metaphor in European literature, going back to Hesiod (fl. c.700 B.C.).

has a large group of men pursuing pure science with unflagging industry, with self-denying zeal, and with high ideals. No secondary motives sway their minds, no cry reaches them in the recesses of their laboratories, "of what practical utility is your work?"[91] but, unhampered by social or theological prejudices, they have been enabled to cherish "the truth which has never been deceived—that complete truth which carries with it the antidote against the bane and danger which follow in the train of half-knowledge." (Helmholtz.)[92]

The leaven of science gives to men habits of mental accuracy, modes of thought which enlarge the mental vision, and strengthens—to use an expression of Epicharmus—"the sinews of the understanding."[93] But is there nothing further? Has science, the last gift of the gods, no message of hope for the race as a whole; can it do no more than impart to the individual imperturbability amid the storms of life, judgment in times of perplexity? Where are the bright promises of the days when "the kindly earth should slumber rapt in universal law"?[94] Are these, then, futile hopes, vain imaginings of the dreamers, who from Plato to Comte[95] have sought for law, for order, for the *civitas Dei*[96] in the *regnum hominis?*[97]

Science has done much, and will do more, to alleviate the unhappy condition in which so many millions of our fellow-creatures live, and in no way more than in mitigating some of the horrors of disease; but we are too apt to forget that apart from and beyond her domain lie those irresistible forces which alone sway the hearts of men. With reason science never parts company, but with feel-

91. This is derived from a Latin phrase used by Cicero. *Cui bono* means "to whose benefit (was something done)?" not "what is the practical use (of something)?" Osler himself, however, seems to have used it in the sense of the latter. Marcus Tullius Cicero, *Pro Milone,* Book 12, sect. 32.

92. Herman Ludwig Ferdinand von *Helmholtz* (1821–1894): German physicist, anatomist, and physiologist, known for numerous contributions. For further information, see "The Old Humanities and the New Science," p. 75, n. 80.

93. *Epicharmus* (c.540–450 B.C.): Greek writer of comedies, of which only fragments remain. Before writing he studied philosophy, both physical and metaphysical, at Megara. The expression evidently comes from the ancient historian Polybius, in *Histories,* book 18, chap. 40, sect. 4, (trans. W. R. Paton [London: Loeb Classical Library Heinemann, 1927], vol. 5, p. 175). It reads: "Be sober and mindful to mistrust; these are the thews of the mind." Polybius attributes it to Epicharmus.

94. Alfred Tennyson, "Locksley Hall," line 130. The text actually says, "lapt," not "rapt."

95. Auguste *Comte* (1798–1857): French philosopher and founder of the positive system of philosophy; author of *Cours de Philosophie Positive* (1830–1842).

96. *civitas Dei:* (Latin) "Concerning the City of God," the exact Latin title of St. Augustine's book. The city of God is the concept of a kingdom in which God's plan or the world's potential for good has come to pass.

97. *regnum hominis:* (Latin) kingdom of man (i.e., the world and time, as distinguished from heaven and eternity).

ing, emotion, passion, what has she to do? They are not of her; they owe her no allegiance. She may study, analyze, and define, she can never control them, and by no possibility can their ways be justified to her. The great philosopher who took such a deep interest in the foundation of this University, chained the lightnings,[98] but who has chained the wayward spirit of man? Strange compound, now wrapt in the ecstasy of the beatific vision, now wallowing in the sloughs of iniquity, no leaven, earthly or divine, has worked any permanent change in him. Listen to the words of a student of the heart of man, a depictor of his emotions: "In all ages the reason of the world has been at the mercy of brute force. The reign of law has never had more than a passing reality, and never can have more than that so long as man is human. The individual intellect, and the aggregate intelligence of nations and races, have alike perished in the struggle of mankind, to revive again, indeed, but as surely to be again put to the edge of the sword. Look where you will throughout the length and breadth of all that was the world, 5000 or 500 years ago; everywhere passion has swept thought before it, and belief, reason. Passion rules the world, and rules alone. And passion is neither of the head nor of the hand, but of the heart. Love, hate, ambition, anger, avarice, either make a slave of intelligence to serve their impulses, or break down its impotent opposition with the unanswerable argument of brute force, and tear it to pieces with iron hands." (Marion Crawford.)[99]

Who runs may read the scroll[100] which reason has placed as a warning over the human menageries: "chained, not tamed."[101] And yet who can doubt that the leaven of science, working in the individual, leavens in some slight degree the whole social fabric. Reason is at least free, or nearly so; the shackles of dogma have been removed, and faith herself, freed from a morganatic alliance,[102] finds in the release great gain.

98. Benjamin *Franklin* (1706–1790): American statesman, scientist, and philosopher. He founded the Academy for the Education of Youth (1751), which preceded the University of Pennsylvania. His experiment with a kite demonstrated the electrical properties of lightning, and in this sense he "chained" or harnessed (controlled) the power of lightning. ("Chained" here does not mean "tamed.")

99. Francis Marion *Crawford* (1854–1909): American novelist whose writings are quite numerous, including *Zoroaster* (1885), *The Heart of Rome* (1903), and novels on various other subjects. We could not find this quote in his writings.

100. See p. 164, n. 65.

101. See p. 171, n. 98.

102. A relation of marriage in which "a man of exalted rank takes to wife a woman of lower station, with the provision that she remains in her former rank, and that the issues of the marriage have no claim to succeed to the possessions or dignities of their father; also, occasionally used to designate the marriage, under similar conditions, of a woman of exalted rank to a man of inferior station" (*OED*).

One of the many fertile fancies of the "laughing philosopher,"[103] a happy anticipation again of an idea peculiarly modern, was that of the influence upon us for weal or woe[104] of Externals,[105] of the idola, images, and effluences which encompass us—of Externals upon which so much of our happiness, yes, so much of our every character depends. The trend of scientific thought in this, as in the atomic theory, has reverted to the Sage of Abdera;[106] and if environment really means so much, how all-important a feature in education must be the nature of these encompassing effluences. This magnificent structure, so admirably adapted to the prosecution of that science from which modern thought has drawn its most fruitful inspirations, gives completeness to the already exhilarating *milieu*[107] of this University. Here at last, and largely owing to your indomitable energy, Mr. Provost,[108] are gathered all the externals which make up a *Schola major*[109] worthy of this great Commonwealth. What, after all, is education but a subtle, slowly affected change, due to the action upon us of the Externals; of the written record of the great minds of all ages, of the beautiful and harmonious surroundings of nature and of art, and of the lives, good or ill, of our fellows—these alone educate us, these alone mould the developing minds. Within the bounds of this campus these influences will lead successive generations of youth from matriculation in the college to graduation in the special school, the complex, varied influences of Art, of Science, and of Charity; of Art, the highest development of which can only come with that sustaining love for ideals which, "burns bright or dim as each are mirrors of the fire for which all thirst;"[110] of Science, the cold logic of which keeps the mind independent and free from toils of self-deception and half-knowledge; of Charity, in which we of the medical profession, to walk worthily, must live and move and have our being.

103. *Democritus* (c.460–c.370 B.C.): See "Physic and Physicians as Depicted in Plato," p. 128, n. 3.

104. *weal or woe:* An old stock phrase meaning "good or evil."

105. Environmental influences.

106. *Democritus* (c.460–c.370 B.C.), who was a native of Abdera, a Greek city on the coast of Thrace.

107. *milieu:* Environment.

108. Polite term for the head of the University.

109. *Schola major:* The curriculum in the Middle Ages, the *quadrivium*, or higher studies (arithmetic, geometry, music, and astronomy). For further information, see "Teacher and Student," p. 000, n. 000.

110. Percy Bysshe Shelley, "Adonais," stanza 54, lines 484–485. This is possibly a reminiscence of Marcus Aurelius, *The Meditations*, Book 9, sect. 9: "Fire indeed has a tendency to rise by reason of the elemental fire. . . . So then all that shares in the Universal Intelligent Nature has a strong affinity towards what is akin, aye, even a stronger." *The Communings with Himself of Marcus Aurelius,* ed. and trans. C. R. Haines (London: Loeb Classical Library, 1930), p. 230. The idea is that natural flames rise because of their affinity with the supposed fiery sphere above the sky, and similarly virtuous minds aspire with good thoughts because of their affinity with the minds of the virtuous immortals in heaven above.

9

TEACHING AND THINKING
The Two Functions of a Medical School

Let us then blush, in this so ample and so wonderful field of nature
(where performance still exceeds what is promised), to credit other men's
traditions only, and thence come uncertain problems to spin out thorny and captious
questions. *Nature* her selfe must be our adviser; the path she chalks must be our
walk: for so while we confer with our own eies, and take our rise from meaner
things to higher, we shall at length be received into her Closet-secrets.
WILLIAM HARVEY, *Anatomical Exercitations Concerning
the Generation of Living Creatures*

THIS ADDRESS AT McGill Medical School in 1895 begins with the assertion that
never before have people enjoyed such *physical* well-being. Osler catalogues the
recent advances in anesthetics, antiseptic surgery, birth procedures, and prevention of plague and epidemics that all contributed to the extension of life expec-
tancy. These have had a big impact on the general public, but are often taken for
granted.

Universities, with their dual functions of teaching and research, have played
a significant role in these medical advances. The teaching function has now been
fully realized at McGill, a relatively new medical school. Osler advocates increasing emphasis on laboratory science and clinical facilities. The laboratory sciences, although time consuming and expensive to teach, are essential to understanding the complex phenomena of diseases.

Osler notes that despite the advances in prevention and treatment of diseases, there is still much criticism of physicians due to a small minority of un-
caring or poorly trained doctors. The number of doctors is increasing with the
demands of specialization and with the increased resort to doctors. Some of the
controversy over drugs is due to patients' demand for inadvisable medications.
There is also a growing realization that each patient shows an individual varia-

tion of the disease. Osler stresses the importance of looking at diet and exercise as treatments. Better education systems and facilities will make graduates better equipped to fight disease. Osler hopes they will be inspired by the same spirit as their predecessors.

Osler then turns to the other function of the University—to contribute to the general store of knowledge. Osler admits that brilliant teachers often lack the time or the inclination for research and that researchers are not always good teachers; yet he stresses the importance of having both. Those who would do research must be up-to-date and knowledgeable and have ideas, ambition, and energy. They alone "confer greatness upon a university" and they must be sought worldwide.

Osler points out that sometimes it is the burden of teaching and laboratory duties that prevents faculty from doing research; so assistantships and fellow-ships are needed to attract students to help in their research. Young researchers will then be trained while stimulating the professors. Osler foresees Montreal as becoming "the Edinburgh of America," a medical center drawing the brightest students and spreading its discoveries to worldwide acclaim, as research gives stature to the medical school. Osler calls for fostering university spirit through devotion to duty and high ideals.

TEACHING AND THINKING

I

MANY THINGS HAVE BEEN urged against our nineteenth century civilization—that political enfranchisement only ends
in anarchy, that the widespread unrest in spiritual matters
leads only to unbelief, and that the best commentary on our
boasted enlightenment is the picture of Europe in arms and the nations everywhere gnarring[1] at each other's heels. Of practical progress in one direction,
however, there can be no doubt; no one can dispute the enormous increase in
the comfort of each individual life. Collectively the human race, or portions of it
at any rate, may in the past have enjoyed periods of greater repose, and longer
intervals of freedom from strife and anxiety; but the day has never been when
the unit has been of such value, when the man, and the man alone, has been
so much the measure, when the individual as a living organism has seemed so
sacred, when the obligations to regard his rights have seemed so imperative. But
even these changes are as nothing in comparison with the remarkable increase
in his physical well-being. The bitter cry of Isaiah that with the multiplication
of the nations their joys have not been increased,[2] still echoes in our ears. The

An address delivered at the opening of the new building at the McGill Medical School, January 8, 1895.
1. *gnarring:* Snarling; growling. This is an echo of Alfred Tennyson, "In Memoriam A.H.H.," part 98,
stanza 5, lines 16–17:

> a thousand wants
> Gnarr at the heels of men.

2. Isaiah 9:3. The exact quotation is: "Thou hast multiplied the nation, *and* not increased the joy: they
joy before thee according to the joy in harvest, and as *men* rejoice when they divide the spoil."

sorrows and troubles of men, it is true, may not have been materially diminished, but bodily pain and suffering, though not abolished, have been assuaged as never before, and the share of each in the *Weltschmerz*[3] has been enormously lessened.

Sorrows and griefs are companions sure sooner or later to join us on our pilgrimage, and we have become perhaps more sensitive to them, and perhaps less amenable to the old time remedies of the physicians of the soul;[4] but the pains and woes of the body, to which we doctors minister, are decreasing at an extraordinary rate, and in a way that makes one fairly gasp in hopeful anticipation.

In his *Grammar of Assent,* in a notable passage on suffering, John Henry Newman[5] asks, "Who can weigh and measure the aggregate of pain which this one generation has endured, and will endure, from birth to death? Then add to this all the pain which has fallen and will fall upon our race through centuries past and to come."[6] But take the other view of it—think of the Nemesis[7] which has overtaken pain during the past fifty years! Anæsthetics and antiseptic surgery have almost manacled the demon, and since their introduction the aggregate of pain which has been prevented far outweighs in civilized communities that which has been suffered. Even the curse of travail[8] has been lifted from the soul of women.

The greatest art is in the concealment of art,[9] and I may say that we of the medical profession excel in this respect. You of the public who hear me, go about the duties of the day profoundly indifferent to the facts I have just mentioned. You do not know, many of you do not care, that for the cross-legged Juno[10] who presided over the arrival of your grandparents, there now sits a benign and straight-legged goddess. You take it for granted that if a shoulder is dislocated

3. *Weltschmerz:* (German) world-weariness (literally); depression about the state of world affairs; sometimes sentimental sadness which one feels and accepts as a necessary portion of one's life.

4. "Physicians of the soul" is usually applied to clergy, at least by older writers, although since Osler's time psychiatrists have appropriated it for themselves.

5. John Henry *Newman* (1801–1890): See "Teacher and Student," p. 112, n. 8.

6. John Henry Newman, *An Essay in Aid of a Grammar of Assent* (1870; Oxford: Clarendon Press, 1985), chap. 10, sect. 1, pp. 256–257.

7. *Nemesis:* Goddess of divine retribution; formidable opponent whom a person cannot conquer; an agent or act of retribution or punishment.

8. *travail:* Labor pains.

9. Latin proverb: *Ars est celare artem* ("Art consists in concealing art").

10. *Juno:* Roman goddess who presided over childbirth. When mortal Alcmene was about to give birth to Hercules, Juno delayed the birth, because Jupiter, her husband, was the father of Hercules. As long as Juno sat cross-legged, the baby could not be born. Homer, *Iliad,* book 19, lines 114 ff; Ovid, *Metamorphoses,* Book 9, lines 290 ff. Osler is thus saying that birth is now much easier, unimpeded by old-fashioned methods.

there is chloroform and a delicious Nepenthe[11] instead of the agony of the pulleys and paraphernalia of fifty years ago. You accept with a selfish complacency, as if you were yourselves to be thanked for it, that the arrows of destruction fly not so thickly, and that the pestilence now rarely walketh in the darkness;[12] still less do you realize that you may now pray the prayer of Hezekiah[13] with a reasonable prospect of its fulfilment, since modern science has made to almost everyone of you the present of a few years.

I say you do not know these things. You hear of them, and the more intelligent among you perhaps ponder them in your hearts, but they are among the things which you take for granted, like the sunshine, and the flowers and the glorious heavens.

'Tis no idle challenge which we physicians throw out to the world when we claim that our mission is of the highest and of the noblest kind, not alone in curing disease but in educating the people in the laws of health, and in preventing the spread of plagues and pestilences; nor can it be gain-said that of late years our record as a body has been more encouraging in its practical results than those of the other learned professions. Not that we all live up to the highest ideals, far from it—we are only men. But we have ideals, which mean much, and they are realizable, which means more. Of course there are Gehazis[14] among us who serve for shekels, whose ears hear only the lowing of the oxen and the jingling of the guineas, but these are exceptions. The rank and file labour earnestly for your good, and self-sacrificing devotion to your interests animates our best work.

The exercises in which we are to-day engaged form an incident in this beneficent work which is in progress everywhere; an incident which will enable me to dwell upon certain aspects of the university as a factor in the promotion of the physical well-being of the race.

11. *Nepenthe:* Ancient potion reported to bring forgetfulness of sorrow or trouble.

12. *the pestilence now rarely walketh in the darkness:* Psalm 91:5–6. The exact quotation is: "Thou shall not be afraid for the terror by night; *nor* for the arrow *that* flieth by day; *Nor* for the pestilence *that* walketh in darkness; *nor* for the destruction *that* wasteth at noonday."

13. *the prayer of Hezekiah:* 2 Kings 20:2–3, Isaiah 38:2–5. The exact quotation is: "Then he turned his face to the wall, and prayed unto the LORD, saying I beseech thee, O LORD, remember now how I have walked before thee in truth and with a perfect heart, and have done *that which* is good in thy sight. And Hezekiah wept sore." His prayer was heard. He was "sick unto death," but the Lord promised that he would be healed and that he would be able to live fifteen more years.

14. *Gehazi:* 2 Kings 5:20–27. Elisha had refused to take any reward from Naaman for curing him of leprosy. Gehazi, Elisha's servant, then ran after Naaman as he was leaving and asked for silver and clothing, giving the impression that Elisha had made the request as an afterthought. When Elisha found out, he transferred the leprosy to Gehazi as a punishment.

II

A great university has a dual function, to teach and to think. The educational aspects at first absorb all its energies, and in equipping various departments and providing salaries, it finds itself hard pressed to fulfil even the first of the duties. The story of the progress of the medical school of this institution [15] illustrates the struggles and difficulties, the worries and vexations attendant upon the effort to place it in the first rank as a teaching body. I know them well, since I was in the thick of them for ten years, and see to-day the realization of many of my day-dreams. Indeed in my wildest flights I never thought to see such a splendid group of buildings as I have just inspected. We were modest in those days, and I remember when Dr. Howard [16] showed me in great confidence the letter of the Chancellor, in which he conveyed his first generous bequest to the Faculty, it seemed so great that in my joy I was almost ready to sing my *Nunc dimittis.*[17] The great advances here, at the Montreal General Hospital, and at the Royal Victoria (both of which institutions form most essential parts of the medical schools of this city) mean increased teaching facilities, and of necessity better equipped graduates, better equipped doctors! Here is the kernel of the whole matter, and it is for this that we ask the aid necessary to build large laboratories and large hospitals in which the student may learn the science and art of medicine. Chemistry, anatomy and physiology give that perspective which enables him to place man and his diseases in their proper position in the scheme of life, and afford at the same time that essential basis upon which alone a trustworthy experience may be built. Each one of these is a science in itself, complicated and difficult, demanding much time and labour for its acquisition, so that in the few years which are given to their study the student can only master the principles and certain of the facts upon which they are founded. Only so far as they bear upon a due understanding of the phenomena of disease do these subjects form part of the medical curriculum, and for us they are but means — essential means it is true — to this end. A man cannot become a competent surgeon without a full knowledge

15. The medical faculty of McGill University.

16. Robert Palmer *Howard* (1823–1889): Osler's teacher and mentor at McGill University. For further information, see "Aequanimitas," p. 28, n. 42, and "The Student Life," pp. 327–328.

17. The canticle of Simeon, which is also known as the *Nunc dimittis* from the opening words of the Latin version. The Anglican *Book of Common Prayer* includes this in the service of Evening Prayer. It begins with the words of Simeon in Luke 2:29–32:

> Lord, now lettest thou thy servant depart in peace, according to thy word:
> For mine eyes have seen thy salvation,
> Which thou hast prepared before the face of all people;
> A light to lighten the Gentiles, and the glory of thy people Israel.

of human anatomy and physiology, and the physician without physiology and chemistry flounders along in an aimless fashion, never able to gain any accurate conception of disease, practising a sort of popgun pharmacy,[18] hitting now the malady and again the patient, he himself not knowing which.

The primary function of this department of the university is to instruct men about disease, what it is, what are its manifestations, how it may be prevented, and how it may be cured; and to learn these things the four hundred young men who sit on these benches have come from all parts of the land. But it is no light responsibility which a faculty assumes in this matter. The task is beset with difficulties, some inherent in the subject and others in the men themselves, while not a few are caused by the lack of common sense in medical matters of the people among whom we doctors work.

The processes of disease are so complex that it is excessively difficult to search out the laws which control them, and, although we have seen a complete revolution in our ideas, what has been accomplished by the new school of medicine is only an earnest of what the future has in store. The three great advances of the century have been a knowledge of the mode of controlling epidemic diseases, the introduction of anæsthetics, and the adoption of antiseptic methods in surgery. Beside them all others sink into insignificance, as these three contribute so enormously to the personal comfort of the individual. The study of the causes of so-called infectious disorders has led directly to the discovery of the methods for their control, for example, such a scourge as typhoid fever becomes almost unknown in the presence of perfect drainage and an uncontaminated water supply. The outlook, too, for specific methods of treatment in these affections is most hopeful. The public must not be discouraged by a few, or even by many failures. The thinkers who are doing the work for you are on the right path, and it is no vain fancy that before the twentieth century is very old there may be effective vaccines against many of the contagious diseases.

But a shrewd old fellow remarked to me the other day, "Yes, many diseases are less frequent, others have disappeared, but new ones are always cropping up, and I notice that with it all there is not only no decrease, but a very great increase in the number of doctors."

The total abolition of the infectious group we cannot expect, and for many years to come there will remain hosts of bodily ills, even among preventable maladies, to occupy our labours; but there are two reasons which explain the relative numerical increase in the profession in spite of the great decrease in the

18. *popgun pharmacy:* Refers contemptuously to an inefficient use or administration of medicines. Osler probably coined the phrase; this quotation is included under the entry "popgun" in the *OED* as the earliest instance of its occurrence.

number of certain diseases. The development of specialties has given employment to many extra men who now do much of the work of the old family practitioner, and again people employ doctors more frequently and so give occupation to many more than formerly.

It cannot be denied that we have learned more rapidly how to prevent than how to cure diseases, but with a definite outline of our ignorance we no longer live now in a fool's Paradise,[19] and fondly imagine that in all cases we control the issues of life and death with our pills and potions. It took the profession many generations to learn that fevers ran their course, influenced very little, if at all, by drugs, and the £60 which old Dover[20] complained were spent in drugs in a case of ordinary fever about the middle of the last century is now better expended on a trained nurse, with infinitely less risk, and with infinitely greater comfort to the patient. Of the difficulties inherent in the art not one is so serious as this which relates to the cure of disease by drugs. There is so much uncertainty and discord even among the best authorities (upon non-essentials it is true) that I always feel the force of a well-known stanza in *Rabbi Ben Ezra*—

> Now, who shall arbitrate?
> Ten men love what I hate,
> Shun what I follow, slight what I receive;
> Ten, who in ears and eyes
> Match me: we all surmise,
> They this thing, and I that: whom shall my soul believe?[21]

One of the chief reasons for this uncertainty is the increasing variability in the manifestations of any one disease. As no two faces, so no two cases are alike in all respects, and unfortunately it is not only the disease itself which is so varied, but the subjects themselves have peculiarities which modify its action.

With the diminished reliance upon drugs, there has been a return with profit to the older measures of diet, exercise, baths, and frictions,[22] the remedies with which the Bithynian Asclepiades[23] doctored the Romans so successfully in

19. *a fool's Paradise:* A proverbial expression meaning illusory happiness based on false beliefs or hopes.

20. Thomas *Dover* (1662–1742): English physician who wrote several medical treatises. The quote here is from *The Ancient Physician's Legacy to his Country* (London: Printed for the author and sold by A. Bettesworth, 1732), p. 140. The exact quotation is: "I must confess, I could never bring an Apothecary's Bill to three Pounds, in a Fever: Whereas I have known some of their Bills, in this Disease, amount to forty, fifty, and sixty Pounds."

21. Robert Browning, "Rabbi Ben Ezra," stanza 22, lines 127–132.

22. *frictions:* The action of rubbing the body, used in medical treatment.

23. *Asclepiades* (124–c.40 B.C.): Greek physician born at Prusa, Bithynia, who practiced at Rome in the first half of the 1st century B.C. He founded his practice on a modification of the atomic (corpuscular)

the first century. Though used less frequently, medicines are now given with infinitely greater skill; we know better their indications and contradictions, and we may safely say (reversing the proportion of fifty years ago) that for one damaged by dosing, one hundred are saved.

Many of the difficulties which surround the subject relate to the men who practise the art. The commonest as well as the saddest mistake is to mistake one's profession, and this we doctors do often enough, some of us, without knowing it. There are men who have never had the preliminary education which would enable them to grasp the fundamental truths of the science on which medicine is based. Others have poor teachers, and never receive that bent of mind which is the all important factor in education; others again fall early into the error of thinking that they know it all, and benefiting neither by their mistakes or their successes, miss the very essence of all experience, and die bigger fools, if possible, than when they started. There are only two sorts of doctors; those who practise with their brains, and those who practise with their tongues. The studious, hard-working man who wishes to know his profession thoroughly, who lives in the hospitals and dispensaries, and who strives to obtain a wide and philosophical conception of disease and its processes, often has a hard struggle, and it may take years of waiting before he becomes successful; but such form the bulwarks of our ranks, and outweigh scores of the voluble Cassios [24] who talk themselves into, and often out of, practice.

Now of the difficulties bound up with the public in which we doctors work, I hesitate to speak in a mixed audience. Common sense in matters medical is rare, and is usually in inverse ratio to the degree of education. I suppose as a body, clergymen are better educated than any other, yet they are notorious supporters of all the nostrums and humbuggery [25] with which the daily and religious papers abound, and I find that the further away they have wandered from the decrees of the Council of Trent,[26] the more apt are they to be steeped in thaumaturgic and Galenical superstition.[27] But know also, man has an inborn craving

---

theory, and his cures aimed at restoring bodily harmony. He recommended simple treatments such as diet, bathing, and exercise.

24. William Shakespeare, *Othello*, I, i, 18–27. Cassio is described as follows: "And what was he? . . . mere prattle without practice." This is ill-intentioned Iago's line.

25. *nostrums and humbuggery:* The practice of a quack remedy.

26. An ecumenical council (1545–1563). Clergy of the Roman Catholic Church met at Trent to counter the attacks by Protestants on Catholicism and defined the doctrines of their church. Osler's point is that the further Christians stray from Catholic dogma as laid down by the Council of Trent, the more prone they are to superstitious credulity, not only in religion but also in medicine.

27. Claudius *Galen* (c.130–c.200): Greek physician who settled in Rome. His views regarding anatomy and physiology were taken as an authority for over one thousand years until Vesalius and Harvey ap-

for medicine. Heroic dosing for several generations has given his tissues a thirst for drugs. As I once before remarked, the desire to take medicine is one feature which distinguishes man, the animal, from his fellow creatures. It is really one of the most serious difficulties with which we have to contend. Even in minor ailments, which would yield to dieting or to simple home remedies, the doctor's visit is not thought to be complete without the prescription. And now that the pharmacists have cloaked even the most nauseous remedies, the temptation is to use medicine on every occasion, and I fear we may return to that state of poly-pharmacy, the emancipation from which has been the sole gift of Hahnemann[28] and his followers to the race. As the public becomes more enlightened, and as we get more sense, dosing will be recognized as a very minor function in the practise of medicine in comparison with the old measures of Asclepiades.[29]

After all, these difficulties—in the subject itself, in us, and in you—are less-ening gradually, and we have the consolation of knowing that year by year the total amount of unnecessary suffering is decreasing at a rapid rate.

In teaching men what disease is, how it may be prevented, and how it may be cured, a University is fulfilling one of its very noblest functions. The wise in-struction and the splendid example of such men as Holmes, Sutherland, Camp-bell, Howard, Ross, Macdonnell, and others[30] have carried comfort into thou-sands of homes throughout this land. The benefits derived from the increased facilities for the teaching of medicine which have come with the great changes made here and at the hospitals during the past few years, will not be confined to

182
TEACHING AND
THINKING

---

peared. He also developed the art or practice of preparing herbal or other vegetable drugs. "He seems to place a more implicit faith in amulets than in medicine, and he is supposed by Cullen to be the originator of the anodyne necklace which was so long famous in England" (*Encyclopedia Americana,* 1969).

28. Samuel Christian *Hahnemann* (1755–1843): German physician and founder of homeopathy, the method of treating disease by drugs, administered in small amounts, which produce in healthy people symptoms similar to those of the disease.

29. *Asclepiades:* See p. 180, n. 23.

30. All McGill professors.

Andrew Fernando *Holmes* (1797–1860): One of the founders of the Medical faculty of McGill, profes-sor of chemistry and materia medica, and later dean. He was a great advocate of research in physiology and pathology. He was loved by his students. Osler dedicated to Dr. Holmes his book *Practice of Medicine.*

William *Sutherland* (1816–1875): Professor of chemistry who helped establish the Montreal School of Medicine and Surgery.

George W. *Campbell* (1810–1882): Professor of surgery and midwifery and dean of the medical faculty when Osler was teaching at McGill. "Deeds, not words" was his motto.

Howard: See p. 000, n. 000.

George *Ross* (1845–1892): Professor of clinical medicine. For further information, see "After Twenty-Five Years," p. 206, n. 18.

Richard Lee *MacDonnell* (1853–1891): Professor of clinical medicine. One of Osler's friends and a mem-ber of the Journal Club for the circulation of French and German journals.

the citizens of this town, but will be widely diffused and felt in every locality to which the graduates of this school may go; and every gift which promotes higher medical education, and which enables the medical faculties throughout the country to turn out better doctors, means fewer mistakes in diagnosis, greater skill in dealing with emergencies, and the saving of pain and anxiety to countless sufferers and their friends.

The physician needs a clear head and a kind heart; his work is arduous and complex, requiring the exercise of the very highest faculties of the mind, while constantly appealing to the emotions and finer feelings. At no time has his influence been more potent than at present, at no time has he been so powerful a factor for good, and as it is one of the highest possible duties of a great University to fit men for this calling, so it will be your highest mission, students of medicine, to carry on the never-ending warfare against disease and death, better equipped, abler men than your predecessors, but animated with their spirit and sustained by their hopes, "for the hope of every creature is the banner that we bear."[31]

III

The other function of a University is to think. Teaching current knowledge in all departments, teaching the steps by which the *status præsens*[32] has been reached, and teaching how to teach, form the routine work of the various college faculties. All this may be done in a perfunctory manner by men who have never gone deeply enough into the subjects to know that really thinking about them is in any way necessary or important. What I mean by the thinking function of a University, is that duty which the professional corps owes to enlarge the boundaries of human knowledge. Work of this sort makes a University great, and alone enables it to exercise a wide influence on the minds of men.

We stand to-day at a critical point in the history of this faculty. The equipment for teaching, to supply which has taken years of hard struggle, is approaching completion, and with the co-operation of the General and the Royal Victoria Hospitals students can obtain in all branches a thorough training. We have now reached a position in which the higher university work may at any rate be discussed, and towards it progress in the future must trend.[33] It may seem to be discouraging, after so much has been done and so much has been so generously given, to say that there remains a most important function to foster and sustain, but this aspect of the question must be considered when a school has

31. *for the hope of every creature is the banner that we bear:* Unknown.
32. *status præsens:* (Latin) medical term meaning "present state."
33. *trend:* "Go in the general direction of."

reached a certain stage of development. In a progressive institution the changes come slowly, the pace may not be perceived by those most concerned, except on such occasions as the present, which serve as land-marks in its evolution. The men and methods of the old Coté street school[34] were better than those with which the faculty started; we and our ways at the new building on University street were better than those of Coté street; and now you of the present faculty teach and work much better than we did ten years ago. Everywhere the old order changeth,[35] and happy those who can change with it. Like the defeated gods in Keats's "Hyperion," too many unable to receive the balm of the truth, resent the wise words of Oceanus[36] (which I quoted here with very different feelings some eighteen years ago in an introductory lecture).

> So on our heels a fresh perfection treads,
> . . . born of us
> And fated to excel us.[37]

Now the fresh perfection which will tread on our heels will come with the opportunities for higher university work. Let me indicate in a few words its scope and aims. Teachers who teach current knowledge are not necessarily investigators; many have not had the needful training; others have not the needful time. The very best instructor for students may have no conception of the higher lines of work in his branch, and contrariwise, how many brilliant investigators have been wretched teachers? In a school which has reached this stage and wishes to do thinking as well as teaching, men must be selected who are not only thoroughly *au courant*[38] with the best work in their department the world over, but who also have ideas, with ambition and energy to put them into force—men who can add each one in his sphere, to the store of the world's knowledge. Men of this stamp[39] alone confer greatness upon a university. They should be sought for far and wide; an institution which wraps itself in Strabo's cloak[40] and does

34. The McGill school was originally on Coté Street. It was moved to the present University grounds in the early 1870s, when Osler spent his two years there.

35. Alfred Tennyson, "Morte d'Arthur," line 240.

36. *Oceanus:* Mythological Titan, the father of the river gods and sea nymphs. John Keats, "Hyperion," Book 2, lines 212–214.

37. Ibid.

38. *au courant:* (French) fully acquainted with matters, up-to-date, conversant on a subject

39. *stamp:* Character, or make.

40. This refers to the world as it was known in those days, not merely Europe. Strabo (54 B.C.–24 A.D.) was a famous Greek geographer who traveled extensively. His work portrayed the world, its customs, and histories as known to its occupants. Thomas Browne, *Religio Medici*, part 1, sect. 56. Osler's allusion is a fanciful way of saying "don't confine the medical world geographically."

not look beyond the college gates in selecting professors may get good teachers, but rarely good thinkers.

One of the chief difficulties in the way of advanced work is the stress of routine class and laboratory duties, which often sap the energies of men capable of higher things. To meet this difficulty it is essential, first, to give the professors plenty of assistance, so that they will not be worn out with teaching; and, secondly, to give encouragement to graduates and others to carry on researches under their direction. With a system of fellowships and research scholarships a university may have a body of able young men, who on the outposts of knowledge are exploring, surveying, defining and correcting. Their work is the outward and visible sign that a university is thinking. Surrounded by a group of bright young minds, well trained in advanced methods, not only is the professor himself stimulated to do his best work, but he has to keep far afield and to know what is stirring in every part of his own domain.

With the wise co-operation of the university and the hospital authorities Montreal may become the Edinburgh of America,[41] a great medical centre to which men will flock for sound learning, whose laboratories will attract the ablest students, and whose teaching will go out into all lands, universally recognized as of the highest and of the best type.

Nowhere is the outlook more encouraging than at McGill. What a guarantee for the future does the progress of the past decade afford! No city on this continent has endowed higher education so liberally. There remains now to foster that undefinable something which, for want of a better term, we call the university spirit, a something which a rich institution may not have, and with which a poor one may be saturated, a something which is associated with men and not with money, which cannot be purchased in the market or grown to order, but which comes insensibly with loyal devotion to duty and to high ideals, and without which *Nehushtan*[42] is written on the portals of any school of Medicine, however famous.

---

41. Edinburgh University was a great medical center where many North American students went to study in the nineteenth century. The McGill School, founded by Scotsmen, closely followed the educational methods of Edinburgh, where the hospitals were closely affiliated with the university.

42. *Nehushtan* is the name of the Brazen Serpent. Moses originally made the Brazen Serpent at God's command, to cure Israelites who had been bitten by serpents (Numbers 21:8–9). But by King Hezekiah's time, the people were treating it as an idol, and he therefore destroyed it (2 Kings 18:4). Osler uses it as a type of treatment that was acceptable given the state of medicine when these treatments were devised, but to which healers have obstinately clung even after better cures were found.

10

NURSE AND PATIENT

I said, I will take heed to my ways, that I offend not in my tongue.
I will keep my mouth as it were with a bridle.
PSALM 34:1–2

If thou hast heard a word, let it die with thee;
and be bold, it will not burst thee.
ECCLESIASTICUS 19:10

Lo, in the vale of years beneath
A grisly troop are seen,
The painful family of death,
More hideous than their queen:
This racks the joints, this fires the veins,
That every labouring sinew strains,
Those in the deeper vitals rage:
THOMAS GRAY, "Ode on a Distant Prospect
of Eton College"

THIS ADDRESS TO NURSES at the graduation exercises in 1897 of Johns Hopkins Hospital Training School for Nurses reveals much about both Victorian views of women and Osler's admiration for the nursing profession. With tongue in cheek, he quips that a sick (i.e., helpless) man resents being ministered to by a woman. But he concludes that except in the "warped judgement" of the sick man, nurses are a blessing, easing the physician's work, often making medications unnecessary and generally "putting all to right."

Osler urges nurses to learn to subdue their emotions and not to become over-involved with patients or their families. Specifically he advises holding confidences sacred, being discreetly silent, and avoiding discussing ailments or using medical jargon.

Addressing the "problem" of the marriage of nurses, Osler holds that it is the natural outcome for a trained nurse. He compares nurses with the female guardians in Plato's *Republic*, saying they are the choicest women in the community and are further enhanced by their hospital experience.

Remember that this was in 1897—Osler advocates nursing as the ideal vocation for spinsters (unmarried women over twenty-five!) to satisfy their hearts and minds, because social engagements and church activities are not enough. He considers nurses a great resource and urges the establishment of a German-style nursing guild to train nurses. This, he believes, could provide good nurses to those hospitals that are not attached to medical schools.

Osler praises nursing as a great blessing to humanity. He warns that the routine work and neverending care of sufferers can have a corroding effect, hardening the "fine edge of sympathy" of nurses and physicians alike. In conclusion, he encourages nurses and physicians to live according to the Golden Rule and to keep their ideals.

Cushing reported that this address "did not entirely please those members of the nursing profession who took themselves too seriously." However, Cushing adds that anyone knowing Osler's eccentricities on the few occasions when he was sufficiently ill to need a nurse "can but smile" (Cushing, p. 452).

NURSE AND PATIENT

THE TRAINED NURSE AS a factor in life may be regarded from many points of view—philanthropic, social, personal, professional and domestic. To her virtues we have been exceeding kind—tongues have dropped manna[1] in their description. To her faults—well let us be blind, since this is neither the place nor the time to expose them. I would rather call your attention to a few problems connected with her of interest to us collectively,—and individually, too, since who can tell the day of her coming.

Is she an added blessing or an added horror in our beginning civilization? Speaking from the point of view of a sick man, I take my stand firmly on the latter view, for several reasons. No man with any self-respect cares to be taken off guard, in *mufti*,[2] so to speak. Sickness dims the eye, pales the cheek, roughens the chin, and makes a man a scarecrow, not fit to be seen by his wife, to say nothing of a strange woman all in white or blue or gray. Moreover she will take such unwarrantable liberties with a fellow, particularly if she catches him with fever; *then* her special virtues could be depicted by King Lemuel[3] alone. So far as she is concerned you are again in swathing bands,[4] and in her hands you are,

An address delivered at the commencement exercises of the Training School for Nurses at the Johns Hopkins Hospital, June 3, 1897.

1. John Milton, *Paradise Lost,* book 2, lines 112–113. *Manna* is the divine food miraculously provided for the Israelites in the wilderness (Exodus 16:14–36).

2. *in mufti:* Not in uniform.

3. Proverbs 31:10–31. King Lemuel describes an ideal woman or wife.

4. *swathing bands* (also, swaddling clothes): Strips of cloth, like bandages, in which infants used to be wrapped. Osler is thinking of Luke 2:12, where the angel announcing the birth of Jesus tells the shepherds: "Ye shall find the babe wrapped in swaddling clothes, lying in a manger"; but the actual phrase he uses

as of yore, a helpless lump of human clay. She will stop at nothing, and between baths and spongings and feeding and temperature-taking you are ready to cry with Job the cry of every sick man—"*Cease then,* and let me alone." [5] For generations has not this been his immemorial privilege, a privilege with vested rights as a deep-seated animal instinct—to turn his face toward the wall, to sicken in peace, and, if he so wishes, to die undisturbed? All this the trained nurse has, alas! made impossible. And more, too. The tender mother, the loving wife, the devoted sister, the faithful friend, and the old servant who ministered to his wants and carried out the doctor's instructions so far as were consistent with the sick man's wishes—all, all are gone, these old familiar faces; [6] and now you reign supreme, and have added to every illness a domestic complication of which our fathers knew nothing. You have upturned an inalienable right in displacing those whom I have just mentioned. You are intruders, innovators, and usurpers, dislocating, as you do, from their tenderest and most loving duties these mothers, wives and sisters. Seriously, you but lightly reck [7] the pangs which your advent may cause. The handing over to a stranger the care of a life precious beyond all computation may be one of the greatest earthly trials. Not a little of all that is most sacred is sacrificed to your greater skill and methodical ways. In the complicated fabric of modern society both our nursing and our charity appear to be better done second-hand, though at the cost in the one case as in the other of many Beatitudes, [8] links of that golden chain, of which the poet sings, [9] let down from heaven to earth.

Except in the warped judgment of the sick man, for which I have the warmest sympathy, but no respect, you are regarded as an added blessing, with, of course, certain limitations. Certainly you have made the practice of medicine easier to the physician; you are more than the equivalent of the old two hourly doses to a fever patient; and as the public grows in intelligence you should save in many instances the entire apothecary's bill. In his chapter on Instinct, in *The Origin of the Species,* Darwin gives a graphic account of the marvellous caretaking capacity of the little Formica fusca—a slave ant. One of these "introduced into a company of her masters who were helpless and actually dying for lack of assistance, instantly set to work, fed and saved the survivors, made some cells,

comes from the well-known Christmas hymn by Nahum Tate (1652–1715) "While Shepherds Watched Their Flocks by Night": "All meanly wrapped in swathing bands,/ And in a manger laid" (stanza 4).

5. Job 10:20.

6. Charles Lamb, "Old Familiar Faces," the refrain.

7. *reck:* Have care, concern, or regard; take heed.

8. Matthew 5:3–11. The eight declarations of blessedness pronounced by Jesus in the Sermon on the Mount, beginning "blessed *are* the poor in spirit: for theirs is the kingdom of heaven."

9. John Milton, *Paradise Lost,* book 2, lines 1051–1052.

and tended the larvae and put all to rights." [10] *Put all to rights!* How often have I thought of this expression and of this incident when at your word I have seen order and quiet replace chaos and confusion, not alone in the sick-room, but in the household.

As a rule, a messenger of joy and happiness, the trained nurse may become an incarnate tragedy. A protracted illness, an attractive and weak Mrs. Ebb-Smith [11] as nurse, and a weak husband—and all husbands are weak—make fit elements for a domestic tragedy which would be far more common were your principles less fixed.

While thus a source of real terror to a wife, you may become a more enduring misery to a husband. In our hurried progress the weak-nerved sisters have suffered sorely, and that deep mysterious undercurrent of the emotions, which flows along silently in each one of us, is apt to break out in the rapids, eddies and whirls of hysteria or neurasthenia. By a finely measured sympathy and a wise combination of affection with firmness, you gain the full confidence of one of these unfortunates, and become to her a rock of defence, to which she clings, and without which she feels again adrift. You become essential in her life, a fixture in the family, and at times a dark shadow between husband and wife. As one poor victim expressed it, "She owns my wife body and soul, and, so far as I am concerned, she has become the equivalent of her disease." [12] Sometimes there develops that occult attraction between women, only to be explained by the theory of Aristophanes as to the origin of the race;[13] but usually it grows out of the natural leaning of the weak upon the strong, and in the nurse the wife may find that "stern strength and promise of control" [14] for which in the husband she looked in vain.

To measure finely and nicely your sympathy in these cases is a very deli-

10. Charles Darwin, *The Origin of Species,* chap. 8, "Special Instincts: Slave-Making Instinct."

11. Osler refers to Mrs. Agnes Ebbsmith in *The Notorious Mrs. Ebbsmith* (1895), a play by A. W. Pinero.

12. Probably Osler's patient's husband complained in this tone.

13. In Plato's *Symposium* Aristophanes claims that there were originally three sexes. Some people were male, some female, and others hermaphrodites (both male and female), each with one head with two faces, four arms, and four legs. In punishment for an attack on the gods, Zeus split each of them down the middle. Those who had been hermaphrodites before became heterosexuals, while those who had been all male or all female became homosexuals, because of "desire for the whole." "And the reason is that human nature was originally one and we were a whole, and the desire and pursuit of the whole is called love." Plato, *Symposium,* 189–193.

14. Matthew Arnold, "A Farewell," lines 21–24. The exact quotation is:

> And women—things that live and move
> Mined by the fever of the soul—
> They seek to find in those they love
> Stern strength, and promise of control.

cate operation. The individual temperament controls the situation, and the more mobile of you will have a hard lesson to learn in subduing your emotions. It is essential, however, and never let your outward action demonstrate the native act and figure of your heart. You are lost irrevocably, should you so far give the reins to your feelings as to "ope the sacred source of sympathetic tears."[15] Do enter upon your duties with a becoming sense of your frailties. Women can fool men always, women only sometimes,[16] and it may be the lot of any one of you to be such a castaway as the nurse of whom I was told a few weeks ago. The patient was one of those Alphonsine Plessis-like creatures[17] whom everybody had to love, and for whom the primrose path of dalliance[18] had ended in a rigid rest cure. After three weary months she was sent to a quiet place in the mountains with the more sedate of the two nurses who had been with her. Miss Blank had had a good training and a large experience, and was a New England woman of the very best type. Alas! hers the greater fall! An accomplishment of this siren, which had produced serious symptoms, was excessive cigarette smoking, and Dr. ——— had strictly forbidden tobacco. Three weeks later, my informant paid a visit to the secluded resort, and to his dismay found patient and nurse on the verandah enjoying the choicest brand of Egyptian cigarette!

While not the recipient of all the wretched secrets of life, as are the parson and the doctor, you will frequently be in households the miseries of which cannot be hid, all the cupboards of which are open to you, and you become the involuntary possessor of the most sacred confidences, known perhaps to no other soul. Nowadays that part of the Hippocratic oath[19] which enjoins secrecy as to the things seen and heard among the sick, should be administered to you at graduation.

Printed in your remembrance, written as headlines on the tablets of your chatelaines,[20] I would have two maxims: "I will keep my mouth as it were with a bridle,"[21] and "If thou hast heard a word let it die with thee."[22] Taciturnity, a dis-

---

15. Thomas Gray, "The Progress of Poesy," III, 1, 94.

16. This is an echo or imitation of "you can fool all the people some of the time, and some of the people all of the time, but you cannot fool all the people all of the time," which has been variously attributed to Abraham Lincoln (1809–1865) and the circus showman P. T. Barnum (1819–1891).

17. The real-life prototype of the heroine of *La Dame aux Camelias* (1848) by Alexandre Dumas, the Younger (1824–1895) and of *La Bohème* (1896), an opera by Giacomo Puccini (1858–1924).

18. *the primrose path of dalliance:* William Shakespeare, *Hamlet*, I, iii, 50.

19. "The Oath," *Hippocratic Writings* (Harmondsworth: Penguin, 1983), pp. 26–27. The original reads: "Whatever I see or hear, professionally or privately, which ought not to be divulged, I will keep secret and tell no one."

20. *chatelaine:* An ornamental device for suspending the bunch of keys, etc., worn at the waist by women.

21. Psalm 39:1.

22. Ecclesiasticus 19:10.

creet silence, is a virtue little cultivated in these garrulous days when the chatter of the bander-log[23] is everywhere about us, when, as some one has remarked, speech has taken the place of thought. As an inherited trait it is perhaps an infirmity, but the kind to which I refer is an acquired faculty of infinite value. Sir Thomas Browne drew the distinction nicely when he said, "Think not silence the wisdom of fools, but, if rightly timed, the honour of wise men, who had not the infirmity but the virtue of taciturnity,"[24] the talent for silence[25] Carlyle calls it.

Things medical and gruesome have a singular attraction for many people, and in the easy days of convalescence a facile-tongued nurse may be led on to tell of "moving incidents" in ward or theatre, and once untied, that unruly member is not apt to cease wagging with the simple narration of events. To talk of diseases is a sort of Arabian Nights' entertainment[26] to which no discreet nurse will lend her talents.

With the growth of one abominable practice in recent days I am not certain you have anything to do, though I have heard your name mentioned in connexion with it. I refer to the habit of openly discussing ailments which should never be mentioned. Doubtless it is in a measure the result of the disgusting publicity in which we live, and to the pernicious habit of allowing the filth of the gutters as purveyed in the newspapers to pollute the stream of our daily lives. This open talk about personal maladies is an atrocious breach of good manners. Not a month ago, I heard two women, both tailor-made, who sat opposite to me in a street-car, compare notes on their infirmities in Fulvian accents[27] audible to everyone. I have heard a young woman at a dinner-table relate experiences which her mother would have blushed to have told to the family physician. Everything nowadays is proclaimed from the house-tops, among them our little bodily woes and worries. This is a sad lapse from the good old practice of our grandfathers, of which George Sand writes, "People knew how to live and die in those days, and kept their infirmities out of sight. You might have the

23. *the bandar-log:* The Monkey People in Rudyard Kipling's *The Jungle Book* (New York: Doubleday, Doran, 1894), pp. 52–54. The exact quotation is: " 'Mowgli,' said Baloo, 'thou hast been talking with the Bandar-log—the Monkey People.' . . . 'They have no speech of their own but use the stolen words which they overhear when they listen and peep and wait up above in the branches.' "

24. Thomas Browne, *Christian Morals,* part 3, sect. 18.

25. Thomas Carlyle, "The Hero as King," in *Heroes and Hero Worship* (1840; Oxford University Press, 1965), p. 294. The exact quotation is: "I hope we English will long maintain our grand talent pour le silence."

26. Shahrazad (also Shaharazade) was married to the sultan, whose habit was to enjoy his wife for one night then have her head cut off and marry a new one. Shahrazad avoided this fate by telling him a series of drawn-out stories. The stories make up *The Arabian Nights' Entertainments.*

27. Fulvia, Mark Antony's wife, was considered to be manipulative and shrewish. William Shakespeare, *Antony and Cleopatra,* I, i, 20.

gout, but you must walk about all the same without making grimaces. It was a point of good breeding to hide one's suffering."[28] We doctors are great sinners in this manner, and among ourselves and with the laity are much too fond of "talking shop."[29]

To another danger I may refer, now that I have waxed bold. With the fullest kind of training you cannot escape from the perils of half-knowledge, of pseudo-science, that most fatal and common of mental states. In your daily work you involuntarily catch the accents and learn the language of science, often without a clear conception of its meaning. I turned incidentally one day to a very fine example of the nurse learned and asked in a humble tone what the surgeon, whom I had failed to meet, had thought of the case, and she promptly replied that "he thought there were features suggestive of an intracanalicular myxoma;" and when I looked anxious and queried, "had she happened to hear if he thought it had an epiblastic or mesoblastic origin?"[30] this daughter of Eve never flinched; "mesoblastic, I believe," was her answer. She would have handed sponges—I mean gauze—with the same *sang froid*[31] at a Waterloo.[32]

It must be very difficult to resist the fascination of a desire to know more, much more, of the deeper depths of the things you see and hear, and often this ignorance must be very tantalizing, but it is more wholesome than an assurance which rests on a thin veneer of knowledge.

A friend, a distinguished surgeon, has written, in the Lady Priestley[33] vein, an essay on "The Fall of the Trained Nurse," which, so far, he has very wisely

28. George Sand, *Histoire de ma vie*, vol. 1, pp. 43–44. In a letter from her grandmother.

29. *talking shop:* Talking about matters pertaining to one's own business and profession (*OED*).

30. *myxoma:* Benign tumor whose parenchyma is composed of connective and mucoid tissue.

   epiblastic: (Embryology) of or like the primordial outer layer of a young embryo before the segregation of the germ layers.

   mesoblastic: (Embryology) of or like the primordial middle layer of a young embryo before the segregation of the germ layers.

31. *sang froid:* (French) the phrase literally means "cold blood," but Osler here means coolness of mind; calmness.

32. Osler's point here is that Waterloo was a very bloody battle, where those tending the wounded faced a huge and daunting task.

33. Lady *Priestley:* Eliza Chambers Priestley (c.1837), who married Charles Priestley, a medical doctor whose great-grand-uncle was Joseph Priestley, the discoverer of oxygen. She met Osler in Philadelphia when she visited the United States. It is likely that she was critical of nurses. She once wrote about her experience during her husband's illness: "These were not the days of trained nurses, and throughout the long fight I only once succeeded in persuading a nurse to come for a few days, but she drank all the brandy and was useless . . . Men nurses were sent on night duty, but this was no relief to me, for I could too plainly hear them sleeping while trying to sleep myself in the adjoining room." *The Story of a Lifetime* (London: K. Paul, Trench, Trubner, 1908), pp. 125, 131.

refrained from publishing, but he has permitted me to make one extract for your delectation. "A fifth common declension[34] is into the bonds of marriage. The facility with which these modern Vestals[35] fall into this commonplace condition is a commentary, shall I not say rather an illustration, of the inconsistency so notorious in the sex. The Association of Superintendents has in hand, I believe, a Collective Investigation dealing with this question, and we shall shortly have accurate figures as to the percentage of lady superintendents, of head-nurses, of graduates and of pupils who have bartered away their heritage for a hoop of gold."[36]

I am almost ashamed to quote this rude paragraph, but I am glad to do so to be able to enter a warm protest against such sentiments. Marriage is the natural end of the trained nurse. So truly as a young man married is a young man marred,[37] is a woman unmarried, in a certain sense, a woman undone. Ideals, a career, ambition, touched though they be with the zeal of St. Theresa,[38] all vanish before "the blind bow-boy's butt shaft."[39] Are you to be blamed and scoffed at for so doing? Contrariwise, you are to be praised, with but this caution—which I insert at the special request of Miss Nutting[40]—that you abstain from philandering during your period of training, and, as much as in you lies, spare your fellow-workers, the physicians and surgeons of the staff. The trained nurse is a modern representative, not of the Roman Vestal,[41] but of the female guardian in Plato's republic[42]—a choice selection from the very best women of the community, who know the laws of health, and whose sympathies have been deepened

34. *declension:* Decline.

35. *Vestals:* Virgin priestesses of Vesta, the ancient Roman goddess of the hearth. She is represented not by a statue but by a symbolic fire, a great necessity and yet difficult to obtain in primitive times, which was kept perpetually burning by the Vestals. Osler here refers to chaste unmarried women.

36. *a hoop of gold:* An engagement ring. Osler was probably remembering Shakespeare's *The Merchant of Venice* (V, i, 146–48), when Portia teasingly asks Graziano, "A quarrel, ho, already! What's the matter?" He answers, "About a hoop of gold, a paltry ring / That she did give me," although the expression is attested at least ninety years earlier (*OED*).

37. *a young man married . . . :* William Shakespeare, *All's Well That Ends Well*, II, iii, 315. The exact quotation is: "A young man married is a man that's marred."

38. St. *Theresa*, (1515–1582): Spanish saint famous for her mystical visions; founder of the Carmelite order (1562).

39. William Shakespeare, *Romeo and Juliet*, II, iv, 16. The *blind bow-boy* means "cupid, the god of love, who was supposed to bestow it by shooting arrows into his victims," and the *butt shaft* means "a blunt arrow, used for target practice."

40. *Mary Adelaide Nutting* (1858–1948): Principal of the Johns Hopkins Hospital School of Nursing, 1894–1907. She wrote *A History of Nursing* (1907) with L. L. Dock.

41. See n. 35.

42. Plato, *Republic*, book 5, 456a–e.

by contact with the best and worst of men. The experiences of hospital and private work, while they may not make her a Martha,[43] enhance her value in many ways as a life-companion, and it is a cause, not for reproach, but for congratulation, that she has not acquired immunity from that most ancient of all diseases—that malady of which the Rose of Sharon sang so plaintively, that sickness "to be stayed not with flagons nor comforted with apples."[44]

A luxury, let us say, in her private capacity, in public the trained nurse has become one of the great blessings of humanity, taking a place beside the physician and the priest, and not inferior to either in her mission. Not that her calling here is in any way new. Time out of mind she has made one of a trinity.[45] Kindly heads have always been ready to devise means for allaying suffering; tender hearts, surcharged with the miseries of this "battered caravanserai,"[46] have ever been ready to speak to the sufferer of a way of peace, and loving hands have ever ministered to those in sorrow, need and sickness. Nursing as an art to be cultivated, as a profession to be followed, is modern; nursing as a practice originated in the dim past, when some mother among the cave-dwellers cooled the forehead of her sick child with water from the brook, or first yielded to the prompting to leave a well-covered bone and a handful of meal by the side of a wounded man left in the hurried flight before an enemy. As a profession, a vocation, nursing has already reached in this country a high development. Graduates are numerous, the directories are full, and in many places there is over-crowding, and a serious complaint that even very capable women find it hard to get employment. This will correct itself in time, as the existing conditions adjust the supply and demand.

A majority of the applicants to our schools are women who seek in nursing a vocation in which they can gain a livelihood in a womanly way; but there is another aspect of the question which may now be seriously taken up in this country. There is a gradually accumulating surplus of women who will not or who cannot fulfil the highest duties for which Nature has designed them. I do not know at what age one dare call a woman a spinster. I will put it, perhaps rashly, at twenty-five. Now, at that critical period a woman who has not to work for her living, who is without urgent domestic ties, is very apt to become a dangerous

196

NURSE AND

PATIENT

43. *Martha:* The sister of Mary and Lazarus, friend of Jesus, known for her active life compared to her contemplative sister (Luke 10:38–42).

44. Song of Solomon 2:1–5. The exact quotation is: "I *am* the rose of Sharon, *and* the lily of the valleys.... Stay me with flagons, comfort me with apples: for I *am* sick of love."

45. The physician, the priest, and the nurse.

46. This refers to this world. *Rubáiyát of Omar Khayyám,* 3rd ed. (1872), trans. Edward Fitzgerald, quatrain 17, line 1.

element unless her energies and emotions are diverted in a proper channel. One skilled in hearts can perhaps read in her face the old, old story;[47] or she calls to mind that tender verse of Sappho[48]—

> As the sweet-apple blushes on the end of the
> bough, the very end of the bough, which the
> gatherers overlooked, nay overlooked not but could
> not reach.[49]

But left alone, with splendid capacities for good, she is apt to fritter away a precious life in an aimless round of social duties, or in spasmodic efforts at Church work. Such a woman needs a vocation, a calling which will satisfy her heart, and she should be able to find it in nursing without entering a regular school or working in ecclesiastical harness.[50]

An organized nursing guild, similar to the German Deaconesses,[51] could undertake the care of large or small institutions, without the establishment of training schools in the ordinary sense of the term. Such a guild might be entirely secular, with St. James, the Apostle of practical religion,[52] as the patron. It would be of special advantage to smaller hospitals, particularly to those unattached to Medical Schools, and it would obviate the existing anomaly of scores of training schools, in which the pupils cannot get an education in any way commensurate with the importance of the profession. In the period of their training, the members of the Nursing Guild could be transferred from one institution to another until their education was complete. Such an organization would be of inestimable service in connexion with District Nursing. The noble work of Theodore Fliedner[53] should be repeated at an early day in this country. The Kaiserswerth

47. Probably Osler refers to some aging woman, such as a maiden aunt, who is disappointed in love and never leaves home but becomes a burden to the family.

48. *Sappho* (c.620–c.565 B.C.): Greek poetess and one of the two great leaders of the Aeolian school of lyric poetry.

49. Sappho, *Sappho: Memoir, Text, Selected Renderings, and a Literal Translation*, trans. Henry Thornton Wharton (London: John Lane, 1885), no. 93, p. 132. In the poem the bride is compared to the apple that has been left unpicked. Osler probably meant virginity.

50. Joining a religious order.

51. Osler refers to the modern revival of Protestant orders of deaconesses, founded in 1836 at Kaiserswerth, Germany, by Pastor Theodor Fliedner (1800–1864). He trained women for Christian service in hospitals and in social work.

52. *St. James*: Half-brother of Jesus and author of "The General Epistle of James" in the New Testament. James writes as follows: "Ye see then how that by works a man is justified, and not by faith only. . . . For as the body without the spirit is dead, so faith without works is dead also" (James 2:24–26).

53. *Theodor Fliedner* (1800–1864): German Protestant theologian and philanthropist who established institutes of deaconesses. See also p. 202, n. 51.

Deaconesses have shown the world the way. I doubt if we have progressed in secularism far enough successfully to establish such guilds apart from church organizations. The Religion of Humanity[54] is thin stuff for women, whose souls ask for something more substantial upon which to feed.

There is no higher mission in this life than nursing God's poor. In so doing a woman may not reach the ideals of her soul; she may fall far short of the ideals of her head, but she will go far to satiate those longings of the heart from which no woman can escape. Romola, the student, helping her blind father, and full of the pride of learning, we admire; Romola, the devotee, carrying in her withered heart woman's heaviest disappointment, we pity; Romola,[55] the nurse, doing noble deeds amid the pestilence, rescuing those who were ready to perish, we love.

On the stepping-stones of our dead selves we rise to higher things,[56] and in the inner life the serene heights are reached only when we die unto those selfish habits and feelings which absorb so much of our lives. To each one of us at some time, I suppose, has come the blessed impulse to break away from all such ties and follow cherished ideals. Too often it is but a flash of youth, which darkens down with the growing years. Though the dream may never be realized, the impulse will not have been wholly in vain if it enables us to look with sympathy upon the more successful efforts of others. In Institutions the corroding effect of routine can be withstood only by maintaining high ideals of work; but these become the sounding brass and tinkling cymbals[57] without corresponding sound practice. In some of us the ceaseless panorama of suffering tends to dull that fine edge of sympathy with which we started. A great corporation cannot have a very fervent charity; the very conditions of its existence limit the exercise. Against this benumbing influence, we physicians and nurses, the immediate agents of the Trust,[58] have but one enduring corrective—the practice towards patients of the Golden Rule of Humanity[59] as announced by Confucius: "What you do not

54. A philosophy advocated by Auguste Comte (1798–1857), a French philosopher. Its aim is the promotion of harmony and well-being of individuals and nations. The basis of the Comtean morality is expressed in the motto "live for others."

55. *Romola:* The heroine in *Romola* (1862–1863), a novel by George Eliot (1819–1880). Failing in marriage, left in utter despair, she later discovered her way in self-sacrifice in nursing.

56. Alfred Tennyson, "In Memoriam A.H.H.," part 1, stanza 1, lines 3–4. The exact quotation is:

> I held it truth . . .
>
> That men may rise on stepping-stones
>
> Of their dead selves to higher things.

57. 1 Corinthians 13:1. The original reads: "Though I speak with the tongues of men and of angels, and have not charity, I am become as sounding brass, or a tinkling cymbal."

58. A body of people engaged in the medical profession.

59. Confucius, *Analects,* book 5, chap. 11; book 12, chap. 2.

like when done to yourself, do not do to others,"—so familiar to us in its positive form as the great Christian counsel of perfection,[60] in which alone are embraced both the law and the prophets.

60. The Golden Rule. Matthew 7:12 and Luke 6:31. The original reads: "Therefore all things whatsoever ye would that men should do to you, do ye even so to them: for this is the law and the prophets." See "L'Envoi," p. 354, n. 15.

11

AFTER TWENTY-FIVE YEARS

For some we loved, the loveliest and the best
That from his Vintage rolling Time has prest,
    Have drunk their Cup a Round or two before,
And one by one crept silently to rest.

OMAR KHAYYAM,
The Rubáiyát of Omar Khayyám

TWENTY-FIVE YEARS after he began his teaching career at McGill University, Osler returned in 1899 to discuss the "revolution" in medical education. Emphasis on laboratory science and clinical experience had supplanted total reliance on lectures. This was a big change from when Osler had been a new teacher and had had to use his own money to buy microscopes to initiate some laboratory teaching in a cloakroom. Although the faculty had grown from seven to fifty-two, increased specialization caused a need for more facilities and equipment. Also, assistants and lighter teaching loads were needed to facilitate research. Clinical work requires medical schools to have relationships with good hospitals, to give students contact with patients.

In a revolutionary vein, Osler suggests eliminating examinations! Instead, he proposes that a student's competence should be certified by the teachers of laboratory and clinical classes. Osler emphasizes that education is a lifelong process. College is only the initial institution to instill principles and to set one on the "right path" for later self-study.

Osler advocates the "happy, contented and useful life," of a general practitioner who relishes learning and working. Outside interests should not be excluded, because success depends on personal qualities as well as medical knowledge. Noting that Browne's *Religio Medici* is a work that greatly influenced his life, he recommends literature so that "when chemistry distresses your soul, seek peace in the great pacifier, Shakespeare."

Osler then gives his favorite advice—to concentrate on today, so that thoughts of the past or future will not absorb one's energy. He reminds each student that his goal is not to become a research scientist but to "recognize and treat disease" as a practical physician. He quotes from Froude, "The knowledge which a man can use is the only real knowledge, the only knowledge which has life and growth in it and converts itself into practical power. The rest hangs like dust about the brain or dries like rain drops off the stones."

AFTER
TWENTY-FIVE YEARS

I

FROM TWO POINTS OF VIEW alone have we a wide and satisfactory view of life—one, as, amid the glorious tints of the early morn, ere the dew of youth has been brushed off,[1] we stand at the foot of the hill, eager for the journey; the other, wider, perhaps less satisfactory, as we gaze from the summit, at the lengthening shadows cast by the setting sun. From no point in the ascent have we the same broad outlook, for the steep and broken pathway affords few halting places with an unobscured view. You remember in the ascent of the Mountain of Purgatory,[2] Dante, after a difficult climb, reached a high terrace encircling the hill, and sitting down turned to the East, remarking to his conductor—"all men are delighted to look back."[3] So on this occasion, from the terrace of a quarter of a century, I am delighted to look back, and to be able to tell you of the prospect.

Twenty-five years ago this Faculty, with some hardihood, selected a young and untried man to deliver the lectures on the Institutes of Medicine.[4] With char-

An address delivered before the faculty and students of the Medical Faculty, McGill University, September 21, 1899.

1. *ere the dew of youth has been brushed off:* This is a reminiscence of Robert Browning, *Pippa Passes,* part 1, "Morning," lines 326, 339. Gottlieb says: "You will have brushed off . . . the bloom of his life . . . I say, you wipe off the very dew of his youth."

2. Purgatory is the second part of Dante's *Divine Comedy,* and a place where repentant sinners are purged of the stain of their sins. Dante Alighieri, "Purgatorio," *La Divina Commedia* (1307–1321), canto 4.

3. Ibid., line 54.

4. Osler's initial teaching position included physiology, pathology, and histology.

acteristic generosity the men who had claims on the position in virtue of service in the school, recognizing that the times were changing, stepped aside in favour of one who had had the advantage of post-graduate training in the subjects to be taught. The experiment of the Faculty, supplemented on my part by enthusiasm, constitutional energy, and a fondness for the day's work, led to a certain measure of success. I have tried to live over again in memory those happy early days, but by no possible effort can I recall much that I would fain remember. The dust of passing years has blurred the details, even in part the general outlines of the picture. The blessed faculty of forgetting is variously displayed in us. In some, as in our distinguished countryman, John Beattie Crozier, it is absent altogether, and he fills chapter after chapter with delightful reminiscences and descriptions of his experiences and mental states.[5] At corresponding periods— we are about the same age—my memory hovers like a shade about the magic circle which Ulysses[6] drew in Hades,[7] but finds no Tiresias[8] to lift the veil with which oblivion has covered the past. Shadowy as are these recollections, which,

> be they what they may
> Are yet the fountain light of all our day,
> Are yet a master light of all our seeing,[9]

they are doubly precious from their association with men who welcomed me into the Faculty, now, alas, a sadly reduced remnant. To them—to their influence, to their example, to the kindly encouragement I received at their hands— I can never be sufficiently grateful. Faithfulness in the day of small things may be said to have been the distinguishing feature of the work of the Faculty in those days. The lives of the senior members taught us youngsters the lesson

5. John Beattie *Crozier* (1849–1921): Canadian author of *The Religion of the Future* (1880) and *Civilization and Progress* (1885). He was one of Osler's classmates. His autobiography , *My Inner Life: Being a Chapter in Personal Evolution and Autobiography* (London: Longmans, Green, 1898), is filled with his personal experiences as well as public ones.

6. *Ulysses:* (Latin name for Odysseus) wisest and shrewdest of the Greek leaders in the Trojan War, immortalized in the epic poem *The Odyssey* by Homer (fl. before 700 B.C.). His ten years of postwar wandering are mainly described in books 1–4.

7. *Hades:* The underworld of the dead.

8. *Tiresias:* Greek seer and prophet who was blinded by Hera and then given special power of prophecy in compensation. He was able to advise Odysseus on how to return from Hades. Homer, *The Odyssey*, book 11.

9. William Wordsworth, "Ode: Intimations of Immortality from Recollections of Early Childhood," stanza 9, line 151. The exact quotation is:

> Those shadowy recollections,
> Which, be they what they may,
> Are yet the fountain light of all our day.

of professional responsibility, and the whole tone of the place was stimulating and refreshing. It was an education in itself, particularly in the amenities of faculty and professional life, to come under the supervision of two such Deans as Dr. George Campbell [10] and Dr. Palmer Howard.[11] How delightful it would be to see the chairs which they adorned in the school endowed in their memories and called by their names!

One recollection is not at all shadowy—the contrast in my feelings to-day only serves to sharpen the outlines. My first appearance before the class filled me with a tremulous uneasiness and an overwhelming sense of embarrassment. I had never lectured, and the only paper I had read before a society was with all the possible vaso-motor accompaniment.[12] With a nice consideration my colleagues did not add to my distress by their presence, and once inside the lecture room the friendly greeting of the boys calmed my fluttering heart, and, as so often happens, the ordeal was most severe in anticipation. One permanent impression of the session abides—the awful task of the preparation of about one hundred lectures. After the ten or twelve with which I started were exhausted I was on the treadmill for the remainder of the session. False pride forbade the reading of the excellent lectures of my predecessor, Dr. Drake,[13] which, with his wonted goodness of heart, he had offered. I reached January in an exhausted condition, but relief was at hand. One day the post brought a brand-new work on physiology by a well-known German professor, and it was remarkable with what rapidity my labours of the last half of the session were lightened. An extraordinary improvement in the lectures was noticed; the students benefited, and I gained rapidly in the facility with which I could translate from the German.

Long before the session was over I had learned to appreciate the value of the position entrusted to me, and sought the means to improve the methods of teaching. I had had the advantage of one of the first systematic courses on practical physiology given at University College, London, a good part of which consisted of lessons and demonstrations in histology.[14] In the first session, with but a single microscope, I was only able to give the stock display of the circulation of the blood, ciliary action, etc., but a fortunate appointment as physician to

10. George W. *Campbell* (1810–1882): See "Teaching and Thinking," p. 182, n. 30.

11. Robert Palmer *Howard* (1823–1889): Osler's teacher and mentor at McGill University. For further information, see "Aequanimitas," p. 28, n. 42 and "The Student Life," pp. 327–328.

12. Osler means here that his blood pressure rose and his heart beat faster with nervousness as he read his paper.

13. Joseph Morely *Drake* (1828–1887): Osler's predecessor and teacher of clinical medicine at McGill College, one of the first faculty members.

14. In 1872–1873 Osler studied physiology at University College, London, with John Burdon Sanderson. It proved to be a profitable and happy seventeen-month period in his laboratory (Cushing, vol. 1, p. 91).

the smallpox department of the General Hospital[15] carried with it a salary which enabled me to order a dozen Hartnack microscopes and a few bits of simple apparatus. This is not the only benefit I received from the old smallpox wards, which I remember with gratitude, as from them I wrote my first clinical papers.[16] During the next session I had a series of Saturday demonstrations, and gave a private course in practical histology. One grateful impression remains—the appreciation by the students of these optional and extra hours. For several years I had to work with very scanty accommodation, trespassing in the chemical laboratory in winter, and in summer using the old cloak room downstairs for the histology. In 1880 I felt very proud when the faculty converted one of the lecture rooms into a physiological laboratory and raised a fund to furnish and equip it. Meanwhile I had found time to take my bearings. From the chair of the Institutes of Medicine both physiology and pathology were taught. It has been a time-honoured custom to devote twenty lectures of the course to the latter, and as my colleagues at the Montreal General Hospital had placed the post-mortem room at my disposal I soon found that my chief interest was in the pathological part of the work. In truth, I lacked the proper technique for practical physiology. For me the apparatus never would go right, and I had not a *Diener*[17] who could prepare even the simplest experiments. Alas! there was money expended (my own usually, I am happy to say, but sometimes my friends', as I was a shocking beggar!) in apparatus that I never could set up, but over which the freshmen firmly believed that I spent sleepless nights in elaborate researches. Still one could always get the blood to circulate, cilia to wave and the fibrin to digest. I do not think that any member of the ten successive classes to which I lectured understood the structure of a lymphatic gland, or of the spleen, or of the placental circulation. To those structures I have to-day an ingrained hatred, and I am always delighted when a new research demonstrates the folly of all preceding views of their formation. Upon no subjects had I harder work to conceal my ignorance. I have learned since to be a better student, and to be ready to say to my fellow students "I do not know." Four years after my college appointment the Governors of the Montreal General Hospital elected me on the visiting staff. What better fortune could a young man desire! I left the same day for London with my dear friend, George Ross,[18] and the happy days we had together working at clinical medicine

15. the Montreal *General Hospital:* One of McGill's three clinical facilities (with University Maternity and Royal Victoria Hospital).

16. Osler reported and published three cases under the care of Dr. D. C. MacCallum, at Montreal General Hospital. The titles are "Fissure of Anus" *Canada M.J.,* 1872; "Angina Ludovici," *Canada M.J.,* 1872; and "Suppurative Nephritis," *Canada M. & S.J.,* 1872.

17. *Diener:* (German) assistant.

18. George *Ross* (1845–1892): Professor of clinical medicine and surgery at McGill, and curator of its

did much to wean me from my first love.[19] From that date I paid more and more attention to pathology and practical medicine, and added to my courses one in morbid anatomy, another in pathological histology, and a summer class in clinical medicine. I had become a pluralist of the most abandoned sort, and at the end of ten years it was difficult to say what I did profess: I felt like the man in Alcibiades II to whom are applied the words of the poet:—

> Full many a thing he knew;
> But knew them all badly.[20]

Weakened in this way, I could not resist when temptation came to pastures new in the fresh and narrower field of clinical medicine.

After ten years of hard work I left this city a rich man not in this world's goods, for such I have the misfortune—or the good fortune—lightly to esteem, but rich in the goods which neither rust nor moth have been able to corrupt,[21]— in treasures of friendship and good fellowship, and in those treasures of widened experience and a fuller knowledge of men and manners which contact with the bright minds in the profession ensures. My heart, or a good bit of it at least, has stayed with those who bestowed on me these treasures. Many a day I have felt it turn towards this city to the dear friends I left there, my college companions, my teachers, my old chums, the men with whom I lived in closest intimacy, and in parting from whom I felt the chordæ tendineæ [22] grow tense.

II

Twenty-five years ago the staff of this school consisted of the historic septenary,[23] with one demonstrator. To-day I find on the roll of the Faculty fifty-two teachers. Nothing emphasizes so sharply the character of the revolution which has gradually and silently replaced in great part for the theoretical, practical teaching, for the distant, cold lecture of the amphitheatre the elbow to elbow personal contact of the laboratory. The school, as an organization, the teacher and the student have been profoundly influenced by this change.

———

medical museum. One of Osler's very close friends who belonged to the monthly dinner club formed by a group of the younger members of the faculty at McGill, and who in 1877 sailed to Europe with Osler.

19. Osler's first professional "love" or interest (probably pathology). He seems to be saying that he became more interested in clinical medicine as opposed to pathological anatomy.

20. Plato, *Alcibiades 2*, 147c.

21. Matthew 6:20.

22. *the chordæ tendineæ:* The "heart-strings," traditionally said to constrict with emotion.

23. *septenary:* A group of seven. The reference is to the body of seven early professors of medicine: anatomy, physiology, chemistry, materia medica, practice, surgery, and obstetrics. See "The Leaven of Science," pp. 154–155.

When I joined the faculty its finances were in a condition of delightful simplicity, so simple indeed that a few years later they were intrusted to my care. The current expenses were met by the matriculation and graduation fees and the government grant, and each professor collected the fees and paid the expenses in his department. To-day the support of the laboratories absorbs a much larger sum than the entire income of the school in 1874. The greatly increased accommodation required for the practical teaching has made endowment a vital necessity. How nobly, by spontaneous gifts and in generous response to appeals, the citizens have aided the efforts of this faculty I need not remind you. Without it McGill could not have kept pace with the growing demands of modern methods. Upon one feature in the organization of a first-class school permit me to dwell for a moment or two. The specialization of to-day means a group of highly trained experts in the scientific branches, men whose entire energies are devoted to a single subject. To attain proficiency of this sort much time and money are required. More than this, these men are usually drawn from our very best students, with minds above the average. For a majority of them the life devoted to science is a sacrifice; not, of course, that it is so felt by them, since the very essence of success demands that in their work should lie their happiness. I wish that the situation could be duly appreciated by the profession at large, and by the trustees, governors and the members of the faculties throughout the country. Owing these men an enormous debt, since we reap where they have sown, and garner the fruits of their husbandry,[24] what do we give them in return? Too often beggarly salaries and an exacting routine of teaching which saps all initiative. Both in the United States and Canada the professoriate as a class, the men who live by college teaching, is wretchedly underpaid. Only a few of the medical schools have reached a financial position which has warranted the establishment of thoroughly equipped laboratories, and fewer still pay salaries in any way commensurate with the services rendered. I am fully aware that with cobwebs in the purse not what a faculty would desire has only too often to be done, but I have not referred to the matter without full knowledge, as there are schools with large incomes in which there has been of late a tendency to cut down salaries

24. *we reap where they have sown, and garner the fruits of their husbandry:* This is a reminiscence of several biblical passages, most notably Micah 6:15, "Thou shalt sow, but thou shalt not reap," and John 4:36–38, "And he that reapeth receiveth wages, and gathereth fruit unto life eternal; that both he that soweth and he that reapeth may rejoice together. And herein is that saying true, One soweth, and another reapeth. I sent you to reap that whereon ye bestowed no labour: other men laboured, and ye are entered into their labours." Osler may also have in mind the Parable of the Tares (Matthew 14:24–30, 36–43), where Jesus compares the angels who will separate the good from the wicked at the Last Judgement to reapers who separate the grain from the weeds, putting the one in their master's garner and burning up the other.

and to fill vacancies too much on Wall Street principles. And not for relief of the pocket alone would I plead. The men in charge of our Canadian laboratories are overworked in teaching. A well organized staff of assistants is very difficult to get, and still more difficult to get paid. The salary of the professor should be in many cases that of the first assistant. When the entire energy of a laboratory is expended on instruction, research, a function of equal importance, necessarily suffers. Special endowments are needed to meet the incessant and urgent calls of the scientific staff. It is gratifying to know that certain of the bequests to this school have of late been of this kind, but I can safely say that no department is as yet fully endowed. Owing to faulty conditions of preliminary education the medical school has to meet certain illegitimate expenses. No one should be permitted to register as a medical student who has not a good preliminary training in chemistry. It is an anomaly that our schools should continue to teach general chemistry, to the great detriment of the subject of medical chemistry, which alone belongs in the curriculum. Botany occupies a similar position.

But *the* laboratories of this medical school are not those directly under its management. McGill College turned out good doctors when it had no scientific laboratories, when the Montreal General Hospital and the University Maternity were its only practical departments. Ample clinical material and good methods of instruction gave the school its reputation more than fifty years ago. Great as has been the growth of the scientific half of the school, the all-important practical half has more than kept pace. The princely endowment of the Royal Victoria Hospital by our large-hearted Canadian Peers [25] has doubled the clinical facilities of this school, and by the stimulus of a healthy rivalry has put the Montreal General Hospital into a condition of splendid efficiency. Among the many changes which have occurred within the past twenty-five years, I would place these first in order of importance, since they assure the continued success of McGill as a school of practical medicine.

Equally with the school as an organization, the teacher has felt deeply the changed conditions in medical education, and many of us are much embarrassed to know what and how to teach. In a period of transition it is not easy to get *orientirt*.[26] In some subjects fortunately there is but the single difficulty—what to teach. The phenomenal strides in every branch of scientific medicine have tended to overload it with detail. To winnow the wheat from the chaff and to prepare it in an easily digested shape for the tender stomachs of first and second year

25. *Canadian Peers:* Canadians who had been ennobled. Osler is probably thinking of Lord Donald A. S. Strathcona (1820–1914) and Lord Mount Stephen (1829–1921) who both lived in Montreal and made fortunes building the Canadian Pacific Railway.

26. *orientirt* (properly *orientiert*): (German, from a Latin root) oriented; having found one's way.

students taxes the resources of the most capable teacher. The devotion to a subject, and the enthusiasm and energy which enables a man to keep abreast with its progress, are the very qualities which often lead him into pedagogic excesses. To reach a right judgment in these matters is not easy, and after all it may be said of teaching as Izaak Walton says of angling, "Men are to be born so, I mean with inclinations to it."[27] For many it is very hard to teach down to the level of beginners. The Rev. John Ward, Vicar of Stratford-on-Avon, shortly after Shakespeare's day made an uncomplimentary classification of doctors which has since become well-known:—"first, those that can talk but doe nothing; secondly, some that can doe but not talk; third, some that can both doe and talk; fourthly, some that can neither doe nor talk—and these get most monie."[28] Professors similarly may be divided into four classes. There is, first, the man who can think but who has neither tongue nor technique. Though useless for the ordinary student, he may be the leaven of a faculty[29] and the chief glory of his university. A second variety is the phonographic professor, who can talk but who can neither think nor work. Under the old régime he repeated year by year the same lecture. A third is the man who has technique but who can neither talk nor think; and a fourth is the rare professor who can do all three—think, talk and work. With these types fairly represented in a faculty, the diversities of gifts only serving to illustrate the wide spirit of the teacher, the Dean at least should feel happy.

But the problem of all others which is perplexing the teacher to-day is not so much what to teach, but how to teach it, more especially how far and in what subjects the practical shall take the place of didactic teaching. All will agree that a large proportion of the work of a medical student should be in the laboratory and in the hospital. The dispute is over the old-fashioned lecture, which has been railed against in good set terms, and which many would like to see abolished altogether. It is impossible, I think, to make a fixed rule, and teachers should be allowed a wide discretion. With the large classes of many schools the abolition of the didactic lecture would require a total reconstruction of the curriculum and indeed of the faculty. Slowly but surely practical methods are everywhere taking the place of theoretical teaching, but there will, I think, always be room in a school for the didactic lecture. It is destined within the next ten years to be much curtailed, and we shall probably, as is usual, go to extremes, but there will

27. Izaak *Walton* (1593–1683): English biographer and naturalist, whose book *The Compleat Angler* (1653) implies that one must be born with an inclination for fishing (or as Osler says, for teaching).

28. John *Ward* (1629–1681): Vicar of Stratford-upon-Avon for thirty years. The quote here is from the *Diary of the Rev. John Ward*, ed. Charles Severn (London: H. Colburn, 1839), p. 265.

29. In several lectures, Osler fondly uses the word "leaven" as a metaphor for an enlivening agent or influence. See "The Leaven of Science," p. 153.

always be men who can present a subject in a more lucid and attractive manner than it can be given in a book. Sir William Gairdner[30] once remarked that the reason why the face and voice of the teacher had so much more power than a book is that one has a more living faith in him. Years ago Murchison[31] (than whom Great Britain certainly never had a more successful teacher of medicine) limited the lecture in medicine to the consideration of rare cases, and the prominent features of a group of cases, and to questions of prognosis which cannot be discussed at the bedside. For the past four years in the subject of medicine I have been making an experiment in teaching only by a weekly examination on a set topic, by practical work in the wards, in the out-patient room and the clinical laboratory, and by a weekly consideration in the amphitheatre of the acute diseases of the season.[32] With a small class I have been satisfied with the results, but the plan would be difficult to carry out with a large body of students.

The student lives a happy life in comparison with that which fell to our lot thirty years ago. Envy, not sympathy, is my feeling towards him. Not only is the *menu*[33] more attractive, but it is more diversified and the viands are better prepared and presented. The present tendency to stuffing and cramming will be checked in part when you cease to mix the milk of general chemistry and botany with the proper dietary of the medical school. Undoubtedly the student tries to learn too much, and we teachers try to teach him too much—neither, perhaps, with great success. The existing evils result from neglect on the part of the teacher, student and examiner of the great fundamental principle laid down by Plato[34]—that education is a life-long process, in which the student can only make a beginning during his college course. The system under which we work asks too much of the student in a limited time. To cover the vast field of medicine in four years is an impossible task. We can only instil principles, put the student in the right path, give him methods, teach him how to study, and early to discern between essentials and non-essentials. Perfect happiness for student and teacher

30. William Tennant *Gairdner* (1824–1907): Scottish physician. George A. Gibson (1854–1913) wrote about him: "He extended to each of his pupils the most respectful consideration for any views which he might express, and the warmest encouragement for all of hearers to question and criticize." *Life of Sir William Tennant Gairdner* (Glasgow: James Maclehose and Sons, 1912), p. 195.

31. Charles *Murchison* (1830–1879): English physician and surgeon. Author of *A Treatise on the Continued Fevers of Great Britain (1862).*

32. In a later address Osler wrote as follows: "When I began clinical work in 1870, the Montreal General Hospital was an old coccus- and rat-ridden building, but with two valuable assets for the student—much acute disease and a group of keen teachers. Pneumonia, phthisis, sepsis and dysentery were rife." "The Medical Clinic," *British Medical Journal,* Jan. 3, 1914.

33. *menu:* The curriculum.

34. Plato, *Republic,* book 6, 498b–c; also, *Protagoras,* 325c.

will come with the abolition of examinations, which are stumbling blocks and rocks of offence[35] in the pathway of the true student. And it is not so Utopian[36] as may appear at first blush. Ask any demonstrator of anatomy ten days before the examinations, and he should be able to give you a list of the men fit to pass. Extend the personal intimate knowledge such as is possessed by a competent demonstrator of anatomy into all the other departments, and the degree could be safely conferred upon certificates of competency, which would really mean a more thorough knowledge of a man's fitness than can possibly be got by our present system of examination. I see no way of avoiding the necessary tests for the license to practise before the provincial or state boards, but these should be of practical fitness only, and not, as is now so often the case, of a man's knowledge of the entire circle of the medical sciences.

III

But what is most important in an introductory lecture remains to be spoken, for dead indeed would I be to the true spirit of this day, were I to deal only with the questions of the curriculum and say nothing to the young men who now begin the serious work of life. Personally, I have never had any sympathy with the oft-repeated sentiment expressed originally by Abernethy,[37] I believe, who, seeing a large class of medical students, exclaimed, "Good God, gentlemen! whatever will become of you?"[38] The profession into which you enter to-day guarantees to each and every one of you a happy, contented, and useful life.[39] I do not know of any other of which this can be said with greater assurance. Many of you have been influenced in your choice by the example and friendship of the doctor in your family, or some country practitioner in whom you have recognized the highest type of manhood and whose unique position in the community has filled you with a laudable ambition. You will do well to make such an one your exem-

35. Isaiah; 8:14. Romans 9:33. The actual word "stumblingblock" is found frequently in the Bible (Leviticus 19:14, etc.), and "stumblingblock," "stumblingstone," and "a stone of stumbling" are interchangeable expressions for an obstacle to one's progress or anything that causes people to offend.

36. Probably Osler was reading Sir Thomas More's *Utopia* (1516), and in the following year (1900) at Albany he began his speech with a happy quotation from Thomas More.

37. John *Abernethy* (1764–1831): English surgeon, anatomist, and physiologist. An eccentric character who is remembered for his brilliant lectures and for the operation involving ligation of the external iliac artery (1797).

38. James Paget, *Selected Essays and Addresses* (New York: Longmans, Green, 1902), chap. 4, p. 27.

39. Osler, in front of the first class of seventeen graduates of the Nurses' Training School at the Johns Hopkins Hospital (1891), predicted that "their lives will be busy, useful, and happy." See "Doctor and Nurse," p. 105.

plar, and I would urge you to start with no higher ambition than to join the noble band of general practitioners. They form the very sinews of the profession — generous-hearted men, with well-balanced, cool heads, not scientific always, but learned in the wisdom not of the laboratories but of the sick room. This school can take a greater pride in her graduates scattered throughout the length and breadth of the continent than in her present splendid equipment; they explain in great part the secret of her strength.

I was much interested the other day in reading a letter of John Locke[40] to the Earl of Peterborough[41] who had consulted him about the education of his son. Locke insisted that the main point in education is to get "a relish of knowledge." "This is putting life into a pupil."[42] Get early this relish, this clear, keen joyance in work, with which languor disappears and all shadows of annoyance flee away. But do not get too deeply absorbed to the exclusion of all outside interests. Success in life depends as much upon the man as on the physician. Mix with your fellow students, mingle with their sports and their pleasures. You may think the latter rash advice, but now-a-days even the pleasures of a medical student have become respectable, and I have no doubt that the "footing supper,"[43] which in old Coté street days[44] was a Bacchanalian orgie,[45] has become a love feast in which even the Principal and the Dean might participate. You are to be members of a polite as well as of a liberal profession and the more you see of life outside the narrow circle of your work the better equipped will you be for

40. John *Locke* (1632–1704): One of Osler's favorite philosophers. The father of English empiricism who studied medicine in France (1675–1679), he was physician, adviser, and live-in tutor for Anthony Ashley Cooper, earl of Shaftesbury.

41. the earl of *Peterborough:* Henry Mordaunt (c.1624–1697), chief adviser on English affairs to King William III (1689–1702). Locke met him in Rotterdam.

42. Osler is fond of this phrase "a relish of knowledge" and often uses it. In answer to a letter from the Earl of Peterborough, who had applied to him to recommend a tutor for his son, Locke writes: "I would have him well-bred, well-tempered; a man that having been conversant with the world and amongst men, would have great application in observing the humour and genius of my Lord your son; and omit nothing that might help to form his mind, and dispose him to virtue, knowledge, and industry. This I look upon as the great business of a tutor; *this is putting life into his pupil,* which when he has got, masters of all kinds are easily to be had; for when a young gentleman has got *a relish of knowledge,* the love and credit of doing well spurs him on; he will, with or without teachers, make great advances in whatever he has a mind to" (italics added by editor). The original is in a letter likely written in February or March of 1690. John Locke, *The Correspondence of John Locke,* ed. E. S. Debeer (Oxford: Clarendon Press, 1979), vol. 4, letter no. 1252, pp. 15–16.

43. Celebration welcoming new students, formerly a rather rowdy event, with overtones of an "initiation." The word "footing" refers to entrance to a new position.

44. The McGill school was founded on Coté street by a Scotsman, James McGill (1744–1813). The school was moved to the present university grounds in the early 1870s, when Osler spent his two years there.

45. A drunken revel, originally one in honor of Bacchus, the Greek god of wine.

the struggle. I often wish that the citizens in our large educational centres would take a little more interest in the social life of the students, many of whom catch but few glimpses of home life during their course.

As to your method of work, I have a single bit of advice, which I give with the earnest conviction of its paramount influence in any success which may have attended my efforts in life—*Take no thought for the morrow.*[46] Live neither in the past nor in the future, but let each day's work absorb your entire energies, and satisfy your widest ambition. That was a singular but very wise answer which Cromwell[47] gave to Bellevire[48]—"No one rises so high as he who knows not whither he is going,"[49] and there is much truth in it. The student who is worrying about his future, anxious over the examinations, doubting his fitness for the profession, is certain not to do so well as the man who cares for nothing but the matter in hand, and who knows not whither he is going!

While medicine is to be your vocation, or calling, see to it that you have also an avocation—some intellectual pastime which may serve to keep you in touch with the world of art, of science, or of letters. Begin at once the cultivation of some interest other than the purely professional. The difficulty is in a selection and the choice will be different according to your tastes and training. No matter what it is—but have an outside hobby. For the hard working medical student it is perhaps easiest to keep up an interest in literature. Let each subject in your year's work have a corresponding outside author. When tired of anatomy refresh your mind with Oliver Wendell Holmes;[50] after a worrying subject in physiology, turn to the great idealists, to Shelley or Keats[51] for consolation; when chemistry distresses your soul, seek peace in the great pacifier, Shakespeare;[52] and when the complications of pharmacology are unbearable, ten minutes with Montaigne[53] will lighten the burden. To the writings of one old physician I can urge your closest attention. There have been, and, happily, there are still in our

46. Matthew 6:34. Sermon on the Mount. Osler frequently quotes this passage. He recommends that we live for the present in "A Way of Life."

47. Oliver *Cromwell* (1599–1658): English general and statesman. He led the Parliamentary forces in the British Civil War (1641–1952), but afterward became Lord Protector (1653–1658) and governed as a dictator.

48. Pierre de *Bellièvre* (1611–1683): French ambassador to England. Thomas Carlyle, *Oliver Cromwell's Letters and Speeches* (New York: Wiley & Putnam, 1845), p. 278.

49. Ibid.

50. Oliver Wendell *Holmes* (1809–1894): See "Sir Thomas Browne," p. 55, n. 170.

51. Percy Bysshe *Shelley* (1792–1822) and John *Keats* (1795–1821): They were both English Romantic poets. Keats, in particular, studied medicine but never practiced. Osler quotes their poems in several places.

52. William *Shakespeare* (1564–1616): In his "Bed-side Library for Medical Students" Osler ranks Shakespeare next to the Old and New Testaments.

53. Michel Eyquem de *Montaigne* (1533–1592): See "Sir Thomas Browne," p. 57, n. 179.

ranks notable illustrations of the intimate relations between medicine and literature, but in the group of literary physicians Sir Thomas Browne [54] stands preeminent. The *Religio Medici*, one of the great English classics, should be in the hands — in the hearts too — of every medical student. As I am on the confessional to-day, I may tell you that no book has had so enduring an influence on my life. I was introduced to it by my first teacher, the Rev. W. A. Johnson, [55] Warden and Founder of the Trinity College School, and I can recall the delight with which I first read its quaint and charming pages. It was one of the strong influences which turned my thoughts towards medicine as a profession, and my most treasured copy — the second book I ever bought — has been a constant companion for thirty-one years, — comes viæ vitæque. [56] Trite but true, is the comment of Seneca — "If you are fond of books you will escape the ennui of life, you will neither sigh for evening, disgusted with the occupations of the day — nor will you live dissatisfied with yourself or unprofitable to others." [57]

And, finally, every medical student should remember that his end is not to be made a chemist or physiologist or anatomist, but to learn how to recognize and treat disease, how to become a practical physician. Twenty years ago during the summer session, I held my first class in clinical medicine at the Montreal General Hospital, and on the title page of a note book I had printed for the students I placed the following sentence, which you will find the alpha and omega [58] of practical medicine, not that it by any means covers the whole field of his education: —

"The knowledge which a man can use is the only real knowledge, the only knowledge which has life and growth in it and converts itself into practical power. The rest hangs like dust about the brain or dries like rain drops off the stones." (Froude.) [59]

54. Thomas *Browne* (1605–1682): English physician and writer. His *Religio Medici* (1643), also in "Bedside Library for Medical Students," was Osler's single favorite book, kept close at hand. Cushing writes about "his bier covered with a plain velvet pall on which lay a single sheaf of lilies and his favourite copy of the 'Religio,' *comes viæ vitæque*" (vol. 2, p. 686).

55. William Arthur *Johnson* (1816–1880): Canadian cleric, schoolmaster, geologist, and naturalist. Osler frequently refers to him in his writings; see "A Way of Life," p. 000, n. 000 and "Sir Thomas Browne," p. 000.

56. *comes viæ vitæque:* Companion for the road and life.

57. Lucius Annaeus *Seneca* (c.4 B.C.–65 A.D.): Roman statesman and philosopher. The translation reads: "If you devote yourself to studies, you will have escaped all your disgust at life." "On Tranquillity of Mind," part 3, sect. 6, *Moral Essays*, book 9, trans. John W. Basore (London: Loeb Classical Library, 1932), vol. 2, p. 225.

58. Revelation 1:8. The phrase means "beginning and end; possessing all power."

59. James Anthony *Froude*, "On Progress," in *Short Studies on Great Subjects* (London: Longmans, Green, 1886), vol. 2, p. 373.

12

BOOKS AND MEN

How easily, how secretly, how safely in books do we make
bare without shame the poverty of human ignorance! These are
the masters that instruct us without rod and ferrule, without words
of anger, without payment of money or clothing. Should ye approach
them, they are not asleep; if ye seek to question them, they do not hide
themselves; should ye err, they do not chide; and should ye show
ignorance, they know not how to laugh. O Books! ye alone are
free and liberal. Ye give to all that seek, and set free
all that serve you zealously.
RICHARD DE BURY, *Philobiblon*

Books delight us when prosperity sweetly smiles; they stay to
comfort us when cloudy fortune frowns. They lend strength to human
compacts, and without them grave judgments may not be propounded.
RICHARD DE BURY, *Philobiblon*

For Books are not absolutely dead things, but do contain a
potency of life in them to be as active as that soul was whose progeny
they are; nay, they do preserve as in a vial the purest efficacy and
extraction of that living intellect that bred them.
JOHN MILTON, *Areopagitica*

OSLER STRESSES THE IMPORTANCE of libraries in this 1901 address at the dedication of a new building for the Boston Medical Library. It can be summarized
by his words: "To study the phenomenon of disease without books is to sail an
uncharted sea, while to study books without patients is not to go to sea at all."

Libraries play a crucial role in medical teaching and research, providing a
window to work done all over the world. Osler advocates learning to read as a
"*sieve*," retaining only the best, as opposed to being a "sponge," which absorbs all
without distinguishing what is important. After one begins a general practice,

the library serves to prevent the premature "senility" that might result from the solitary life of a self-centred, self-taught physician. Those who do not read and keep intellectually keen will become uninformed, apathetic, and incompetent. Osler suggests that a young doctor can build his reputation by utilizing the fresh knowledge found in current scientific journals.

Then Osler cites several benefits of reading for pleasure: perspective, sense of historical continuity, inspiration, and improvement of character. He praises the library as a great catalyst to accelerate the progress of medicine.

BOOKS AND
MEN

BOOKS AND MEN

T HOSE OF US FROM OTHER CITIES who bring congratulations this evening can hardly escape the tinglings of envy when we see this noble
treasure house; but in my own case the bitter waters of jealousy which
rise in my soul are at once diverted by two strong sensations. In the
first place I have a feeling of lively gratitude towards this library. In 1876 as a
youngster interested in certain clinical subjects to which I could find no reference in our library at McGill, I came to Boston, and I here found what I wanted,
and I found moreover a cordial welcome and many friends. It was a small matter
I had in hand but I wished to make it as complete as possible, and I have always
felt that this library helped me to a good start. It has been such a pleasure in recurring visits to the library to find Dr. Brigham[1] in charge, with the same kindly
interest in visitors that he showed a quarter of a century ago. But the feeling
which absorbs all others is one of deep satisfaction that our friend, Dr. Chadwick,[2] has at last seen fulfilled the desire of his eyes. To few is given the tenacity
of will which enables a man to pursue a cherished purpose through a quarter of
a century—"*Ohne Hast, aber ohne Rast*"[3] ('tis his favourite quotation); to fewer

An address delivered at the opening of the new building of the Boston Medical Library, January 12, 1901.
1. Edwin Howard *Brigham* (1840–1926): Head of the Boston Medical Library for thirty-four years and
member of the Boston Library Association. Although he received his M.D. from the Harvard Medical
School he never practiced medicine, but devoted most of his life to the collection and preservation of
medical literature.
2. James Read *Chadwick* (1844–1905): Specialist in gynecology, founder of the American Gynecological
Society and a librarian of the Boston Medical Library.
3. *Ohne Hast, aber ohne Rast:* (German) "without haste, but without rest." Johann Wolfgang von Goethe,

still is the fruition granted. Too often the reaper is not the sower.[4] Too often the fate of those who labour at some object for the public good is to see their work pass into other hands, and to have others get the credit for enterprises which they have initiated and made possible. It has not been so with our friend, and it intensifies a thousandfold the pleasure of this occasion to feel the fitness, in every way, of the felicitations which have been offered to him.

It is hard for me to speak of the value of libraries in terms which would not seem exaggerated. Books have been my delight these thirty years, and from them I have received incalculable benefits. To study the phenomena of disease without books is to sail an uncharted sea, while to study books without patients is not to go to sea at all. Only a maker of books can appreciate the labours of others at their true value. Those of us who have brought forth fat volumes should offer hecatombs[5] at these shrines of Minerva Medica.[6] What exsuccous, attenuated offspring they would have been but for the pabulum furnished through the placental circulation of a library. How often can it be said of us with truth, *"Das beste was er ist verdankt er Andern!"*[7]

For the teacher and the worker a great library such as this is indispensable. They must know the world's best work and know it at once. They mint and make current coin the ore so widely scattered in journals, transactions and monographs. The splendid collections which now exist in five or six of our cities and the unique opportunities of the Surgeon-General's Library[8] have done much to give to American medicine a thoroughly eclectic character.

But when one considers the unending making of books, who does not sigh for the happy days of that thrice happy Sir William Browne[9] whose pocket library sufficed for his life's needs; drawing from a Greek testament[10] his

---

"Zahme Xenien," part 2, stanza 6, lines 2–3. According to Benham's *Book of Quotations* (1907), this was Goethe's motto.

4. *Too often the reaper is not the sower:* See "After Twenty-Five Years," p. 208, n. 24.

5. *hecatombs:* Originally in ancient Greece, sacrifices of one hundred bulls; later, sacrifices of any large number of victims, and finally, any great sacrifice or slaughter.

6. *Minerva:* (Roman myth.) goddess of wisdom, arts, and war (identified with the Greek goddess Athena). She was one of the three chief divinities, along with Jupiter and Juno.

7. *Das beste was er ist verdankt er Andern:* (German) "he owes to others what is best in him." The quote has not been identified.

8. Now the National Library of Medicine in Washington, D.C.

9. William Browne (1692–1774): English physician. Elzevir's *Horace* was his favorite book, kept close to hand. Osler's original note reads: "In one of the Annual Orations at the Royal College of Physicians he said: 'Behold an instance of human ambition! not to be satisfied but by the conquest, as it were, of three worlds, lucre in the country, honour in the college, pleasure in the medicinal springs.'"

10. The New Testament in the original Greek.

divinity, from the aphorisms of Hippocrates[11] his medicine, and from an Elzevir Horace[12] his good sense and vivacity. There should be in connection with every library a corps of instructors in the art of reading, who would, as a labour of love, teach the young idea how to read. An old writer says that there are four sorts of readers: "Sponges which attract all without distinguishing; Howre-glasses which receive and powre out as fast; Bagges which only retain the dregges of the spices and let the wine escape, and Sives which retaine the best onely."[13] A man wastes a great many years before he reaches the "sive" stage.

For the general practitioner a well-used library is one of the few correctives of the premature senility which is so apt to overtake him. Self-centred, self-taught, he leads a solitary life, and unless his every-day experience is controlled by careful reading or by the attrition of a medical society it soon ceases to be of the slightest value and becomes a mere accretion of isolated facts, without correlation. It is astonishing with how little reading a doctor can practise medicine, but it is not astonishing how badly he may do it. Not three months ago a physician living within an hour's ride of the Surgeon-General's Library brought to me his little girl, aged twelve. The diagnosis of infantile myxœdema required only a half glance. In placid contentment he had been practising twenty years in "Sleepy Hollow"[14] and not even when his own flesh and blood was touched did he rouse from an apathy deep as Rip Van Winkle's sleep.[15] In reply to questions: No, he had never seen anything in the journals about the thyroid gland; he had seen no pictures of cretinism or myxœdema; in fact his mind was a blank on the whole subject. He had not been a reader, he said, but he was a practical man with very little time. I could not help thinking of John Bunyan's remarks on the elements of success in the practice of medicine. "Physicians," he says, "get neither name nor fame by the pricking of wheals or the picking out thistles, or by laying of plaisters to the scratch of a pin; every old woman can do this. But if they would have a name and a fame, if they will have it quickly, they must do some great and desperate cures. Let them fetch

11. The best-known work of the Hippocrates' empirical method and his high ethical standard. Browne often quotes Hippocrates in his writings.

12. Louis *Elzevir* (also *Elzevier*) (c.1546–1617) and his sons and grandson: Famous Dutch booksellers and publishers who issued beautiful editions of classical authors from 1581 to 1712.

   Horace (in full, Quintus Horatius Flaccus) (65–68 B.C.): Latin lyric poet and satirist. Osler refers to works of Horace printed by the Elzeviers.

13. John Donne, *Biathanatos* (1646 and 1648), preface.

14. Washington Irving, *The Sketch Book of Geoffrey Crayon, Gent.* (1819–1820). The volume includes "The Legend of Sleepy Hollow" and "Rip Van Winkle."

15. Rip Van Winkle is a ne'er-do-well who falls asleep and awakens after twenty years to find his wife dead, his house in ruins, and everything changed.

one to life that was dead, let them recover one to his wits that was mad, let them make one that was born blind to see, or let them give ripe wits to a fool—these are notable cures, and he that can do thus, if he dost thus first, he shall have the name and fame he deserves; he may lie abed till noon."[16] Had my doctor friend been a reader he might have done a great and notable cure and even have given ripe wits to a fool! It is in utilizing the fresh knowledge of the journals that the young physician may attain quickly to the name and fame he desires.

There is a third class of men in the profession to whom books are dearer than to teachers or practitioners—a small, a silent band, but in reality the leaven of the whole lump. The profane call them bibliomaniacs, and in truth they are at times irresponsible and do not always know the difference between *meum* and *tuum*.[17] In the presence of Dr. Billings[18] or of Dr. Chadwick[19] I dare not further characterize them. Loving books partly for their contents, partly for the sake of the authors, they not alone keep alive the sentiment of historical continuity in the profession, but they are the men who make possible such gatherings as the one we are enjoying this evening. We need more men of their class, particularly in this country, where every one carries in his pocket the tape-measure of utility. Along two lines their work is valuable. By the historical method alone can many problems in medicine be approached profitably. For example, the student who dates his knowledge of tuberculosis from Koch[20] may have a very correct, but he has a very incomplete, appreciation of the subject. Within a quarter of a century our libraries will have certain alcoves devoted to the historical consideration of the great diseases, which will give to the student that mental perspective which is so valuable an equipment in life. The past is a good nurse, as Lowell remarks,[21] particularly for the weanlings of the fold.

16. John Bunyan, *The Jerusalem Sinner Saved; or Good News for the Vilest of Men*, *The Complete Works of John Bunyan*, ed. Henry Stebbing (1688; New York: Johnson Reprint Corp, 1970), vol. 2, p. 462.

17. *meum and tuum:* (Latin) "mine and thine." Osler is referring to people's bad habit of not returning borrowed books.

18. John Shaw *Billings* (1838–1913): American physician and librarian who fostered the growth of the Surgeon General's Library (the National Library of Medicine) in Washington, D.C., and the Public Library in New York. With Dr. Robert Fletcher he prepared *Index Medicus* (1879–1895), a monthly guide to current medical literature. He designed the Johns Hopkins Hospital and served as its medical advisor.

19. Dr. *Chadwick:* See p. 219, n. 2.

20. Robert *Koch* (1843–1910): German physician and pioneering bacteriologist. He isolated the tubercle bacillus (1882) and produced tuberculin, of value in diagnosing tuberculosis (1890).

21. James Russell Lowell, *The Biglow Papers*, "The Debate in the Sennit: Sot to a Nusry Rhyme," preface to no. 5. The full quotation is: "The Past is a good nurse, but we must be weaned from her sooner or later, even though, like Plotinus, we should run home from school to ask the breast, after we are tolerably well-grown youths."

'Tis man's worst deed
To let the things that have been, run to waste
And in the unmeaning Present sink the Past.[22]

But in a more excellent way these *laudatores temporis acti*[23] render a royal service. For each one of us to-day, as in Plato's time, there is a higher as well as a lower education.[24] The very marrow and fitness of books may not suffice to save a man from becoming a poor, mean-spirited devil, without a spark of fine professional feeling, and without a thought above the sordid issues of the day. The men I speak of keep alive in us an interest in the great men of the past and not alone in their works, which they cherish, but in their lives, which they emulate. They would remind us continually that in the records of no other profession is there to be found so large a number of men who have combined intellectual pre-eminence with nobility of character. This higher education so much needed to-day is not given in the school, is not to be bought in the market place, but it has to be wrought out in each one of us for himself; it is the silent influence of character on character and in no way more potent than in the contemplation of the lives of the great and good of the past, in no way more than in "the touch divine of noble natures gone."[25]

I should like to see in each library a select company of the Immortals set apart for special adoration. Each country might have its representatives in a sort of alcove of Fame, in which the great medical classics were gathered. Not necessarily books, more often the epoch-making contributions to be found in ephemeral journals. It is too early, perhaps, to make a selection of American medical classics, but it might be worth while to gather suffrages in regard to the contributions which ought to be placed upon our Roll of Honour.[26] A few years ago I made out a list of those I thought the most worthy which I carried down to 1850, and it has a certain interest for us this evening. The native modesty of the Boston physician is well known, but in certain circles there has been associated with it a curious psychical phenomenon, a conviction of the utter worthlessness of the *status præsens*[27] in New England, as compared with conditions existing elsewhere. There is a variety to-day of the Back Bay Brahmin[28] who delights in

22. Charles Lamb, "Sonnet," 9.

23. *laudatores temporis acti:* (Latin) "those who praise time past." Horace, *Ars Poetica* (13–8 B.C.), line 173.

24. Plato, *Republic,* book 7, 537 foll.

25. James Russell Lowell, "Memoriæ Positum," part 1, stanza 2, lines 9–10.

26. List of the most praiseworthy things in life (books, people, etc.).

27. *status præens:* "The present state of affairs," used medically

28. A person of great cultural pretensions living in the Back Bay, a fashionable residential district of Boston (named after the adjacent part of the Charles River estuary) then occupied by the city's most established families.

cherishing the belief that medically things are everywhere better than in Boston, and who is always ready to predict "an Asiatic removal of candlesticks,"[29] to borrow a phrase from Cotton Mather. Strange indeed would it have been had not such a plastic profession as ours felt the influences which moulded New England into the intellectual centre of the New World. In reality, nowhere in the country has the profession been adorned more plentifully with men of culture and of character—not voluminous writers or exploiters of the products of other men's brains—and they manage to get a full share on the Roll of Fame which I have suggested. To 1850, I have counted some twenty contributions of the first rank, contributions which for one reason or another deserve to be called American medical classics. New England takes ten. But in medicine the men she has given to the other parts of the country have been better than books. Men like Nathan R. Smith, Austin Flint, Willard Parker, Alonzo Clark, Elisha Bartlett, John C. Dalton, and others[30] carried away from their New England homes a

29. *an Asiatic removal of candlesticks:* Cotton Mather, "General Introduction," *Magnalia Christi Americana* (New York: Russell & Russell, 1967), sect. 3, p. 27. The exact quotation is: "And, let us humbly speak it, it shall be profitable for you to consider the *light* which, from the midst of this 'outer darkness,' is now to be darted over unto the other side of the Atlantick Ocean. But we must therewithal ask your Prayers, that these 'golden Candlesticks' may not quickly be 'removed out of their place!' " Mather is remembering Revelation 2:5. Osler uses "Asiatic" because the seven churches addressed in Revelation chaps. 1 & 2 were in Asia. But he seems to be misremembering Mather's "Atlantick."

30. Nathan Ryno *Smith* (1797–1877): American surgeon and teacher of anatomy and surgery. He was a member of the first faculty of Jefferson Medical College in Philadelphia, one of his pupils being Osler's friend, Dr. Samuel D. Gross. He later taught at the University of Maryland, and he was also the founder of Dartmouth and Yale College medical schools. His invention, the anterior splint, was his chief contribution to surgery.

Austin *Flint* (1812–1886): American physician. He was one of the founders of Buffalo Medical College (1847) and was a professor at the University of Louisville, New Orleans Medical College, and Long Island College Hospital. In 1861 he founded Bellevue Hospital Medical College and taught there until his death. Because of his openness to innovative ideas, he advocated the bacterial theory of disease.

Willard *Parker* (1800–1884): American surgeon known for the first successful operation on an abscessed appendix in 1867. Professor at the College of Physicians and Surgeons, New York.

Alonzo *Clark* (1807–1887): American professor of pathology at the College of Physicians and Surgeons, New York. He studied in London and Paris and returned to New York with a keen interest in pathology and use of the microscope. He was esteemed for his skill as a diagnostician. His contributions to medicine include auscultatory percussion, his management of typhus fever, and his treatment of peritonitis with opium. He also contributed to the development of American medical education.

Elisha *Bartlett* (1804–1855): American physician and educator. Professor of anatomy at Berkshire Medical Institution, Mass.; Transylvania University, Lexington, Ky.; the University of Maryland, Baltimore.; the University of Louisville, Ky.; New York University; and the College of Physicians and Surgeons, New York. Osler wrote a brief biography of Bartlett, "Elisha Bartlett, a Rhode Island Philosopher" (1900).

John Call *Dalton* (1825–1889): American physiologist. Professor and president of the College of Physicians and Surgeons, 1884–1889. He had previously taught at the University of Buffalo and the Univer-

love of truth, a love of learning and above all a proper estimate of the personal character of the physician.

Dr. Johnson [31] shrewdly remarked that ambition was usually proportionate to capacity,[32] which is as true of a profession as it is of a man. What we have seen to-night reflects credit not less on your ambition than on your capacity. A library after all is a great catalyser, accelerating the nutrition and rate of progress in a profession, and I am sure you will find yourselves the better for the sacrifice you have made in securing this home for your books, this workshop for your members.

————

sity of Vermont. His "Treatise on Human Physiology" (1st edition 1859; 7th edition 1882) was used as a standard medical textbook in American medical schools.

31. Samuel *Johnson* (1709–1784): See "A Way of Life," p. 5, n. 14.

32. *ambition was usually proportionate to capacity:* "Boerhaave," in *The Works of Samuel Johnson* (London: J. Nichols and Son, 1810), vol. 12, p. 17.

13

CHAUVINISM IN MEDICINE

I feel not in myself those common antipathies that I can discover
in others: those national repugnances do not touch me, nor do I behold
with prejudice the French, Italian, Spaniard, or Dutch: but where I find their
actions in balance with my countrymen's, I honour, love, and embrace them in
the same degree. I was born in the eighth climate, but seem for to be framed
and constellated unto all: I am no plant that will not prosper out of a
garden; all places, all airs, make unto me one country; I am in
England, everywhere, and under any meridian.

SIR THOMAS BROWNE, *Religio Medici*

All's not offence that indiscretion finds
And dotage terms so.

WILLIAM SHAKESPEARE, *King Lear*

Still in thy right hand carry gentle peace,
To silence envious tongues.

WILLIAM SHAKESPEARE, *King Henry VIII*

IN THIS ADDRESS IN 1902 to the Canadian Medical Association, Osler laments
that even the medical profession, for all its accomplishments, is not free of the
failings of smugness, various forms of provincialism, and chauvinism. These are
all unworthy of the noble beginnings of medicine. The ancient Greek physicians
of the Hippocratic school fought superstition and based their work on skepticism and careful observation as well as high moral ideals. Medicine was viewed
as the profession for cultivated gentlemen. No other field has had such an unbroken continuity of methods and ideals and such a remarkable worldwide solidarity. Medicine is progressive because of its scientific basis and its eagerness
for improvements. Recent advances such as anaesthesia, sanitation, and aseptic
conditions for surgery significantly contribute toward solving the problems of
human suffering.

At the start of the twentieth century, these advances, along with better training and equipment, give medicine a bright outlook. However, growth also causes some problems for the medical profession. Osler lists these problems as extremes of nationalism, provincialism, sectionalism, and—on a more personal level—parochialism.

Osler happily notes a lessening of the problems caused by nationalism, thanks to the growth of international medical groups, studies abroad, and increasing acceptance of scientific literature from other countries. Unfortunately, no decrease is seen in provincialism. Licensing boards, in effect, penalize those who wish to practice in a certain state or province but who were trained elsewhere. Osler argues that more uniform training has made such a rigid system of licensing unnecessary. He says that such boards are often not up-to-date and should, at most, only administer practical examinations, because they cannot accurately assess scientific competence.

Parochialism, as distinguished from "proper" pride in one's university, is especially dangerous when it degenerates into intolerance, especially in basing faculty appointments on criteria other than merit. Although proponents of the scientific areas of medicine have become more aware of the harm of "inbreeding" in faculty, they retain the problem of, distrust of results of research done elsewhere.

Chauvinism causes general practitioners to neglect the continuing training needed to keep up in their field. This neglect also sacrifices mental independence and leads to self-deception as well as to susceptibility to drug advertisers. The greatest ignorance is thinking that one knows when one does not. A particularly virulent form of chauvinism is not getting aid for a difficult diagnosis. Osler admonishes physicians to rely more on diagnosis and less on drugs, especially pharmaceutical fads. He urges the mentoring of younger doctors by their elders, who then benefit from their students' newer knowledge while sharing their own long experience.

To avoid narrowness, a physician needs the "culture" given by a liberal education as well as medical learning. Osler advises his audience to ignore both gossip and overblown praise, to be charitable to fellow practitioners, and to actively pursue good relations, especially with potential rivals. In his conclusion, he stresses that there is little room in medicine for chauvinism. He urges open minds, receptiveness to new ideas, and cultivation of friendly relationships with others.

CHAUVINISM IN MEDICINE

A RARE AND PRECIOUS GIFT is the Art of Detachment,[1] by which a man may so separate himself from a life-long environment as to take a panoramic view of the conditions under which he has lived and moved: it frees him from Plato's den[2] long enough to see the realities as they are, the shadows as they appear. Could a physician attain to such an art he would find in the state of his profession a theme calling as well for the exercise of the highest faculties of description and imagination as for the deepest philosophic insight. With wisdom of the den only and of my fellow-prisoners, such a task is beyond my ambition and my powers, but to emphasize duly the subject that I wish to bring home to your hearts I must first refer to certain distinctive features of our profession.

I. Four Great Features of the Guild

Its noble ancestry. — Like everything else that is good and durable in this world, modern medicine is a product of the Greek intellect, and had its origin when that

An address delivered at the Canadian Medical Association, Montreal, September 17, 1902. Regarding *chauvinism*, Osler's original note reads: "Definition: a narrow, illiberal spirit in matters national, provincial, collegiate or personal." This word is often used to express exaggerated patriotism of an aggressive type, jingoism, etc. This French word was originally derived from Nicolas Chauvin (fl. 1790–1810), a soldier of the French Republic and of the 1st Empire who was a passionate admirer of Napoleon. The word "chauvinism" was coined to signify a feeling of exaggerated devotion, especially of patriotism.

1. Osler previously advised medical students to cultivate this art. See "Teacher and Student," p. 118.

2. Osler is recalling *Republic*, book 7, 514–515c, where Plato compares those who see only images of the truth to prisoners in a cave who can see only the shadows cast on its walls, not the realities of the outer world.

wonderful people created positive or rational science, and no small credit is due to the physicians who, as Professor Gomperz[3] remarks (in his brilliant chapter "On the Age of Enlightenment," *Greek Thinkers*, vol. 1), very early brought to bear the spirit of criticism on the arbitrary and superstitious views of the phenomena of life. If science was ever to acquire "steady and accurate habits instead of losing itself in a maze of phantasies, it must be by quiet methodical research."[4] "It is the undying glory of the school of Cos[5] that it introduced this innovation into the domain of its Art, and thus exercised the most beneficial influence on the whole intellectual life of mankind. Fiction to the right! Reality to the left! was the battle cry of this school in the war it was the first to wage against the excesses and defects of the nature philosophy" (Gomperz).[6] The critical sense and sceptical attitude of the Hippocratic school laid the foundations of modern medicine on broad lines, and we owe to it: *first,* the emancipation of medicine from the shackles of priestcraft and of caste; *secondly,* the conception of medicine as an art based on accurate observation, and as a science, an integral part of the science of man and of nature; *thirdly,* the high moral ideals, expressed in that most "memorable of human documents" (Gomperz), the Hippocratic oath;[7] and *fourthly,* the conception and realization of medicine as the profession of a cultivated gentleman.[8] No other profession can boast of the same unbroken continuity of methods and of ideals. We may indeed be justly proud of our apostolic succession. Schools and systems have flourished and gone, schools which have swayed for generations the thought of our guild, and systems that have died before their founders; the philosophies of one age have become the absurdities of the next, and the foolishness of yesterday has become the wisdom of to-morrow; through long ages which were slowly learning what we are hurrying to forget— amid all the changes and chances of twenty-five centuries, the profession has never lacked men who have lived up to these Greek ideals. They were those of

3. Theodor *Gomperz* (1832–1912): German philosopher and classical scholar. Author of *Greek Thinkers: A History of Ancient Philosophy* (London: John Murray, 1901–1912).

4. Theodor *Gomperz*, "On the Age of Enlightenment," in *Greek Thinkers*, vol. 1, book 3, chap. 1, sect. 5, p. 296.

5. The medical school of Hippocrates.

6. Theodor Gomperz, *Greek Thinkers*.

7. *"memorable of human documents"* (the Hippocratic oath): Theodor Gomperz, *Greek Thinkers*, sect. 2, p. 281. The exact quotation is: "This oath brings the memorable document to a close, with repeated solemn adjurations to the gods."

8. Osler's original note reads: "Nowhere in literature do we have such a charming picture illustrating the position of a cultivated physician in society as that given in Plato's *Dialogues* of Eryximachus, himself the son of a physician, Acumenus. In that most brilliant age the physician was the companion and friend, and in intellectual intercourse the peer of its choicest spirits."

Galen[9] and of Aretæus,[10] of the men of the Alexandrian and Byzantine schools, of the best of the Arabians, of the men of the Renaissance, and they are ours to-day.

A second distinctive feature is the *remarkable solidarity*. Of no other profession is the word universal applicable in the same sense. The celebrated phrase used of the Catholic Church is in truth much more appropriate when applied to medicine. It is not the prevalence of disease or the existence everywhere of special groups of men to treat it that betokens this solidarity, but it is the identity throughout the civilized world of our ambitions, our methods and our work. To wrest from nature the secrets which have perplexed philosophers in all ages, to track to their sources the causes of disease, to correlate the vast stores of knowledge, that they may be quickly available for the prevention and cure of disease—these are our ambitions. To carefully observe the phenomena of life in all its phases, normal and perverted, to make perfect that most difficult of all arts, the art of observation, to call to aid the science of experimentation, to cultivate the reasoning faculty, so as to be able to know the true from the false—these are our methods. To prevent disease, to relieve suffering and to heal the sick—this is our work. The profession in truth is a sort of guild or brotherhood, any member of which can take up his calling in any part of the world and find brethren whose language and methods and whose aims and ways are identical with his own.

Thirdly, *its progressive character.*—Based on science, medicine has followed and partaken of its fortunes, so that in the great awakening which has made the nineteenth memorable among centuries, the profession received a quickening impulse more powerful than at any period in its history. With the sole exception of the mechanical sciences, no other department of human knowledge has undergone so profound a change—a change so profound that we who have grown up in it have but slight appreciation of its momentous character. And not only in what has been actually accomplished in unravelling the causes of disease, in perfecting methods of prevention, and in wholesale relief of suffering, but also in the unloading of old formulæ and in the substitution of the scientific spirit of free inquiry for cast-iron dogmas we see a promise of still greater achievement and of a more glorious future.

And lastly, the profession of medicine is distinguished from all others by

9. Claudius *Galen* (c.130–c.200): See "Teaching and Thinking," p. 181, n. 27.

10. *Aretæus* of Cappadocia (c.1st to 2nd cent. A.D.): Greek physician who followed the Hippocratic tradition of bedside observation. His works were long lost, but two of his manuscripts were rediscovered in 1554: *On the Causes and Indications of Acute and Chronic Diseases* and *On the Treatment of Acute and Chronic Diseases*. These included a wealth of accurate and valuable information of his descriptions of diseases and their cures including those of diabetes, epilepsy, etc.

its *singular beneficence.* It alone does the work of charity in a Jovian [11] and God-like way, dispensing with free hand truly Promethean gifts. There are those who listen to me who have seen three of the most benign endowments granted to the race since the great Titan stole fire from the heavens.[12] Search the scriptures of human achievement and you cannot find any to equal in beneficence the introduction of Anæsthesia, Sanitation, with all that it includes, and Asepsis— a short half-century's contribution towards the practical solution of the problems of human suffering, regarded as eternal and insoluble. We form almost a monopoly or trust in this business. Nobody else comes into active competition with us, certainly not the other learned professions which continue along the old lines. Every few years sees some new conquest, so that we have ceased to wonder. The work of half a dozen men, headed by Laveran,[13] has made waste places of the earth habitable and the wilderness to blossom as the rose. The work of Walter Reed [14] and his associates will probably make yellow fever as scarce in the Spanish Main as is typhus fever with us. There seems to be no limit to the possibilities of scientific medicine, and while philanthropists are turning to it as to the hope of humanity, philosophers see, as in some far-off vision, a science from which may come in the prophetic words of the Son of Sirach, "Peace over all the earth." [15]

Never has the outlook for the profession been brighter. Everywhere the physician is better trained and better equipped than he was twenty-five years ago. Disease is understood more thoroughly, studied more carefully and treated more skilfully. The average sum of human suffering has been reduced in a way to make the angels rejoice. Diseases familiar to our fathers and grandfathers have disappeared, the death rate from others is falling to the vanishing point, and public health measures have lessened the sorrows and brightened the lives of millions. The vagaries and whims, lay and medical, may neither have diminished in number nor lessened in their capacity to distress the faint-hearted who do not appreciate that to the end of time people must imagine vain things, but they are dwarfed by comparison with the colossal advance of the past fifty years.

11. "Jovian" is derived from "Jove," which is an alternative name for Jupiter. It means "cheerfully bountiful," as Jove was supposed to be.

12. (Greek myth.) Prometheus, who is fabled to have stolen fire for men from Olympus and to have taught them various arts.

13. Charles Alphonse *Laveran* (1845–1922): French physician who discovered in 1880 that the causative factor of malaria was a plasmodium. This brought him the Nobel Prize in physiology and medicine in 1907.

14. Walter *Reed* (1851–1902): American military surgeon and bacteriologist who proved that the causative agent of yellow fever was a filterable virus carried by mosquitoes.

15. Ecclesiasticus 38:8. *Ecclesiasticus* (or "Sirach") is one of the *Apocrypha,* the fourteen biblical books not universally accepted as canonical.

So vast, however, and composite has the profession become, that the physiological separation, in which dependent parts are fitly joined together, tends to become pathological, and while some parts suffer necrosis and degeneration, others, passing the normal limits, become disfiguring and dangerous outgrowths on the body medical. The dangers and evils which threaten harmony among the units, are internal, not external. And yet, in it more than in any other profession, owing to the circumstances of which I have spoken, is complete organic unity possible. Of the many hindrances in the way time would fail me to speak, but there is one aspect of the question to which I would direct your attention in the hope that I may speak a word in season.

Perhaps no sin so easily besets us as a sense of self-satisfied superiority to others. It cannot always be called pride, that master sin, but more often it is an attitude of mind which either leads to bigotry and prejudice or to such a vaunting conceit in the truth of one's own beliefs and positions, that there is no room for tolerance of ways and thoughts which are not as ours are. To avoid some smirch of this vice is beyond human power; we are all dipped in it, some lightly, others deeply grained. Partaking of the nature of uncharitableness, it has not the intensity of envy, hatred and malice,[16] but it shades off in fine degrees from them. It may be a perfectly harmless, even an amusing trait in both nations and individuals, and so well was it depicted by Charlet,[17] Horace Vernet,[18] and others, under the character of an enthusiastic recruit named Chauvin,[19] that the name Chauvinism has become a by-word, expressing a bigoted, intolerant spirit. The significance of the word has been widened, and it may be used as a synonym for a certain type of nationalism, for a narrow provincialism, or for a petty parochialism. It does not express the blatant loudness of Jingoism,[20] which is of the

16. *uncharitableness, it has not the intensity of envy, hatred and malice:* This is an echo of the Litany in the *Book of Common Prayer:* "From envy, hatred, and malice, and all uncharitableness, Good Lord deliver us."

17. Nicolas Toussaint *Charlet* (1762–1845): French painter and engraver. His sketches of children and military incidents were very popular.

18. Jean-Emile-Horace *Vernet* (1789–1863): French historical painter who depicted battles in the wars of the Revolution and the Empire.

19. Nicolas *Chauvin* (fl. 1790–1810): French soldier whose fanatical patriotism and devotion to Napoleon led to the coining of the word "chauvinism." See p. 000, n. 000.

20. *Jingoism:* Blatant patriotism, especially practices of people who brag of their country's preparedness for war. "Jingoism" derives from a popular song of the time of the Russo-Turkish War (1877–1878), beginning

> We don't want to fight, but, by jingo, if we do,
>
> We've got the ships, we've got the men, we've got the money too,

by one G. W. Hunt, who is otherwise obscure. "By jingo" is said to have originally been gibberish used by stage conjurers—an appeal to a fictitious spirit.

tongue, while Chauvinism is a condition of the mind, an aspect of character much more subtle and dangerous. The one is more apt to be found in the educated classes, while the other is pandemic in the fool multitude—"that numerous piece of monstrosity which, taken asunder, seem men and reasonable creatures of God, but confused together, make but one great beast, and a monstrosity more prodigious than Hydra"[21] (*Religio Medici*).[22] Wherever found, and in whatever form, Chauvinism is a great enemy of progress and of peace and concord among the units. I have not the time, nor if I had, have I the ability to portray this failing in all its varieties; I can but touch upon some of its aspects, national, provincial and parochial.

II. Nationalism in Medicine

Nationalism has been the great curse of humanity. In no other shape has the Demon of Ignorance[23] assumed more hideous proportions; to no other obsession do we yield ourselves more readily. For whom do the hosannas[24] ring higher than for the successful butcher of tens of thousands of poor fellows who have been made to pass through the fire to this Moloch[25] of nationalism? A vice of the blood,[26] of the plasm rather, it runs riot in the race, and rages to-day as of yore in spite of the precepts of religion and the practice of democracy. Nor is there any hope of change; the pulpit is dumb, the press fans the flames, literature panders to it and the people love to have it so. Not that all aspects of nationalism are bad. Breathes there a man with soul so dead[27] that it does not glow at the thought

21. *Hydra:* (Greek myth.) a monstrous serpent with nine heads. When Hercules fought it, two heads grew back for every one he cut off, but eventually he killed it. It came to represent a blind force or ignorant opinion that is hard to root out or destroy.

22. Thomas Browne, *Religio Medici*, part 2, sect. 1.

23. *the Demon of Ignorance:* Osler is here comparing chauvinism to the Demon of Ignorance, the personification of ignorance.

24. *hosannas:* Osler is likely to have been thinking of Jesus' triumphant entry into Jerusalem riding on a donkey, when the crowds cried, "Hosanna!" (Mark 12:9, etc). The chorus of a very well known hymn for Palm Sunday, is

> All glory, laud and honour
> To thee, Redeemer King,
> To whom the lips of children
> Made sweet hosannas ring.

(trans. John Mason Neale from the Latin of St. Theodulph of Orleans).

25. *Moloch:* A deity worshipped by the Israelites who demanded the sacrifice of children.

26. Alfred Tennyson, "In Memoriam A.H.H.," part 3, stanza 4, line 3.

27. Walter Scott, "The Lay of the Last Minstrel," canto 6, stanza 1, line 1. The exact quotation is:

> Breathes there the man, with soul so dead,

of what the men of his blood have done and suffered to make his country what it is? There is room, plenty of room, for proper pride of land and birth. What I inveigh against is a cursed spirit of intolerance, conceived in distrust and bred in ignorance,[28] that makes the mental attitude perennially antagonistic, even bitterly antagonistic to everything foreign, that subordinates everywhere the race to the nation, forgetting the higher claims of human brotherhood.

While medicine is everywhere tinctured with national characteristics, the wider aspects of the profession, to which I have alluded—our common lineage and the community of interests—should always save us from the more vicious aspects of this sin, if it cannot prevent it altogether. And yet I cannot say, as I wish I could, that we are wholly free from this form of Chauvinism. Can we say, as English, French, German or American physicians, that our culture is always cosmopolitan, not national, that our attitude of mind is always as frankly open and friendly to the French as to the English, to the American as to the German, and that we are free at all times and in all places from prejudice, at all times free from a self-satisfied feeling of superiority the one over the other? There has been of late years a closer union of the profession of the different countries through the International Congress and through the international meetings of the special societies; but this is not enough, and the hostile attitude has by no means disappeared. Ignorance is at the root. When a man talks slightingly of the position and work of his profession in any country, or when a teacher tells you that he fails to find inspiration in the work of his foreign colleagues, in the words of the Arabian proverb—he is a fool, shun him![29] Full knowledge, which alone disperses the mists of ignorance, can only be obtained by travel or by a thorough acquaintance with the literature of the different countries. Personal, first-hand intercourse with men of different lands, when the mind is young and plastic, is the best vaccination against the disease. The man who has sat at the feet of Virchow,[30] or has listened to Traube, or Helmholtz, or Cohnheim,[31] can never look with unfriendly eyes at German medicine or German methods. Who ever

235

CHAUVINISM

IN MEDICINE

Who never to himself hath said,

This is my own, my native land?

28. *conceived in distrust and bred in ignorance:* This may be an echo of Psalm 51:5: "Behold, I was shapen in iniquity; and in sin did my mother conceive me."

29. Arabic proverb. "He who knows not and knows not that he knows not, is a fool. Shun him."

30. Rudolf *Virchow* (1821–1902): See "The Old Humanities and the New Science," p. 75, n. 80.

31. Ludwig *Traube* (1818–1876): See "The Old Humanities and the New Science," p. 75, n. 80.

Hermann Ludwig Ferdinand von *Helmholtz* (1821–1894): See "The Old Humanities and the New Science," p. 75, n. 80.

Julius Friedrich *Cohnheim* (1839–1884): German pathologist. His experiments with the induction of tuberculosis into a rabbit's eye helped lead Koch to the discovery of the tuberculosis baccillus.

met with an English or American pupil of Louis or of Charcot,[32] who did not love French medicine, if not for its own sake, at least for the reverence he bore his great master? Let our young men, particularly those who aspire to teaching positions, go abroad. They can find at home laboratories and hospitals as well equipped as any in the world, but they may find abroad more than they knew they sought—widened sympathies, heightened ideals and something perhaps of a *Welt-cultur*[33] which will remain through life as the best protection against the vice of nationalism.

Next to a personal knowledge of men, a knowledge of the literature of the profession of different countries will do much to counteract intolerance and Chauvinism. The great works in the department of medicine in which a man is interested, are not so many that he cannot know their contents, though they be in three or four languages. Think of the impetus French medicine gave to the profession in the first half of the last century, of the debt we all owe to German science in the latter half, and of the lesson of the practical application by the English of sanitation and asepsis! It is one of our chief glories and one of the unique features of the profession that, no matter where the work is done in the world, if of any value, it is quickly utilized. Nothing has contributed more to the denationalization of the profession of this continent than, on the one hand, the ready reception of the good men from the old countries who have cast in their lot with us, and, on the other, the influence of our young men who have returned from Europe with sympathies as wide as the profession itself. There is abroad among us a proper spirit of eclecticism, a willingness to take the good wherever found, that augurs well for the future. It helps a man immensely to be a bit of a hero-worshipper, and the stories of the lives of the masters of medicine do much to stimulate our ambition and rouse our sympathies. If the life and work of such men as Bichat and Laënnec[34] will not stir the blood of a young man and make him feel proud of France and of Frenchmen, he must be a dull and muddy mettled rascal.[35] In reading the life of Hunter, of Jenner,[36] who thinks

32. Pierre Charles Alexandre *Louis* (1787–1872): French physician who introduced the statistical method for the clinical investigation of disease.

Jean Martin *Charcot* (1825–1893): French physician who specialized in the treatment of mental and nervous disorders, and who used the techniques of hypnosis and mental suggestion. One of his students, Sigmund Freud (1856–1939), further developed his technique to treat patients with such disorders.

33. *Welt-cultur* (now Weltkultur): (German) world culture; that is, a culture that crosses national boundaries. Johann Wolfgang von Goethe, *Unterhaltungen mit Müller*, August 23, 1827.

34. Marie François Xavier *Bichat* (1771–1802): French physician and pioneer in scientific histology and pathological anatomy.

Théophile René Hyacinthe *Laënnec* (1781–1826): French physician who invented the stethoscope. His specialty was diseases of the chest.

35. *a dull and muddy mettled rascal:* William Shakespeare, *Hamlet*, II, ii, 594.

of the nationality which is merged and lost in our interest in the man and in his work? In the halcyon days [37] of the Renaissance there was no nationalism in medicine, but a fine catholic spirit made great leaders like Vesalius, Eustachius, Stensen [38] and others at home in every country in Europe. While this is impossible to-day, a great teacher of any country may have a world-wide audience in our journal literature, which has done so much to make medicine cosmopolitan.

III. Provincialism in Medicine

While we may congratulate ourselves that the worst aspects of nationalism in medicine are disappearing before the broader culture and the more intimate knowledge brought by ever-increasing intercourse, yet in English-speaking countries conditions have favoured the growth of a very unpleasant subvariety, which may be called provincialism or sectionalism. In one sense the profession of this continent is singularly homogeneous. A young man may be prepared for his medical course in Louisiana and enter McGill College, or he may enter Dalhousie College, Halifax, from the State of Oregon, and in either case he will not feel strange or among strangers so soon as he has got accustomed to his environment. In collegiate life there is a frequent interchange of teachers and professors between all parts of the country. To better his brains the scholar goes freely where he wishes—to Harvard, McGill, Yale, or Johns Hopkins; there are no restrictions. The various medical societies of the two countries are, without exception, open to the members of the profession at large. The President of the Association of American Physicians this year (Dr. James Stewart),[39] is a resident of this city, which gave also last year I believe, presidents to two of the special societies. The chief journals are supported by men of all sections. The

36. John *Hunter* (1728–1793): See "The Old Humanities and the New Science," p. 93, n. 214.

Edward *Jenner* (1749–1823): English physician and one of Hunter's students. He founded the science of immunology by the vaccination of smallpox. He is known first for vaccinating based on the observation that milkers who had contracted cowpox did not get the disease smallpox.

37. Halcyon days are in midwinter, a calm period before the storm when the halcyon or kingfisher (a bird) is seen; hence, days of peace and happiness.

38. Andreas *Vesalius* (1514–1564): See "The Leaven of Science," p. 163, n. 62.

Bartolommeo *Eustachio* (c.1510–1574): Italian anatomist known for his anatomical illustrations and his discovery of the eustachian tube, a narrow canal connecting the ear and throat, and the eustachian valve of the heart.

Nielo *Stensen* (also Niels Steensen or Niels Stenson) (1638–1686): Danish anatomist and geologist known for his observations and discoveries concerning the glands, the muscles (especially the heart), the brain, the embryo, etc. He also contributed to comparative anatomy.

39. James A. *Stewart* (1846–1906): Professor of medicine at McGill University and physician to the Royal Victoria Hospital.

text-books and manuals are everywhere in common; there is, in fact, a remarkable homogeneity in the English-speaking profession, not only on this continent but throughout the world. Naturally, in widely scattered communities sectionalism — a feeling or conviction that the part is greater than the whole — does exist, but it is diminishing, and one great function of the national associations is to foster a spirit of harmony and brotherhood among the scattered units of these broad lands. But we suffer sadly from a provincialism which has gradually enthralled us, and which sprang originally from an attempt to relieve conditions insupportable in themselves. I have praised the unity of the profession of this continent, in so many respects remarkable, and yet in another respect it is the most heterogeneous ever known. Democracy in full circle touches tyranny, and as Milton remarks, the greatest proclaimers of liberty may become its greatest engrossers (or enslavers).[40] The tyranny of labour unions, of trusts, and of an irresponsible press may bear as heavily on the people as autocracy in its worst form. And, strange irony of fate! the democracy of Provincial and State Boards has imposed in a few years a yoke more grievous than that which afflicts our brethren in Great Britain, which took generations to forge.

The delightful freedom of intercourse of which I spoke, while wide and generous, is limited to intellectual and social life, and on the practical side, not only are genial and courteous facilities lacking, but the bars of a rigid provincialism are put up, fencing each State as with a Chinese wall.[41] In the Dominion of Canada there are eight portals of entry to the profession, in the United States almost as many as there are States, in the United Kingdom nineteen, I believe, but in the latter the license of any one of these bodies entitled a man to registration anywhere in the kingdom. Democracy in full circle has reached on this hemisphere a much worse condition than that in which the conservatism of many generations has entangled the profession of Great Britain. Upon the origin and growth of the Provincial and State Boards I do not propose to touch. The ideal has been reached so far as organization is concerned, when the profession elects its own Parliament, to which is committed the control of all matters relating to

40. This is not an exact quote, but a reminiscence of the following passage: "What should ye doe then, should ye suppresse all this flowry crop of knowledge and new light sprung up and yet springing daily in this City, should ye set an *Oligarchy* of twenty ingrossers over it, to bring a famin upon our minds again, when we shall know nothing but what is measur'd to us by their bushel." John Milton, *Areopagitica,* ed. William Haller, *The Works of John Milton* (1644; New York: Columbia University Press, 1931), vol. 4, p. 345. Milton is arguing against a proposal to establish a board of twenty censors. He compares them to engrossers, who are monopolists — those who try to buy up all there is of a commodity, so that they can control its price and distribution. Osler's point is rather different: namely that those who are loudest in their demand for liberty may, when they come to power, only extend it to their own faction.
41. The Great Wall of China.

the license. The recognition, in some form, of this democratic principle, has been one great means of elevating the standard of medical education, and in a majority of the States of the Union it has secured a minimum period of four years of study, and a State Examination for License to Practise. All this is as it should be. But it is high time that the profession realized the anomaly of eight boards in the Dominion and some scores in the United States. One can condone the iniquity in the latter country more readily than in Canada, in which the boards have existed for a longer period, and where there has been a greater uniformity in the medical curriculum. After all these years that a young man, a graduate of Toronto and a registered practitioner in Ontario, cannot practise in the Province of Quebec, his own country, without submitting to vexatious penalties of mind and pocket, or that a graduate from Montreal and a registered practitioner of this province cannot go to Manitoba, his own country again, and take up his life's work without additional payments and penalties, is, I maintain, an outrage; it is provincialism run riot. That this pestiferous condition should exist throughout the various provinces of this Dominion and so many States of the Union, illustrates what I have said of the tyranny of democracy and how great enslavers of liberty its chief proclaimers may be.

That the cure of this vicious state has to be sought in Dominion bills [42] and National examining boards, indicates into what debasing depths of narrow provincialism we have sunk. The solution seems to be so simple, particularly in this country, with its uniformity of methods of teaching and length of curriculum. A generous spirit that will give to local laws a liberal interpretation, that limits its hostility to ignorance and viciousness, that has regard as much or more for the good of the guild as a whole as for the profession of any province—could such a spirit brood over the waters,[43] the raging waves of discord would soon be stilled. With the attitude of mind of the general practitioner in each province rests the solution of the problem. Approach it in a friendly and gracious spirit and the difficulties which seem so hard will melt away. Approach it in a Chauvinistic mood, fully convinced that the superior and unparalleled conditions of your province

42. *Dominion bills:* Proposals for legislation by the Dominion (national) Parliament to override provincial particularism. No such legislation was ever enacted.

43. *spirit brood over the waters:* This is an echo of Genesis 1:1: "In the beginning . . . the Spirit of God moved upon the face of the waters," where the *Revised Version* (1885) has "was brooding" as a marginal alternative to "moved." Osler could also have been thinking of Milton's invocation of the Holy Spirit at the beginning of *Paradise Lost* (book 1, lines 19–22):

> Thou from the first
> Wast present, and with mighty wings outspread
> Dove-like satst brooding on the vast Abyss
> And mad'st it pregnant.

will be jeopardized by reciprocity or by Federal legislation, and the present antiquated and disgraceful system must await for its removal the awakening of a younger and more intelligent generation.

It would ill become me to pass from this subject—familiar to me from my student days from the interest taken in it by that far-sighted and noble-minded man, Dr. Palmer Howard[44]—it would ill become me, I say, not to pay a tribute of words to Dr. Roddick[45] for the zeal and persistence with which he has laboured to promote union in the compound, comminuted fracture of the profession of this Dominion.[46] My feeling on the subject of international, intercolonial, and interprovincial registration is this—a man who presents evidence of proper training, who is a registered practitioner in his own country and who brings credentials of good standing at the time of departure, should be welcomed as a brother, treated as such in any country, and registered upon payment of the usual fee. The ungenerous treatment of English physicians in Switzerland, France, and Italy, and the chaotic state of internecine[47] warfare existing on this continent, indicate how far a miserable Chauvinism can corrupt the great and gracious ways which should characterize a liberal profession.

Though not germane to the subject, may I be allowed to refer to one other point in connexion with the State Boards—a misunderstanding, I believe, of their functions. The profession asks that the man applying for admission to its ranks shall be of good character and fit to practise the science and art of medicine. The latter is easily ascertained if practical men have the place and the equipment for practical examinations. Many of the boards have not kept pace with the times, and the questions set too often show a lack of appreciation of modern methods. This has, perhaps, been unavoidable since, in the appointment of examiners, it has not always been possible to select experts. The truth is, that however well organized and equipped, the State Boards cannot examine properly in the scientific branches, nor is there need to burden the students with additional examinations in anatomy, physiology and chemistry. The Provincial and State Boards have done a great work for medical education on this continent, which they would crown and extend by doing away at once with all theoretical examinations and limiting the tests for the license to a rigid practical examination in medicine, surgery, and midwifery, in which all minor subjects could be included.

44. Robert Palmer *Howard* (1823–1889): Osler's teacher and mentor. For further information, see "Aequanimitas," p. 28, n. 42 and "The Student Life," p. 327.

45. Thomas George *Roddick* (1846–1923): Professor of surgery and dean of the Medical Faculty at McGill University.

46. A fracture in which the splintered or crushed end of the bone has penetrated the skin. Hence, figuratively, Dr. Roddick has expended a great deal of effort on a fracture that is very difficult to repair.

47. *internecine:* (Latin) mutually destructive conflict, aiming at each other's extermination.

IV. Parochialism in Medicine

Of the parochial and more personal aspects of Chauvinism I hesitate to speak; all of us, unwittingly as a rule, illustrate its varieties. The conditions of life which round us and bound us, whether in town or country, in college or institution, give to the most liberal a smack of parochialism, just as surely as we catch the tic of tongue of the land in which we live. The dictum put into the mouth of Ulysses, "I am a part of all that I have met,"[48] expresses the truth of the influence upon us of the social environment, but it is not the whole truth, since the size of the parish, representing the number of points of contact, is of less moment than the mental fibre of the man. Who has not known lives of the greatest freshness and nobility hampered at every turn and bound in chains the most common-place and sordid, lives which illustrate the liberty and freedom enjoyed by minds innocent and quiet, in spite of stone walls and iron bars. On the other hand, scan the history of progress in the profession, and men the most illiberal and narrow, reeking of the most pernicious type of Chauvinism, have been among the teachers and practitioners in the large cities and great medical centres; so true is it, that the mind is its own place and in itself can make a man independent of his environment.

There are shades and varieties which are by no means offensive. Many excellent features in a man's character may partake of its nature. What, for example, is more proper than the pride which we feel in our teachers, in the university from which we have graduated, in the hospital at which we have been trained? He is a "poor sort" who is free from such feelings, which only manifest a proper loyalty. But it easily degenerates into a base intolerance which looks with disdain on men of other schools and other ways. The pride, too, may be in inverse proportion to the justness of the claims. There is plenty of room for honest and friendly rivalry between schools and hospitals, only a blind Chauvinism puts a man into a hostile and intolerant attitude of mind at the mention of a name. Alumni and friends should remember that indiscriminate praise of institutions or men is apt to rouse the frame of mind illustrated by the ignorant Athenian who, so weary of hearing Aristides always called the Just, very gladly took up the oyster shell for his ostracism, and even asked Aristides[49] himself, whom he did not know, to mark it.

48. Alfred Tennyson, "Ulysses," line 18.

49. *Aristides* (also *Aristeides*) (c.530–c.468 B.C.): Athenian statesman and general, called "The Just." Plutarch in his *Lives* relates that an illiterate voter asked Aristides, whom he did not know, to write "Aristides" on his tablet for ostracism, not because Aristides had ever injured him but because "I am tired of hearing him everywhere called 'the Just!' " Aristides was ostracized in 483 B.C. Plutarch, "Aristides," in *The Lives of the Noble Grecians and Romans,* trans. John Dryden (New York: Modern Library, n.d.), p. 396.

A common type of collegiate Chauvinism is manifest in the narrow spirit too often displayed in filling appointments. The professoriate of the profession, the most mobile column of its great army, should be recruited with the most zealous regard to fitness, irrespective of local conditions that are apt to influence the selection. Inbreeding is as hurtful to colleges as to cattle. The interchange of men, particularly of young men, is most stimulating, and the complete emancipation of the chairs which has taken place in most of our universities should extend to the medical schools. Nothing, perhaps, has done more to place German medicine in the forefront to-day than a peripatetic professoriate, owing allegiance only to the profession at large, regardless of civic, sometimes, indeed, of national limitations and restrictions. We acknowledge the principle in the case of the scientific chairs, and with increasing frequency act upon it, but an attempt to expand it to other chairs may be the signal for the display of rank parochialism.

Another unpleasant manifestation of collegiate Chauvinism is the outcome, perhaps, of the very keen competition which at present exists in scientific circles. Instead of a generous appreciation of the work done in other places, there is a settled hostility and a narrowness of judgment but little in keeping with the true spirit of science. Worse still is the "lock and key" laboratory in which suspicion and distrust reign, and everyone is jealous and fearful lest the other should know of or find out about his work. Thank God! this base and bastard spirit is not much seen, but it is about, and I would earnestly entreat any young man who unwittingly finds himself in a laboratory pervaded with this atmosphere, to get out ere the contagion sinks into his soul.

Chauvinism in the unit, in the general practitioner, is of much more interest and importance. It is amusing to read and hear of the passing of the family physician. There never was a time in our history in which he was so much in evidence, in which he was so prosperous, in which his prospects were so good or his power in the community so potent. The public has even begun to get sentimental over him! He still does the work; the consultants and the specialists do the talking and the writing; and take the fees! By the work, I mean that great mass of routine practice which brings the doctor into every household in the land and makes him, not alone the adviser, but the valued friend. He is the standard by which we are measured. What he is, we are; and the estimate of the profession in the eyes of the public is their estimate of him. A well-trained, sensible doctor is one of the most valuable assets of a community, worth to-day, as in Homer's time, many another man. To make him efficient is our highest ambition as teachers, to save him from evil should be our constant care as a guild. I can only refer here to certain aspects in which he is apt to show a narrow Chauvinism hurtful to himself and to us.

In no single relation of life does the general practitioner show a more illiberal spirit than in the treatment of himself. I do not refer so much to careless
habits of living, to lack of routine in work, or to failure to pay due attention to
the business side of the profession—sins which so easily beset him—but I would
speak of his failure to realize *first,* the need of a lifelong progressive personal
training, and *secondly,* the danger lest in the stress of practice he sacrifice that
most precious of all possessions, his mental independence. Medicine is a most
difficult art to acquire. All the college can do is to teach the student principles,
based on facts in science, and give him good methods of work. These simply start
him in the right direction, they do not make him a good practitioner—that is
his own affair. To master the art requires sustained effort, like the bird's flight
which depends on the incessant action of the wings, but this sustained effort is
so hard that many give up the struggle in despair. And yet it is only by persis-
tent intelligent study of disease upon a methodical plan of examination that a
man gradually learns to correlate his daily lessons with the facts of his previous
experience and of that of his fellows, and so acquires clinical wisdom. Nowadays it is really not a hard matter for a well-trained man to keep abreast of the
best work of the day. He need not be very scientific so long as he has a true appreciation of the dependence of his art on science, for, in a way, it is true that
a good doctor may have practice and no theory, art and no science. To keep up
a familiarity with the use of instruments of precision is an all-important help
in his art, and I am profoundly convinced that as much space should be given
to the clinical laboratory as to the dispensary. One great difficulty is that while
waiting for the years to bring the inevitable yoke,[50] a young fellow gets stale and
loses that practised familiarity with technique which gives confidence. I wish
the older practitioners would remember how important it is to encourage and
utilize the young men who settle near them. In every large practice there are a
dozen or more cases requiring skilled aid in the diagnosis, and this the general
practitioner can have at hand. It is his duty to avail himself of it, and failing to
do so he acts in a most illiberal and unjust way to himself and to the profession
at large. Not only may the older man, if he has soft arteries in his grey cortex,
pick up many points from the young fellow, but there is much clinical wisdom
afloat in each parish which is now wasted or dies with the old doctor, because he
and the young men have never been on friendly terms.

In the fight which we have to wage incessantly against ignorance and quackery among the masses and follies of all sorts among the classes, *diagnosis,* not

50. *the inevitable yoke:* William Wordsworth, "Ode: Intimations of Immortality from Recollections of
Early Childhood," stanza 8, line 124.

drugging, is our chief weapon of offence. *Lack of systematic personal training in the methods of the recognition of disease leads to the misapplication of remedies, to long courses of treatment when treatment is useless, and so directly to that lack of confidence in our methods which is apt to place us in the eyes of the public on a level with empirics and quacks.*

Few men live lives of more devoted self-sacrifice than the family physician, but he may become so completely absorbed in work that leisure is unknown; he has scarce time to eat or to sleep, and, as Dr. Drummond remarks in one of his poems, "He's the only man, I know me, don't get no holiday."[51] There is danger in this treadmill life lest he lose more than health and time and rest—his intellectual independence. More than most men he feels the tragedy of isolation—that inner isolation so well expressed in Matthew Arnold's line "We mortal millions live *alone.*"[52] Even in populous districts the practice of medicine is a lonely road which winds up-hill all the way and a man may easily go astray and never reach the Delectable Mountains unless he early finds those shepherd guides of whom Bunyan tells, *Knowledge, Experience, Watchful,* and *Sincere.*[53] The circumstances of life mould him into a masterful, self-confident, self-centered man, whose worst faults often partake of his best qualities. The peril is that should he cease to think for himself he becomes a mere automaton, doing a penny-in-the-slot business which places him on a level with the chemist's clerk who can hand out specifics for every ill, from the "pip" to the pox.[54] The salt of life for him is a judicious scepticism, not the coarse, crude form, but the sober sense of honest doubt expressed in the maxim of the sly old Sicilian Epicharmus, "Be sober and distrustful; these are the sinews of the understanding."[55] A great advantage, too, of a sceptical attitude of mind is, as Green the historian remarks, "One is never very surprised or angry to find that one's oppo-

51. William Henry Drummond (1854–1907): Canadian poet and physician. "The Canadian Country Doctor," stanza 2, line 4.

52. Matthew Arnold, "To Marguerite—Continued," line 4.

53. John Bunyan, *The Pilgrim's Progress* (1678), part 1. In this allegory, Christian journeys from the City of Destruction to the City of Zion, situated amid the Delectable Mountains.

54. From merely feeling out of sorts to having a serious illness, such as syphilis or smallpox. The "pip" is physical lethargy accompanied by mental depression.

55. *Epicharmus* (c.540–c.450 B.C.): See "The Leaven of Science," p. 170, n. 93. Theodor Gomperz (1832–1912) also writes:

> A sober sense of honest doubt
> Keeps human reason hale and stout.

This maxim was taken as the guiding star by those who wanted to be free from mythical thought and take positive methods of scientific research. *Greek Thinkers.* trans. Laurie Magnus (New York: Charles Scribner's Sons, 1901), p. 313.

244

CHAUVINISM

IN MEDICINE

nents are in the right."[56] It may keep him from self-deception and from falling into that medical slumber into which so many drop, deep as the theological slumber so lashed by Erasmus,[57] in which a man may write letters, debauch himself, get drunk, and even make money—a slumber so deep at times that no torpedo-touch can waken him.

It may keep the practitioner out of the clutches of the arch enemy of his professional independence—the pernicious literature of our camp-followers, a literature increasing in bulk, in meretricious attractiveness, and in impudent audacity. To modern pharmacy we owe much, and to pharmaceutical methods we shall owe much more in the future, but the profession has no more insidious foe than the large borderland pharmaceutical houses. No longer an honoured messmate, pharmacy in this form threatens to become a huge parasite, eating the vitals of the body medical. We all know only too well the bastard literature which floods the mail, every page of which illustrates the truth of the axiom, the greater the ignorance the greater the dogmatism. Much of it is advertisements of nostrums foisted on the profession by men who trade on the innocent credulity of the regular physician, quite as much as any quack preys on the gullible public. Even the most respectable houses are not free from this sin of arrogance and of ignorant dogmatism in their literature. A still more dangerous enemy to the mental virility of the general practitioner, is the "drummer" of the drug house.[58] While many of them are good, sensible fellows, there are others, voluble as Cassio, impudent as Autolycus, and senseless as Caliban,[59] who will tell you glibly of the virtues of extract of the coccygeal gland in promoting pineal metabolism, and are ready to express the most emphatic opinions on questions about which the greatest masters of our art are doubtful. No class of men with which we have to deal illustrates more fully that greatest of ignorance—the ignorance which is the conceit that a man knows what he does not know; but the enthralment of the practitioner by the manufacturing chemist and the revival of a pseudo-scientific polypharmacy are too large questions to be dealt with at the end of an address.

56. John Richard *Green* (1837–1883): English historian and frequent contributor to the *Saturday Review*. Author of *A Short History of the English People* (1874), *The History of the English People* (1877–1880), and many other works.

57. J. A. Froude, *Life and Letters of Erasmus* (New York: Charles Scribner's Sons, 1895), p. 69. The passage is from Erasmus' letter no. 85 to his student Grey. The original reads: "Hush! You do not understand the theological slumber. You can write letters in it. You can debauch yourself and get drunk in it."

    Desiderius *Erasmus* (c.1467–1536): See "The Old Humanities and the New Science," p. 66, n. 11.

58. Commercial traveler and propagator of medicines.

59. All characters in Shakespeare's plays: Cassio in *Othello*, Autolycus in *The Winter's Tale*, and Caliban in *The Tempest*.

But there is a still greater sacrifice which many of us make, heedlessly and thoughtlessly forgetting that "Man does not live by bread alone."[60] One cannot practise medicine alone and practise it early and late, as so many of us have to do, and hope to escape the malign influences of a routine life. The incessant concentration of thought upon one subject, however interesting, tethers a man's mind in a narrow field. The practitioner needs culture as well as learning. The earliest picture we have in literature of a scientific physician, in our sense of the term, is as a cultured Greek gentleman;[61] and I care not whether the young man labours among the beautiful homes on Sherbrooke Street,[62] or in the slums of Caughnawauga,[63] or in some sparsely settled country district, he cannot afford to have learning only. In no profession does culture count for so much as in medicine, and no man needs it more than the general practitioner, working among all sorts and conditions of men, many of whom are influenced quite as much by his general ability, which they can appreciate, as by his learning of which they have no measure. The day has passed for the "practiser of physic"[64] to be like Mr. Robert Levet,[65] Dr. Johnson's friend, "Obscurely wise and coarsely kind."[66] The wider and freer a man's general education the better practitioner is he likely to be, particularly among the higher classes to whom the reassurance and sympathy of a cultivated gentleman of the type of Eryximachus,[67] may mean much more than pills and potions. But what of the men of the type of Mr. Robert Levet, or "Ole Docteur Fiset,"[68] whose virtues walk a narrow round, the men who do the hard

60. Deuteronomy 8:3.

61. Osler probably refers to Eryximachus (4th cent. B.C.). See p. 246, n. 67.

62. *Sherbrooke Street* is one of the main streets of Montreal and was a fashionable residential area in Osler's day.

63. *Caughnawauga,* Quebec, is the site of an Indian reserve on the south bank of the St. Lawrence River, near the Lachine Rapids, opposite Lachine.

64. *"Physic"* here means the art and skill of healing.

65. Robert *Levet* (also Levett or Levit) (1705–1782): English physician and faithful friend of Samuel Johnson. James Boswell (1740–1795), autobiographer famed for his *Life of Samuel Johnson* (1791), which presented both Johnson's virtues and his foibles and documented their long friendship.

66. Samuel Johnson (1649–1703) wrote a verse to honor his physician's memory. "On the Death of Dr. Robert Levet," line 10. Quoted in Boswell's *Life of Samuel Johnson,* Sunday, January 20, 1782.

67. *Eryximachus* (4th cent. B.C.): Greek physician. Plato describes him as telling Aristophanes how to cure hiccups while making a speech on love or harmony (*Symposium,* 185d–e). For further information, see "Physic and Physicians as Depicted in Plato," p. 148.

68. William Henry Drummond, "Ole Docteur Fiset," in *The Habitant,* stanza 1, lines 1–5. The original reads:

> Ole Docteur Fiset of Saint Anicet,
> Sapré tonnerre! he was leev long tam!
> I'm sure he's got ninety year or so,

general practices in the poorer districts of the large cities, in the factory towns and in the widely scattered rough agricultural regions—what, I hear you say, has culture to do with them? Everything! It is the bichloride which may prevent the infection and may keep a man sweet and whole amid the most debasing surroundings. Of very little direct value to him in his practice—though the poor have a pretty keen appreciation of a gentleman—it may serve to prevent the degeneration so apt to overtake the overworked practitioner, whose nature is only too prone to be subdued like the dyer's hand to what it works in. If a man does not sell his soul, if he does not part with his birthright of independence for a mess of pottage[69] to the Ishmaelites[70] who harass our borders with their clubs and oppress us with their exactions, if he can only keep *free*, the conditions of practice are nowhere incompatible with St. Paul's noble Christian[71] or Aristotle's true gentleman (Sir Thomas Browne).[72]

Whether a man will treat his professional brethren in a gentlemanly way or in a narrow illiberal spirit is partly a matter of temperament, partly a matter of training. If we had only to deal with one another the difficulties would be slight, but it must be confessed that the practice of medicine among our fellow creatures is often a testy and choleric business. When one has done his best or when a mistake has arisen through lack of special knowledge, but more particularly when, as so often happens, our heart's best sympathies have been engaged, to be misunderstood by the patient and his friends, to have evil motives imputed and to be maligned, is too much for human endurance and justifies a righteous indignation. Women, our greatest friends and our greatest enemies, are the chief sinners, and while one will exhaust the resources of the language in describing

---

Beat all on de Parish 'cept Pierre Courteau,

An' day after day he work all de sam'.

69. *pottage:* A thick soup. There is a complex of biblical references here, all from Genesis. Esau, Isaac's elder son, came in famished from hunting one day and found his younger brother Jacob making pottage. Esau begged Jacob to give him some, but Jacob slyly required him first to make over to him his birthright (his right to the largest share of their father's inheritance) (Genesis 25:29–34). Hence "to sell one's birthright for a mess of pottage" is a proverb for parting with one's dearest possession for a trifling and transitory reward.

70. Osler refers to a group of wandering tribes who traced their descent from Ishmael (Genesis 25:18–19), suggesting outcasts from society.

71. Philippians 4:8. Osler is thinking of nobility of character.

72. Referring to persecution, Browne examines "the circumstances and requisites which Aristotle requires for true and perfect valour" and mentions Aristotle's pupil, Alexander the Great, and then Julius Caesar. Thomas Browne, *Religio Medici*, part 1, sect. 25.

   St. Paul's noble Christian and Aristotle's true gentleman: Osler got the pairing from Thomas Browne in "A Letter to a Friend," in *The Works of Sir Thomas Browne*, ed. Geoffrey Keynes (Chicago: University of Chicago Press, 1964), vol. 1, p. 117.

our mistakes and weaknesses, another will laud her pet doctor so indiscriminately that all others come under a sort of oblique condemnation. "Feminæ sunt medicorum tubæ"[73] is an old and true saying. It is hard to say whether as a whole we do not suffer just as much from the indiscriminate praise. But against this evil we are helpless. Far otherwise, when we do not let the heard word die; not to listen is best, though that is not always possible, but silence is always possible, than which we have no better weapon in our armoury against evil-speaking, lying, and slandering. The bitterness is when the tale is believed and a brother's good name is involved. Then begins the worst form of ill-treatment that the practitioner receives—and at his own hands! He allows the demon of resentment to take possession of his soul, when five minutes' frank conversation might have gained a brother. In a small or a large community what more joyful than to see the brethren dwelling together in unity. The bitterness, the rancour, the personal hostility which many of us remember in our younger days has been largely replaced by a better feeling and while the golden rule[74] is not always, as it should be, our code of ethics, we have certainly become more charitable the one towards the other.

To the senior man in our ranks we look for an example, and in the smaller towns and country districts if he would remember that it is his duty to receive and welcome the young fellow who settles near him, that he should be willing to act as his adviser and refuse to regard him as a rival, he may make a good friend and perhaps gain a brother. In speaking of professional harmony, it is hard to avoid the trite and commonplace, but neglecting the stale old chaps whose ways are set and addressing the young, to whom sympathy and encouragement are so dear, and whose way of life means so much to the profession we love, upon them I would urge the practice of St. Augustine,[75] of whom it is told in the *Golden Legend*[76] that "he had these verses written at his table:

Quisquis amat dictis absentum rodere vitam,
Hanc mensam indignam noverit esse sibi.

73. *Fœminæ sunt medicorum tubæ:* (Latin) "women are the trumpets of doctors." *Diary of the Rev. John Ward*, ed. Charles Severn (London: H. Colburn, 1839), p. 241.

74. *the golden rule:* Matthew 7:12 and Luke 6:31. Also, Confucius, (*Analects*, book 5, chap. 11, and book 12, chap. 2): "What you do not like when done to yourself, do not do to others."

75. *St. Augustine* (354–430): Early Christian Church father and philosopher who exerted enormous influence throughout the Christian world. Author of *De Civitate Dei* (The City of God, completed in twenty-two books by 426) and his autobiography *The Confessions*. His doctrines reaffirmed and developed those of St. Paul.

76. A medieval collection of saints' lives, arranged in the calendar order in which their feasts come in the Christian year. It was compiled by Jacobus de Voragine (c.1229–1298).

That is to say: Whosoever loves to missay any creature that is absent, it may be said that this table is denied to him at all."[77]

With our History, Traditions, Achievements, and Hopes, there is little room for Chauvinism in medicine. The open mind, the free spirit of science, the ready acceptance of the best from any and every source, the attitude of rational receptiveness rather than of antagonism to new ideas, the liberal and friendly relationship between different nations and different sections of the same nation, the brotherly feeling which should characterize members of the oldest, most beneficent and universal guild that the race has evolved in its upward progress—these should neutralize the tendencies upon which I have so lightly touched.

I began by speaking of the art of detachment as that rare and precious quality demanded of one who wished to take a philosophical view of the profession as a whole. In another way and in another sense this art may be still more precious. There is possible to each one of us a higher type of intellectual detachment, a sort of separation from the vegetative life of the work-a-day world—always too much with us—which may enable a man to gain a true knowledge of himself and of his relations to his fellows. Once attained, self-deception is impossible, and he may see himself even as he is seen—not always as he would like to be seen—and his own deeds and the deeds of others stand out in their true light. In such an atmosphere pity for himself is so commingled with sympathy and love for others that there is no place left for criticism or for a harsh judgment of his brother. But as Sir Thomas Browne—most liberal of men and most distinguished of general practitioners—so beautifully remarks: "These are Thoughts of things which Thoughts but tenderly touch,"[78] and it may be sufficient to remind this audience, made up of practical men, *that the word of action is stronger than the word of speech.*[79]

77. Jacobus de Voragine, *The Golden Legend: Readings on the Saints* (Princeton, N.J.: Princeton University Press, 1993), pp. 122–123. Probably these verses are not really by St. Augustine but were merely attributed to him by Jacobus de Voragine.

78. *These are Thoughts of things which Thoughts but tenderly touch:* Thomas Browne; probably in one of his letters, but we could not find it.

79. A Latin proverb: The usual form of the maxim is "Actions speak louder than words." The Latin form *"facta non verba,"* literally means "deeds, not words."

14

THE MASTER-WORD IN MEDICINE

If any one is desirous of carrying out in detail the Platonic education of after-life, some such counsels as the following may be offered to him: That he shall choose the branch of knowledge to which his own mind most distinctly inclines, and in which he takes the greatest delight, either one which seems to connect with his own daily employment, or, perhaps, furnishes the greatest contrast to it. He may study from the speculative side the profession or business in which he is practically engaged. He may make Homer, Dante, Shakespeare, Plato, Bacon the friends and companions of his life. He may find opportunities of hearing the living voice of a great teacher. He may select for inquiry some point of history, or some unexplained phenomenon of nature. An hour a day passed in such scientific or literary pursuits will furnish as many facts as the memory can retain, and will give him "a pleasure not to be repented of." Only let him beware of being the slave of crotchets, or of running after a Will o' the Wisp in his ignorance, or in his vanity of attributing to himself the gifts of a poet, or assuming the air of a philosopher. He should know the limits of his own powers. Better to build up the mind by slow additions, to creep on quietly from one thing to another, to gain insensibly new powers and new interests in knowledge, than to form vast schemes which are never destined to be realized.

BENJAMIN JOWETT, *Introduction to Plato's* Republic

> Contend, my soul, for moments and for hours;
> Each is with service pregnant, each reclaimed
> Is like a Kingdom conquered, where to reign.
> ROBERT LOUIS STEVENSON

> In the case of our habits we are only masters of the beginning,
> their growth by gradual stages being imperceptible,
> like the growth of disease.
> ARISTOTLE, *Ethics*

OSLER GAVE THIS LONG but well-received speech to medical students in 1903. It was at the dedication of new laboratories for Physiology and Pathology at the

University of Toronto, thirty-five years after he had studied there. He praises the school's faculty and its recent merger with a rival school.

Obviously the changes in medical schools since then make some of his comments of historical interest only. At the time of this speech, Osler was well known for his influence on medical education, having founded the medical school at Johns Hopkins. He extols Toronto's new facilities as making possible excellent medical education and research. He reminds listeners that the faculty, not the buildings, create true greatness, so he urges more assistants to give the faculty time for research.

Osler reveals "the secret of life," that the "master-word" is *work*. It is work that is responsible for all advances in medicine in the past twenty-five centuries. He extols the value of work, order, and aiming for perfection.

Osler entreats the students to form good work habits. He urges them to strive to balance the two parts of their education, the technical study of diseases and the inner education, to be truly good human beings. Even though they have many required subjects to study, they must maintain enthusiasm and a sense of proportion. They must avoid becoming too involved in one subject at the expense of others. A degree is not the goal sought but the beginning of a lifelong process of education.

To maximize one's capabilities with the least possible strain, he recommends cultivating *systematic habits* of order, concentration, and tenacity. Physicians especially need attention to detail, desire for perfection, and willingness to be self-critical.

Overwork must be avoided by keeping healthy. Osler observes that worry, not overwork, is the cause of most students' problems. Worry can be minimized by *focusing on what needs to be done today*. Osler also advocates avoiding romantic entanglements during the student years and keeping religious concerns separate from those of science.

Apathy and complete concentration on professional work both lead to a dangerous narrowmindedness. To prevent this from happening and to deal with the intimate personal nature of medical work, medical students need a lifelong liberal education. He recommends reading the classics briefly each day, to help one rise above daily problems and discouragements.

Medicine is not a business but a calling that requires love and charity for fellow practitioners and patients alike. Osler advises students to ignore gossip about other doctors and to mend any misunderstandings immediately. He reminds them of the noble heritage of their field, and of their duty in "the great army of quiet workers" who minister in sorrow and sickness. Humanity, high principles, and sound judgement are needed in addition to medical knowledge and skills.

Finally, Osler wishes the students the happiness that he has found in the profession. He acknowledges his debt to his teachers who set "forth a true and lively word to the great enlightenment of our darkness." He especially credits Dr. James Bovell of Toronto and the Rev. W. A. Johnson for his success. He defines success as "getting what you want and being satisfied with it."

THE MASTER-WORD
IN MEDICINE

I

BEFORE PROCEEDING TO the pleasing duty of addressing the undergraduates, as a native of this province and as an old student of this school, I must say a few words on the momentous changes inaugurated with this session, the most important, perhaps, which have taken place in the history of the profession in Ontario. The splendid laboratories which we saw opened this afternoon, a witness to the appreciation by the authorities of the needs of science in medicine, make possible the highest standards of education in the subjects upon which our Art is based. They may do more. A liberal policy, with a due regard to the truth that the greatness of a school lies in brains not bricks, should build up a great scientific centre which will bring renown to this city and to our country. The men in charge of the departments are of the right stamp. See to it that you treat them in the right way by giving skilled assistance enough to ensure that the vitality of men who could work for the world is not sapped by the routine of teaching. One regret will, I know, be in the minds of many of my younger hearers. The removal of the department of anatomy and physiology from the biological laboratory of the university breaks a connexion which has had an important influence on medicine in this city. To Professor Ramsay Wright[1] is due much of the inspiration which has made possible these fine new laboratories. For years he has encouraged in every way the cultivation of the

An address delivered at the opening of the new laboratories for physiology and pathology at the University of Toronto, October 1, 1903.

1. Ramsay *Wright* (1852–1933): The first professor of biology at the University of Toronto. The Zoological Laboratories at the University of Toronto are now named in his honor.

scientific branches of medicine and has unselfishly devoted much time to promoting the best interests of the Medical Faculty. And in passing let me pay a tribute to the ability and zeal with which Dr. A. B. Macallum[2] has won for himself a world-wide reputation by intricate studies which have carried the name of this University to every nook and corner of the globe where the science of physiology is cultivated. How much you owe to him in connexion with the new buildings I need scarcely mention in this audience.

But the other event which we celebrate is of much greater importance. When the money is forthcoming it is an easy matter to join stone to stone in a stately edifice, but it is hard to find the market in which to buy the precious cement which can unite into an harmonious body the professors of medicine of two rival medical schools in the same city.[3] That this has been accomplished so satisfactorily is a tribute to the good sense of the leaders of the two faculties, and tells of their recognition of the needs of the profession in the province. Is it too much to look forward to the absorption or affiliation of the Kingston and London schools into the Provincial University? The day has passed in which the small school without full endowment can live a life beneficial to the students, to the profession or to the public. I know well of the sacrifice of time and money which is freely made by the teachers of those schools; and they will not misunderstand my motives when I urge them to commit suicide, at least so far as to change their organizations into clinical schools in affiliation with the central university, as part, perhaps, of a widespread affiliation of the hospitals of the province. A school of the first rank in the world, such as this must become, should have ample clinical faculties under its own control. It is as much a necessity that the professors of medicine and surgery, etc., should have large hospital services under their control throughout the year, as it is that professors of pathology and physiology should have laboratories such as those in which we here meet. It should be an easy matter to arrange between the provincial authorities and the trustees of the Toronto General Hospital to replace the present antiquated system of multiple small services by modern well-equipped clinics—three in medicine and three in surgery to begin with. The increased efficiency of the service would be a substantial *quid pro quo*,[4] but there would have to be a self-denying ordinance on the part of many of the attending physicians. With the large number of students in the combined school no one hospital can furnish in practical medicine, surgery and the specialties a training in the art an equivalent of that which the student

2. Archibald B. *Macallum* (1858–1934): Professor of biology at the University of Toronto.

3. Medical schools of the University of Toronto and the University of Trinity College, where Osler had been a student before going to McGill. When Trinity College agreed to affiliate with the University of Toronto, the two medical schools were merged.

4. *quid pro quo:* (Latin) something in return for something else.

will have in the science in the new laboratories. An affiliation should be sought with every other hospital in the city and province of fifty beds and over, in each of which two or three extra-mural teachers could be recognized, who would receive for three or more months a number of students proportionate to the beds in the hospital. I need not mention names. We all know men in Ottawa, Kingston, London, Hamilton, Guelph and Chatham, who could take charge of small groups of the senior students and make of them good practical doctors. I merely throw out the suggestion. There are difficulties in the way; but is there anything worth struggling for in this life which does not bristle with them?

Students of Medicine: May this day be to each of you, as it was to me when I entered this school thirty-five years ago, the beginning of a happy life in a happy calling. Not one of you has come here with such a feeling of relief as that which I experienced at an escape from conic sections and logarithms and from Hooker and Pearson.[5] The dry bones became clothed with interest, and I felt that I had at last got to work. Of the greater advantages with which you start I shall not speak. Why waste my words on what you cannot understand. To those of us only who taught and studied in the dingy old building which stood near here is it given to feel the full change which the years have wrought, a change which my old teachers, whom I see here to-day—Dr. Richardson, Dr. Ogden, Dr. Thorburn and Dr. Oldright[6]—must find hard to realize. One looks about in vain for some accustomed object on which to rest the eye in its backward glance—all, all are gone, the old familiar places.[7] Even the landscape has altered, and the sense of loneliness and regret, the sort of homesickness one

256

5. Osler is referring to his first term at Trinity College, where he was studying for the Anglican ministry. These are two classic Anglican theologians, whose works he would then have had to read.

Richard *Hooker* (c.1554–1600): Author of *The Laws of Ecclesiastical Polity* (1594–1597). John *Pearson* (1613–1686): Bishop of Chester, author of *An Exposition of the Creed* (1659).

Canon Arthur Jarvis, who was Osler's classmate at both Trinity College School and Trinity College, wrote that Osler decided to become a medic rather than a clergyman after a quarrel with Dr. George Whitaker, the provost (i.e., head) of Trinity College. See "The Reminiscences of Canon Arthur Jarvis, UE," ed. Patrick Cain and Sean Morley, *Trinity College Historical Society* 1 (1992), p. 19.

6. James Henry *Richardson* (1823–1910): The first graduate in medicine at the University of Toronto. He studied in England, being the first Canadian to obtain his diploma at the Royal College of Surgeons in 1847. After that he was a professor of anatomy at the University of Toronto.

Uzziel *Ogden* (1828–1910): Professor of physiology, materia medica, and midwifery and gynecology, as well as dean of Victoria College (1880–1892).

James *Thorburn* (1830–1905): Professor of pharmacology and therapeutics at the University of Toronto, and president of the Canadian Medical Association (1895).

William *Oldright* (1842–1917): Professor of hygiene at the University of Toronto, and the first chairman of the Ontario Provincial Board of Health.

7. *all, all are gone, the old familiar places:* Osler is thinking of the refrain of "Old Familiar Faces," a poem by Charles Lamb (1775–1834). The original reads: "all, all are gone, these old familiar faces."

experiences on such occasions, is relieved by a feeling of thankfulness that at least some of the old familiar faces have been spared to see this day. To me at least the memory of those happy days is a perpetual benediction, and I look back upon the two years I spent at this school with the greatest delight. There were many things that might have been improved—and we can say the same of every medical school of that period—but I seem to have got much more out of it than our distinguished philosopher friend, J. Beattie Crozier,[8] whose picture of the period seems hardly drawn. But after all, as someone has remarked, instruction is often the least part of an education, and, as I recall them, our teachers in their life and doctrine set forth a true and lively word[9] to the great enlightenment of our darkness. They stand out in the background of my memory as a group of men whose influence and example were most helpful. In William R. Beaumont and Edward Mulberry Hodder,[10] we had before us the highest type of the cultivated English surgeon. In Henry H. Wright[11] we saw the incarnation of faithful devotion to duty—too faithful, we thought, as we trudged up to the eight o'clock lecture in the morning. In W. T. Aikins,[12] a practical surgeon of remarkable skill and an ideal teacher for the general practitioner. How we wondered and delighted in the anatomical demonstrations of Dr. Richardson,[13] whose infective enthusiasm did much to make anatomy the favourite subject among the students. I had the double advantage of attending the last course of Dr. Ogden[14] and the first of Dr. Thorburn[15] on materia medica and therapeutics.

8. John Beattie *Crozier* (1849–1921): Canadian writer, a classmate of Osler's at the University of Toronto. According to him, he felt uncomfortable in the surroundings, perhaps owing to his preoccupation with literature and philosophy. He described the professors as "pompous and fussy . . . deprecating and solicitous of our good opinion . . . so easily offended . . . callous and indifferent." Regarding the lectures, "the ordinary contents of the text books . . . being flung at us pell-mell without word of guidance, and leaving us standing helpless, bewildered, and starved in the midst of what seemed a superabundance of wealth." "The University," in *My Inner Life: Being a Chapter in Personal Evolution and Autobiography* (London: Longmans, Green, 1898), part 1, book 2, chap. 12, pp. 225–226.

9. *true and lively word:* This is an echo of the Prayer for the Church in the Communion service in the *Book of Common Prayer.*

10. William R. *Beaumont* (1803–1875): English surgeon who came to Toronto to teach ophthalmology. He was the first professor of surgery at the University of Toronto in 1841 and dean in 1851.

Edward Mulberry *Hodder* (1810–1878): English surgeon who came to Toronto to teach surgery (gynecology). He was one of the founders of the Upper Canada School of Medicine, where he was professor of midwifery and diseases of women. He served as dean fron 1870 to 1878.

11. Henry Hover *Wright* (1816–1899): Professor of medicine at the University of Toronto. Known as an enthusiastic teacher and scientific practitioner.

12. William T. *Aikins* (1827–1895): Surgeon who was also engaged in medical education in Toronto.

13. *Richardson:* See p. 256, n. 6.

14. *Ogden:* Ibid.

15. *Thorburn:* Ibid.

And Dr. Oldright [16] had just begun his career of unselfish devotion to the cause of hygiene.

To one of my teachers I must pay in passing the tribute of filial affection. There are men here to-day who feel as I do about Dr. James Bovell [17] — that he was of those finer spirits, not uncommon in life, touched to finer issues only in a suitable environment. Would the Paul of evolution have been Thomas Henry Huxley [18] had the Senate elected the young naturalist to a chair in this university in 1851? Only men of a certain metal rise superior to their surroundings, and while Dr. Bovell had that all-important combination of boundless ambition with energy and industry, he had that fatal fault of diffuseness, in which even genius is strangled. With a quadrilateral mind, which he kept spinning like a teetotum,[19] one side was never kept uppermost for long at a time. Caught in a storm which shook the scientific world with the publication of *The Origin of Species*,[20] instead of sailing before the wind, even were it with bare poles, he put about and sought a harbour of refuge in writing a work on Natural Theology, which you will find on the shelves of second-hand book shops in a company made respectable at least by the presence of Paley.[21] He was an omnivorous reader and transmutor, he could talk pleasantly, even at times transcendentally, upon anything in the

16. *Oldright:* Ibid.

17. James *Bovell* (1817–1880): One of Osler's three most admired teachers. In this passage Osler pays him the "tribute of filial affection": "Three years of association with Dr. Bovell were most helpful. Books and the Man! The best the human mind has afforded was on his shelves, and in him all that one could desire in a teacher, a clear head and a loving heart. Infected with the Aesculapian spirit, he made me realize the truth of those memorable words in the Hippocratic oath, 'I will honour as my father the man who teaches me the Art.'" "Introduction," *Bibliotheca Osleriana* (1929; Montreal: McGill-Queen's University Press, 1969), p. xxiii.

18. Thomas Henry *Huxley* (1825–1895): English zoologist, one of the first to defend Darwin. *Paul* (d.67 A.D.): An apostle in the New Testament (i.e., Huxley is to Darwin's theory as St. Paul was to the spread of Christianity). Osler is blaming Bovell's responsibilities at the university for his indifference or lack of focus and his lack of recognition. Bovell helped Dr. Hodder to organize a medical department for Trinity College in 1850 and later joined the Toronto Medical School Faculty, where he served until 1875.

19. *teetotum:* A kind of die with each of its four sides marked with an initial letter, used in games of chance.

20. Charles Robert Darwin (1809–1882): Author of *On the Origin of Species by Means of Natural Selection* (1859), which was highly controversial when published.

21. William *Paley* (1743–1805): Archdeacon of Carlisle and author of *Natural Theology; or Evidences of the Existence and Attributes of the Deity Collected from the Appearances of Nature* (1802), in which he argued that the order observable in nature proved that it must have been created by God. This book was widely read before the appearance of Darwin's theory. Osler's point is that Paley's book was worth taking seriously, but that many later books along the same lines are not.

A.B. McKillop, in *A Disciplined Intelligence* (Montreal: McGill-Queen's University Press, 1979), pp. 75–76, pointed out that Osler's severe criticisms of James Bovell's book *Outlines of Natural Theology* (1859) were somewhat unfair, in that Bovell wrote it before Darwin published *The Origin of Species*.

science of the day, from protoplasm to evolution; but he lacked concentration and that scientific accuracy which only comes with a long training (sometimes, indeed, never comes,) and which is the ballast of the boat. But the bent of his mind was devotional, and early swept into the Tractarian movement,[22] he became an advanced Churchman, a good Anglican Catholic. As he chaffingly remarked one day to his friend, the Rev. Mr. Darling,[23] he was like the waterman in *Pilgrim's Progress*,[24] rowing one way towards Rome, but looking steadfastly in the other direction towards Lambeth.[25] His *Steps to the Altar* and his *Lectures on the Advent* attest the earnestness of his convictions; and later in life, following the example of Linacre,[26] he took orders and became another illustration of what Cotton Mather calls the angelic conjunction of medicine with divinity.[27] Then, how well I recall the keen love with which he would engage in metaphysical discussions, and the ardour with which he studied Kant, Hamilton, Reed, and Mill.[28] At that day, to the Rev. Prof. Bevan[29] was intrusted the rare privilege of directing the minds of the thinking youths at the Provincial University into

22. *Tractarians:* A body of clergy within the Church of England who stressed its continuity with the ancient and mediaeval Catholic Church and urged a stricter adherence to its official doctrines and to the directions for worship in the *Book of Common Prayer*. They issued many *Tracts for the Times* at Oxford between 1833 and 1841. The more extreme or "advanced" members wished for a speedy reunion with the Roman Catholic Church and imitated many of its ceremonies.

23. William Stewart *Darling* (1818–1886): Rector of the Church of the Holy Trinity, Toronto.

24. The Waterman is the great-grandfather of By-ends who came from the town of Fair-speech. By-ends says about his family: "The parson of our parish, Mr. Two-tongues, was my mother's own brother by father's side; and to tell you the truth, I am become a gentleman of good quality, yet my great-grandfather was but a waterman, looking one way and rowing another, and I got most of my estate by the same occupation." John Bunyan, *Pilgrim's Progress* (1678; London: George Routledge and Son, n.d.), p. 154.

25. *Lambeth* Palace: The official south London residence of archbishops of Canterbury.

26. Thomas *Linacre* (c.1460–1524): See "The Old Humanities and the New Science," p. 66, n. 8.

27. Cotton *Mather* (1663–1728): American Congregationalist minister and author of pamphlets in science, *Essays to Do Good* (1710; London: J. Dennett, 1808), pp. 84f. He urged clergymen to "unite your counsels" with physicians on medical problems.

28. Immanuel *Kant* (1724–1804): German metaphysician and transcendental philosopher.

  William *Hamilton* (1788–1856): English philosopher born in Scotland who dealt with the association of ideas, and the relation of perception and sensation.

  Sampson *Reed* (1800–1880): American philosopher, author of *Observations on the Growth of the Mind* (1826), which influenced many, including Emerson.

  John Stuart *Mill* (1806–1873): English philosopher and economist, author of *On Liberty* (1859).

29. James *Bevan* (also Beaven) (1801–1875): Clergyman and professor of metaphysics at the University of Toronto. Bevan's contemporaries had different opinions about him; his "slow prosaic manner" often irritated his students, although his learning was highly respected in his clerical circle. Daniel Wilson, president of the University of Toronto, in a moment of irritation, once described his colleague as "a stupid dry old stick that we would be well rid of." T. R. Millman, *Dictionary of Canadian Biography* (1871–1880), vol. 10, p. 40.

proper philosophical channels. It was rumoured that the hungry sheep looked up and were not fed.[30] I thought so at least, for certain of them, led by T. Wesley Mills,[31] came over daily after Dr. Bovell's four o'clock lecture to reason high and long with him.

On Providence, Foreknowledge, Will and Fate,
Fixed Fate, Freewill, Foreknowledge absolute.[32]

Yet withal, his main business in life was as a physician, much sought after for his skill in diagnosis, and much beloved for his loving heart. He had been brought up in the very best practical schools. A pupil of Bright and of Addison,[33] a warm personal friend of Stokes and of Graves,[34] he maintained loyally the traditions of Guy's,[35] and taught us to reverence his great masters. As a teacher he had grasped the fundamental truth announced by John Hunter[36] of the unity of physiological and pathological processes, and, as became the occupant of the chair of the Institutes of Medicine, he would discourse on pathological processes in lectures on physiology, and illustrate the physiology of bioplasm in lectures on the pathology of tumours to the bewilderment of the students. When in September, 1870, he wrote to me that he did not intend to return from the West Indies I felt that I had lost a father and a friend; but in Robert Palmer Howard,[37] of Mon-

30. John Milton (1608–1674), "Lycidas," line 125. The original reads:
   The hungry Sheep look up, and are not fed,
   But swoln with wind, and the rank mist they draw,
   Rot inwardly, and foul contagion spread.

31. T. Wesley *Mills* (1847–1915): Canadian physiologist and veterinarian. He was a classmate of Osler's in Toronto (1867–1869) and later became his colleague at McGill.

32. John Milton, *Paradise Lost*, book 2, lines 559–560. The original reads: "Of Providence" instead of "On Providence" "On" is a mistake by either the printer or Osler. The line which follows is: "And found no end, in wand'ring mazes lost."

33. Richard *Bright* (1789–1858) and Thomas *Addison* (1793–1860): English physicians and researchers at Guy's Hospital and medical school, London. Both described diseases that were later named after them.

34. William *Stokes* (1804–1878): Irish physician known for the study of the stethoscope.
   Robert James *Graves* (1796–1853): Irish physician known for the hyperthyroid disease named after him.
   James Bovell spent a few years in Dublin under Stokes and Graves. He was stricken with typhus, and after recovering from it he returned to Canada.

35. Guy's Hospital: A well-known medical school in London that was active in research.

36. John *Hunter* (1728–1793): Scottish anatomist and surgeon who sharply changed the progress of medicine by his use of postmortem anatomy and human pathology to correlate symptoms with actual causes. Previously, medical research had focused on animal physiology to learn about healthy systems. Hunter's approach was empirical, based on observation. For his biographical information, See "The Old Humanities and the New Science," p. 93, n. 214.

37. Robert Palmer *Howard* (1823–1889): Osler's teacher, mentor, and father figure at McGill University. For further information, see "Aequanimitas," p. 28, n. 42 and "The Student Life," p. 327.

treal, I found a noble step-father, and to these two men, and to my first teacher, the Rev. W. A. Johnson,[38] of Weston, I owe my success in life—if success means getting what you want and being satisfied with it.

II

Of the value of an introductory lecture I am not altogether certain. I do not remember to have derived any enduring benefit from the many that I have been called upon to hear, or from the not a few that I have inflicted in my day. On the whole, I am in favour of abolishing the old custom, but as this is a very special occasion, with special addresses, I consider myself most happy to have been selected for this part of the programme. To the audience at large I fear that what I have to say will appear trite and commonplace, but bear with me, since, indeed, to most of you how good soever the word, the season is long past in which it could be spoken to your edification. As I glance from face to face the most striking single peculiarity is the extraordinary diversity that exists among you. Alike in that you are men and white, you are unlike in your features, very unlike in your minds and in your mental training, and your teachers will mourn the singular inequalities in your capacities. And so it is sad to think will be your careers; for one success, for another failure; one will tread the primrose path to the great bonfire,[39] another the straight and narrow way to renown; some of the best of you will be stricken early on the road, and will join that noble band of youthful martyrs who loved not their lives to the death; others, perhaps the most brilliant among you, like my old friend and comrade, Dick Zimmerman[40] (how he would have rejoiced to see this day!), the Fates will overtake and whirl to destruction just as success seems assured. When the iniquity of oblivion has blindly scattered her poppy over us,[41] some of you will be the trusted counsellors of this

38. William Arthur *Johnson* (1816–1880): Osler's teacher at Trinity College School, a private high school in Weston, where Osler studied for eighteen months. Under the influence of Johnson, Osler developed his interest in natural science, thus choosing the profession of medicine instead of the ministry. For further information, see "A Way of Life," p. 6, n. 17, and "Sir Thomas Browne," p. 33.

39. *tread the primrose path to the great bonfire:* William Shakespeare, *Macbeth,* II, iii, 20–21. The drunken porter talks of those who follow: "go the primrose way to the everlasting bonfire." "The primrose way" means the path of pleasure that leads to Hell, the "everlasting bonfire."

40. Richard *Zimmerman* (1851–1888): Demonstrator in histology, pathology, and surgery. One of Osler's classmates at the Toronto School of Medicine; Osler mourns his untimely death at age thirty-seven.

41. The poppy, because of its narcotic properties, is a symbol of forgetting or sleeping. By "blindly scattered" Osler means that as the poppy seeds are scattered at random, so some students will be forgotten and others remembered, not necessarily in keeping with their merits. Thomas Browne, *Hydriotaphia, Urn-Burial,* in *The Works of Sir Thomas Browne,* ed. Geoffrey Keynes (1658; Chicago: The University of Chicago Press, 1964), vol. 1, p. 167.

community, and the heads of the departments of this Faculty; while for the large majority of you, let us hope, is reserved the happiest and most useful lot given to man—to become vigorous, whole-souled, intelligent, general practitioners.

It seems a bounden duty on such an occasion to be honest and frank, so I propose to tell you the secret of life as I have seen the game played, and as I have tried to play it myself. You remember in one of the Jungle Stories that when Mowgli wished to be avenged on the villagers he could only get the help of Hathi and his sons by sending them the master-word.[42] This I propose to give you in the hope, yes, in the full assurance, that some of you at least will lay hold upon it to your profit. Though a little one, the master-word looms large in meaning. It is the open sesame[43] to every portal, the great equalizer in the world, the true philosopher's stone, which transmutes all the base metal of humanity into gold. The stupid man among you it will make bright, the bright man brilliant, and the brilliant student steady. With the magic word in your heart all things are possible, and without it all study is vanity and vexation. The miracles of life are with it; the blind see by touch, the deaf hear with eyes, the dumb speak with fingers. To the youth it brings hope, to the middle-aged confidence, to the aged repose. True balm of hurt minds, in its presence the heart of the sorrowful is lightened and consoled. It is directly responsible for all advances in medicine during the past twenty-five centuries. Laying hold upon it Hippocrates[44] made observation and science the warp and woof[45] of our art. Galen[46] so read its meaning that fifteen centuries stopped thinking, and slept until awakened by the *De Fabrica* of Vesalius,[47] which is the very incarnation of the master-word. With its inspiration Harvey[48] gave an impulse to a larger circulation than he

---

42. Rudyard Kipling, "Letting in the Jungle," in *The Second Jungle Book* (1895; New York: Doubleday, Doran, 1929), p. 96. The original reads: "I have a Master-word for him now. Bid him come to Mowgli, the Frog, and if he does not hear at first, bid him come because of the Sack of the Fields of Bhurtpore." Osler here alludes to the Master-word of medicine, instead of the Master-word of the Jungle in the original. Kipling was one of Osler's favorite authors. When he was dying of bronchial pneumonia, among the books he enjoyed having read to him he especially asked for something from the *Jungle Books* (Cushing, vol. 2, p. 684).

43. *open sesame:* The magic words that open the thieves' treasury in the tale of "Ali Baba and the Forty Thieves" in *The Arabian Nights*.

44. *Hippocrates* (c.460–c.375 B.C.): Osler, at the end of this speech, refers to the Hippocratic oath as a guideline to medical students. See p. 274, n. 108.

45. *warp and woof:* The lengthwise and crosswise threads, respectively, in weaving; hence, the very essence or substance of anything.

46. Claudius *Galen* (c.130–c.200 A.D.): His observations of animal anatomy contained many errors that were not questioned due to his authority. See "Teaching and Thinking," p. 181, n. 27.

47. Andreas *Vesalius* (1514–1564): See "The Leaven of Science," p. 163, n. 62.

48. William *Harvey* (1578–1657): See "Teacher and Student," p. 116, n. 22.

wot of,[49] an impulse which we feel to-day. Hunter [50] sounded all its heights and depths, and stands out in our history as one of the great exemplars of its virtue. With it Virchow [51] smote the rock, and the waters of progress gushed out;[52] while in the hands of Pasteur [53] it proved a very talisman to open to us a new heaven in medicine and a new earth in surgery. Not only has it been the touchstone of progress, but it is the measure of success in every-day life. Not a man before you but is beholden to it for his position here, while he who addresses you has that honour directly in consequence of having had it graven on his heart when he was as you are to-day. And the master-word is *Work*, a little one, as I have said, but fraught with momentous sequences if you can but write it on the tablets of your hearts, and bind it upon your foreheads. But there is a serious difficulty in getting you to understand the paramount importance of the work-habit as part of your organization. You are not far from the Tom Sawyer stage with its philosophy "that work consists of whatever a body is obliged to do, and that play consists of whatever a body is not obliged to do."[54]

A great many hard things may be said of the work-habit. For most of us it means a hard battle; the few take to it naturally; the many prefer idleness and never learn to love labour. Listen to this: "Look at one of your industrious fellows for a moment, I beseech you,"[55] says Robert Louis Stevenson. "He sows hurry and reaps indigestion; he puts a vast deal of activity out to interest, and receives a large measure of nervous derangement in return. Either he absents himself entirely from all fellowship, and lives a recluse in a garret, with carpet slippers and a leaden inkpot, or he comes among people swiftly and bitterly, in a contraction of his whole nervous system, to discharge some temper before he returns to work. I do not care how much or how well he works, this fellow is an evil feature in other people's lives."[56] These are the sentiments of an over-

49. *wot:* To know. Osler has incorrectly used "he wot" as a past tense, instead of "he wist."

50. *Hunter:* See p. 260, n. 36.

51. Rudolf *Virchow* (1821–1902): See "The Old Humanities and the New Science," p. 75, n. 80.

52. Psalm 78:20. The exact quotation is: "Behold, he smote the rock, that the waters gushed out, and the streams overflowed." This text refers to the passage in Exodus 18:6, where Moses strikes a rock with his rod and water gushes out.

53. Louis *Pasteur* (1822–1895): French chemist who developed and used a curative and preventive treatment for hydrophobia in men and for rabies in dogs. he was founder of the science of bacteriology and known for his work on preventative medicine.

54. Mark Twain, *The Adventures of Tom Sawyer* (1876; London: the Penguin Group, 1986), p. 17, in the famous episode of the whitewashed fence.

55. Robert Louis Stevenson, "An Apology for Idlers," in *Virginibus Puerisque* (1881; New York: Charles Scribner's Sons, 1924), vol. 13, p. 77.

56. Ibid.

worked, dejected man; let me quote the motto of his saner moments: "To travel hopefully is better than to arrive, and the true success is in labour."[57] If you wish to learn of the miseries of scholars in order to avoid them, read part I, section 2, member 3, subsection 15, of that immortal work, the *Anatomy of Melancholy;*[58] but I am here to warn you against these evils, and to entreat you to form good habits in your student days.

At the outset appreciate clearly the aims and objects each one of you should have in view—a knowledge of disease and its cure, and a knowledge of yourself. The one, special education, will make you a practitioner of medicine; the other, an inner education, may make you a truly good man, four square and without a flaw. The one is extrinsic and is largely accomplished by teacher and tutor, by text and by tongue; the other is intrinsic and is the mental salvation to be wrought out by each one for himself. The first may be had without the second; any one of you may become an active practitioner, without ever having had sense enough to realize that through life you have been a fool; or you may have the second without the first, and, without knowing much of the art, you may have the endowments of head and heart that make the little you do possess go very far in the community. With what I hope to infect you is a desire to have a due proportion of each.

So far as your professional education is concerned, what I shall say may make for each one of you an easy path easier. The multiplicity of the subjects to be studied is a difficulty, and it is hard for teacher and student to get a due sense of proportion in the work. We are in a transition stage in our methods of teaching, and have not everywhere got away from the idea of the examination as the "be-all and end-all;"[59] so that the student has constantly before his eyes the magical letters of the degree he seeks. And this is well, perhaps, if you will remember that having, in the old phrase, commenced Bachelor of Medicine, you have only reached a point from which you can begin a life-long process of education.

So many and varied are the aspects presented by this theme that I can only lay stress upon a few of the more essential. The very first step towards success

57. Ibid., "El Dorado," p. 109. The last sentence of the essay.

58. Robert Burton, "Marsilius Ficinus," in *Anatomy of Melancholy* (1621; Boston: William Veazie, 1859), vol. 1, p. 399–400. The original reads: "Hard students are commonly troubled with gouts, catarrhs, rheums, cachexia, bradypepsia, bad eyes, stone, and colic, crudities, oppilations, vertigo, winds, consumptions, and all such diseases as come by overmuch sitting; they are most part lean, dry, ill-coloured, spend their fortunes, lose their wits, and many times their lives, and all through immoderate pains and extraordinary studies."

59. William Shakespeare, *Macbeth*, I, vii, 5.

in any occupation is to become interested in it. Locke[60] put this in a very happy way when he said, give a pupil "a relish of knowledge"[61] and you put life into his work. And there is nothing more certain than that you cannot study well if you are not interested in your profession. Your presence here is a warrant that in some way you have become attracted to the study of medicine, but the speculative possibilities so warmly cherished at the outset are apt to cool when in contact with the stern realities of the class-room. Most of you have already experienced the all-absorbing attraction of the scientific branches, and nowadays the practical method of presentation has given a zest which was usually lacking in the old theoretical teaching. The life has become more serious in consequence, and medical students have put away many of the childish tricks with which we used to keep up their bad name. Compare the picture of the "sawbones"[62] of 1842, as given in the recent biography of Sir Henry Acland,[63] with the representatives to-day, and it is evident a great revolution has been effected, and very largely by the salutary influences of improved methods of education. It is possible now to fill out a day with practical work, varied enough to prevent monotony, and so arranged that the knowledge is picked out by the student himself, and not thrust into him, willy-nilly,[64] at the point of the tongue. He exercises his wits and is no longer a passive Strasbourg goose, tied up and stuffed to repletion.

How can you take the greatest possible advantage of your capacities with the least possible strain? By cultivating system. I say cultivating advisedly, since some of you will find the acquisition of systematic habits very hard. There are minds congenitally systematic; others have a life-long fight against an inherited tendency to diffuseness and carelessness in work. A few brilliant fellows try to dispense with it altogether, but they are a burden to their brethren and a sore trial

60. John *Locke* (1632–1704): See "After Twenty-Five Years," p. 213, n. 40.

61. *a relish of knowledge:* See "After Twenty-Five Years," p. 213, n. 42.

62. *sawbones:* A disparaging term for surgeons, particularly ships' surgeons, who in old times were often the least skilled of their profession. Osler here is contrasting the state of surgical skill at the time when he was writing to what was common sixty years earlier. He might well have got the word from his father, who was in the navy before he went into the church. Osler is referring to the account of Acland's time at St. George's Hospital, London. James Beresford Atlay, *Sir Henry Wentworth Acland* (London: Smith Elder, 1903), pp. 81ff.

63. Henry Wentworth *Acland* (1815–1900): Oxford professor of sanitation and medicine (1858–1894) who tried to introduce biology and chemistry into the ordinary curriculum at Oxford. He studied the relations between the practice of medicine and the state of the natural sciences. It was in Acland's library that Osler first saw the panel of three portraits—Linacre, Harvey, and Sydenham. "He made such an ado about it that Mrs. Osler subsequently asked Sir Henry if they might not be copied for him as a birthday present. This was done, and in turn the triumvirate came to adorn the mantel of his own library and office" (Cushing, vol. 1, p. 401).

64. *willy-nilly:* willingly or unwillingly.

to their intimates. I have heard it remarked that order is the badge of an ordinary mind.[65] So it may be, but as practitioners of medicine we have to be thankful to get into that useful class. Let me entreat those of you who are here for the first time to lay to heart what I say on this matter. Forget all else, but take away this counsel of a man who has had to fight a hard battle, and not always a successful one, for the little order he has had in his life; take away with you a profound conviction of the value of system in your work. I appeal to the freshmen especially, because you to-day make a beginning, and your future career depends very much upon the habits you will form during this session. To follow the routine of the classes is easy enough, but to take routine into every part of your daily life is a hard task. Some of you will start out joyfully as did Christian and Hopeful, and for many days will journey safely towards the Delectable Mountains, dreaming of them and not thinking of disaster until you find yourselves in the strong captivity of Doubt and under the grinding tyranny of Despair.[66] You have been over-confident. Begin again and more cautiously. No student escapes wholly from these perils and trials; be not disheartened, expect them. Let each hour of the day have its allotted duty, and cultivate that power of concentration which grows with its exercise, so that the attention neither flags nor wavers, but settles with a bull-dog tenacity on the subject before you. Constant repetition makes a good habit fit easily in your mind, and by the end of the session you may have gained that most precious of all knowledge—the power to work. Do not underestimate the difficulty you will have in wringing from your reluctant selves the stern determination to exact the uttermost minute on your schedule. Do not get too interested in one study at the expense of another, but so map out your day that due allowance is given to each. Only in this way can the average student get the best that he can out of his capacities. And it is worth all the pains and trouble he can possibly take for the ultimate gain—if he can reach his doctorate with system so ingrained that it has become an integral part of his being. The artistic sense of perfection in work is another much-to-be-desired quality to be cultivated. No matter how trifling the matter on hand, do it with a feeling that it demands the best that is in you, and when done look it over with a criti-

65. *order is the badge of an ordinary mind:* Osler may be somewhat vaguely remembering a dictum of Ralph Waldo Emerson, "A foolish consistency is the hobgoblin of little minds." "Self-Reliance," in *Essays: First Series,* no. 2, *The Collected Works of Ralph Waldo Emerson* (Cambridge, Mass.: Harvard University Press, 1979), vol. 2, p. 33.

66. John Bunyan, *Pilgrim's Progress* (1678; London: George Routledge and Son, n.d.), part 1. The Giant Despair finds Christian and Hopeful asleep in his grounds and carries them off to his dungeon in Doubting Castle, where he beats them, tries to make them kill themselves, and threatens to pull them to pieces. When Christian at last finds that his Key of Promise will unlock the dungeon door, they escape and soon arrive at the Delectable Mountains.

cal eye, not sparing a strict judgment of yourself. This it is that makes anatomy a student's touchstone.[67] Take the man who does his "part" to perfection, who has got out all there is in it, who labours over the tags of connective tissue and who demonstrates Meckel's ganglion[68] in his part—this is the fellow in after years who is apt in emergencies, who saves a leg badly smashed in a railway accident, or fights out to the finish, never knowing when he is beaten, in a case of typhoid fever.

Learn to love the freedom of the student life, only too quickly to pass away; the absence of the coarser cares of after days, the joy in comradeship, the delight in new work, the happiness in knowing that you are making progress. Once only can you enjoy these pleasures. The seclusion of the student life is not always good for a man, particularly for those of you who will afterwards engage in general practice, since you will miss that facility of intercourse upon which often the doctor's success depends. On the other hand sequestration is essential for those of you with high ambitions proportionate to your capacity. It was for such that St. Chrysostom gave his famous counsel, "Depart from the highways and transplant thyself into some enclosed ground, for it is hard for a tree that stands by the wayside to keep its fruit till it be ripe."[69]

Has work no dangers connected with it? What of this bogie of overwork of which we hear so much? There are dangers, but they may readily be avoided with a little care. I can only mention two, one physical, one mental. The very best students are often not the strongest. Ill-health, the bridle of Theages,[70] as Plato called it in the case of one of his friends whose mind had thriven at the expense of his body, may have been the diverting influence towards books or the profession. Among the good men who have studied with me there stands out in my remembrance many a young Lycidas, "dead ere his prime,"[71] sacrificed to

67. A test or criterion for judging the qualities of a student.

68. The sphenopalatine ganglion, which was named after Johann Friedrich Meckel (the elder) (1724–1774), a German anatomist.

69. St. John *Chrysostom* (347–407): One of the Fathers of the Greek Church and archbishop of Constantinople, famed for his eloquence, influential writings, and charity to hospitals. Osler has quoted this metaphor from John Donne, *Biathanatos* (1644), part 1, distinction 2, sect. 2, lines 1695–1697. According to M. Rudick in his edition of Donne (1982, p. 214), there is nothing like this metaphor in Chrysostom's homily; so this may be Donne's own embroidery on certain moralizations of scriptural passages on roads and marketplaces given by Chrysostom.

70. Plato, *Republic*, book 6, 496b. "The bridle of Theages" suggests that the bad health of Theages, pupil of Socrates, kept him out of politics and saved him for philosophy. Osler often quotes this expression in his memo book, giving examples of his patients.

71. John Milton, "Lycidas," line 8. This is a memorial poem in honor of Milton's scholarly friend, Edward King of Christ's College, Cambridge, who drowned in 1637. The name Lycidas is taken from "Idyll 7: Harvest Home" of Theocritus (fl. 270 B.C.), the founder of pastoral poetry.

carelessness in habits of living and neglect of ordinary sanitary laws. Medical students are much exposed to infection of all sorts, to combat which the body must be kept in first-class condition. Grosseteste,[72] the great Bishop of Lincoln, remarked that there were three things necessary for temporal salvation—food, sleep and a cheerful disposition. Add to these suitable exercise and you have the means by which good health may be maintained. Not that health is to be a matter of perpetual solicitation, but habits which favour the *corpus sanum* foster the *mens sana*,[73] in which the joy of living and the joy of working are blended in one harmony. Let me read you a quotation from old Burton,[74] the great authority on *morbi eruditorum*.[75] There are "many reasons why students dote more often than others. The first is their negligence; other men look to their tools, a painter will wash his pencils, a smith will look to his hammer, anvil, forge; a husbandman will mend his plough-irons, and grind his hatchet, if it be dull; a falconer or huntsman will have an especial care of his hawks, hounds, horses, dogs, etc.; a musician will string and unstring his lute, etc.; only scholars neglect that instrument, their brain and spirits (I mean) which they daily use."[76]

Much study is not only believed to be a weariness of the flesh,[77] but also an active cause of ill-health of mind, in all grades and phases. I deny that work, legitimate work, has anything to do with this. It is that foul fiend Worry[78] who is responsible for a large majority of the cases. The more carefully one looks into the causes of nervous breakdown in students, the less important is work *per se* as

72. Robert *Grosseteste* (c.1175–1253): English theologian and bishop of Lincoln (1235–1253). He was a staunch defender of church rights against both the pope and the king and a pioneer experimenter in the natural sciences. His translation of Aristotle's *Nicomachean Ethics* was the first known complete translation into Latin and gained a major place in medieval philosophy. As is shown in this passage, he did not approve of excessive strictness. *Monumenta Franciscana*, ed. John Sherren Brewer (London: R. S., 1858), p. 64.

73. *the corpus sanum foster the mens sana:* (Latin) "the sound body fosters the sane mind." Juvenal, *The Satires*, satire 10, line 356. The original reads: "Orandum est ut sit mens sana in corpore sano," ("Your prayer must be for a sound mind in a sound body").

74. Robert Burton, *Anatomy of Melancholy* (1621; Boston: William Veazie, 1859).

75. *morbi eruditorum:* (Latin) diseases of educated people.

76. Osler's original note reads: "Quotation mainly from *Marsilius Ficinus*." Burton is citing Marsilius Ficinus, an Italian philosopher of the fifteenth century. Burton, *Anatomy of Melancholy* (1621; Boston: William Veazie, 1859), p. 303.

77. *much study is not only believed to be a weariness of the flesh:* Ecclesiastes 12:12. The exact quotation is: "Of making many books there *is* no end; and much study *is* a weariness of the flesh."

78. Osler probably refers to Edgar's warning to King Lear when he first puts on the disguise: "Away! The foul fiend follows me!", and also his further warning to the King: "Take heed o' the foul fiend." William Shakespeare, *King Lear*, III, iv, 45, 82. Here Osler is talking about students' nervous breakdown, referring to Lear's madness.

a factor. There are a few cases of genuine overwork, but they are not common. Of the causes of worry in the student life there are three of prime importance to which I may briefly refer.

An anticipatory attitude of mind, a perpetual forecasting, disturbs the even tenor of his way and leads to disaster. Years ago a sentence in one of Carlyle's essays made a lasting impression on me: "Our duty is not to *see* what lies dimly at a distance, but to *do* what lies clearly at hand."[79] I have long maintained that the best motto for a student is, "Take no thought for the morrow."[80] Let the day's work suffice; live for it, regardless of what the future has in store, believing that to-morrow should take thought for the things of itself. There is no such safeguard against the morbid apprehensions about the future, the dread of examinations and the doubt of the ultimate success. Nor is there any risk that such an attitude may breed carelessness. On the contrary, the absorption in the duty of the hour is in itself the best guarantee of ultimate success. "He that observeth the wind shall not sow; and he that regardeth the clouds shall not reap,"[81] which means you cannot work profitably with your mind set upon the future.

Another potent cause of worry is an idolatry by which many of you will be sore let and hindered.[82] The mistress of your studies should be the heavenly Aphrodite,[83] the motherless daughter of Uranus. Give her your whole heart, and she will be your protectress and friend. A jealous creature, brooking no second, if she finds you trifling and coquetting with her rival, the younger, earthly Aphrodite, daughter of Zeus and Dione, she will whistle you off and let you down the wind to be a prey, perhaps to the examiners, certainly to the worm regret. In plainer language, put your affections in cold storage for a few years, and you will take them out ripened, perhaps a bit mellow, but certainly less subject to those frequent changes which perplex so many young men. Only a grand passion, an all-absorbing devotion to the elder goddess can save the man with a congenital tendency to philandering, the flighty Lydgate who sports with Celia

79. This is Osler's motto. Thomas Carlyle, *Signs of the Times* (1829), the opening passage, in *Critical and Miscellaneous Essays* (New York: C. Scribner's Sons, 1900), vol. 2, p. 56. Osler here substitutes "our duty" for "our grand business" in the original. He quotes and explains how he came across this passage in "A Way of Life," p. 6.

80. Matthew 6:34. Sermon on the Mount. Osler elaborates this philosophy in "A Way of Life," pp. 6–9.

81. Ecclesiastes 11:4.

82. *sore let and hindered:* This is a reminiscence of the collect for the fourth Sunday in Advent in the *Book of Common Prayer.* The word "let" here means "obstructed" or "impeded."

83. According to Socrates in Plato's *Symposium* (180d–181c), the Greek goddess of love and beauty had a dual aspect: Aphrodite *Pandemos,* patroness of physical love, and the older Aphrodite *Titania,* patroness of spiritual and intellectual love; the latter is the one Osler is referring to as the elder goddess.

and Dorothea, and upon whom the judgment ultimately falls in a basil-plant of a wife like Rosamond.[84]

And thirdly, one and all of you will have to face the ordeal of every student in this generation who sooner or later tries to mix the waters of science with the oil of faith. You can have a great deal of both if you only keep them separate. The worry comes from the attempt at mixture. As general practitioners you will need all the faith you can carry, and while it may not always be of the conventional pattern, when expressed in your lives rather than on your lips, the variety is not a bad one from the standpoint of St. James;[85] and may help to counteract the common scandal alluded to in the celebrated diary of that gossipy old pastor-doctor, the Rev. John Ward:[86] "One told the Bishop of Gloucester that he imagined physicians of all other men the most competent judges of all other affairs of religion—and his reason was because they were wholly unconcerned with it."[87]

III

Professional work of any sort tends to narrow the mind, to limit the point of view and to put a hall-mark on a man of a most unmistakable kind. On the one hand are the intense, ardent natures, absorbed in their studies and quickly losing interest in everything but their profession, while other faculties and interests "fust" unused.[88] On the other hand are the bovine[89] brethren, who think of nothing but the treadmill and the corn. From very different causes, the one from concentration, the other from apathy, both are apt to neglect those outside studies that widen the sympathies and help a man to get the best there is out of life. Like art, medicine is an exacting mistress, and in the pursuit of one of the scien-

84. *Lydgate, Celia, Dorothea,* and *Rosamond* are characters in *Middlemarch* (1871), written by George Eliot (1819–1880). Lydgate, a physician and medical reformer, got married to Rosamond, a selfish and ambitious woman. It is said that Sir Henry Acland, professor of medicine at Oxford, is the model for this hero.

85. The author of the Epistle of James in the New Testament. He writes as follows: "Ye see then how that by works a man is justified, and not by faith only" (James 2:24).

86. John *Ward* (1629–1681): Vicar of Stratford-upon-Avon. His diary extends from 1648 to 1679, and was edited by Charles Severn, M.D., in 1839.

87. John Ward, *Diary of the Rev. John Ward* (1648–1679; London: H. Colburn, 1839), p. 100.

88. William Shakespeare, *Hamlet,* IV, iv, 39. To "fust" means to "grow musty." The exact quotation is:

> Sure, He that made us with such large discourse,
> Looking before and after, gave us not
> That capability and godlike reason
> To fust in us unused.

89. *bovine:* Like cattle; dull, stolid.

tific branches, sometimes, too, in practice, not a portion of a man's spirit may be left free for other distractions, but this does not often happen. On account of the intimate personal nature of his work, the medical man, perhaps more than any other man, needs that higher education of which Plato speaks,—"that education in virtue from youth upwards, which enables a man eagerly to pursue the ideal perfection."[90] It is not for all, nor can all attain to it, but there is comfort and help in the pursuit, even though the end is never reached. For a large majority the daily round and the common task furnish more than enough to satisfy their heart's desire, and there seems no room left for anything else. Like the good, easy man whom Milton scores in the *Areopagitica*, whose religion was a "traffic so entangled that of all mysteries he could not skill to keep a stock going upon that trade" and handed it over with all the locks and keys to "a divine of note and estimation," so it is with many of us in the matter of this higher educa-tion. No longer intrinsic, wrought in us and ingrained, it has become, in Milton's phrase, a "dividual movable,"[91] handed over nowadays to the daily press or to the haphazard instruction of the pulpit, the platform or the magazines. Like a good many other things, it comes in a better and more enduring form if not too consciously sought. The all-important thing is to get a relish[92] for the good com-pany of the race in a daily intercourse with some of the great minds of all ages. Now, in the spring-time of life, pick your intimates among them, and begin a systematic cultivation of their works. Many of you will need a strong leaven[93] to raise you above the dough in which it will be your lot to labour. Uncongenial surroundings, an ever-present dissonance between the aspirations within and the actualities without, the oppressive discords of human society, the bitter tragedies of life, the *lacrymae rerum*,[94] beside the hidden springs of which we sit in sad despair—all these tend to foster in some natures a cynicism quite foreign to our vocation, and to which this inner education offers the best antidote. Personal contact with men of high purpose and character will help a man to make a start—to have the desire, at least, but in its fulness this culture—for that word best expresses it—has to be wrought out by each one for himself. Start at once a bed-side library[95] and spend the last half hour of the day in communion with the saints of humanity. There are great lessons to be learned from Job and from

90. Plato, *Laws*, book 1, 643e.

91. John Milton, *Areopagitica*, in *The Works of John Milton*, ed. William Haller (1644; New York: Colum-bia University Press, 1931), vol. 4, pp. 333–334.

92. *get a relish:* See "After Twenty-Five Years", p. 213, n. 42.

93. *leaven:* See "The Leaven of Science," p. 153, n.

94. *lacrymae rerum:* (Latin) the innate sadness of human life. The phrase literally means "tears for things." Virgil, *Aeneid*, book 1, line 462.

95. Osler's suggested list of ten books for medical students is printed at the end of this volume.

David, from Isaiah and St. Paul. Taught by Shakespeare you may take your intellectual and moral measure with singular precision. Learn to love Epictetus and Marcus Aurelius. Should you be so fortunate as to be born a Platonist, Jowett will introduce you to the great master through whom alone we can think in certain levels, and whose perpetual modernness startles and delights. Montaigne will teach you moderation in all things, and to be "sealed of his tribe"[96] is a special privilege. We have in the profession only a few great literary heroes of the first rank, the friendship and counsel of two of whom you cannot too earnestly seek. Sir Thomas Browne's *Religio Medici* should be your pocket companion, while from the Breakfast Table Series of Oliver Wendell Holmes you can glean a philosophy of life peculiarly suited to the needs of a physician. There are at least a dozen or more works which would be helpful in getting wisdom in life which only comes to those who earnestly seek it.[97]

A conscientious pursuit of Plato's ideal perfection[98] may teach you the three great lessons of life. *You may learn to consume your own smoke.*[99] The atmosphere is darkened by the murmurings and whimperings of men and women over the non-essentials, the trifles that are inevitably incident to the hurly burly of the day's routine. Things cannot always go your way. Learn to accept in silence the minor aggravations, cultivate the gift of taciturnity and consume your own smoke with an extra draught of hard work, so that those about you may not be annoyed with the dust and soot of your complaints. More than any other the practitioner of medicine may illustrate the second great lesson, *that we are here not to get all we can out of life for ourselves, but to try to make the lives of others happier.*[100] This is the essence of that oft-repeated admonition of Christ, "He that findeth his life shall lose it: and he that loseth his life for my sake shall find it,"[101] on which hard saying if the children of this generation would only lay hold, there would be less misery and discontent in the world. It is not possible for anyone to have better opportunities to live this lesson than you will enjoy. The practice of medicine is an art, not a trade; a calling, not a business; a calling in which your

96. Ben Jonson (1572–1637): poet, playwright, and contemporary of Shakespeare, "An Epistle 49," line 78. The exact quotation is: "Sir, you are Sealed of the Tribe of *Ben,*"—which means counted among his friends. This is also an echo of Revelation 7:5–8.

97. See "Bed-side Library for Medical Students," p. 371.

98. Plato: See p. 271, n. 90.

99. James Russell Lowell, "Chaucer," in *My Study Windows* (1871; Boston: Houghton, Osgood, 1880), p. 228. The exact quotation is: "Poets have forgotten that the first lesson of literature, no less than of life, is the learning how to burn your own smoke."

100. Previously, in "Doctor and Nurse," Osler said, "we are here to add what we can *to*, not to get what we can *from*, life" (p. 105).

101. Matthew 10:39.

heart will be exercised equally with your head. Often the best part of your work will have nothing to do with potions and powders, but with the exercise of an influence of the strong upon the weak, of the righteous upon the wicked, of the wise upon the foolish. To you, as the trusted family counsellor, the father will come with his anxieties, the mother with her hidden grief, the daughter with her trials, and the son with his follies. Fully one-third of the work you do will be entered in other books than yours. Courage and cheerfulness will not only carry you over the rough places of life, but will enable you to bring comfort and help to the weak-hearted and will console you in the sad hours when, like Uncle Toby, you have "to whistle that you may not weep."[102]

And the third lesson you may learn is the hardest of all—that *the law of the higher life is only fulfilled by love, i.e. charity.*[103] Many a physician whose daily work is a daily round of beneficence will say hard things and think hard thoughts of a colleague. No sin will so easily beset you as uncharitableness towards your brother practitioner. So strong is the personal element in the practice of medicine, and so many are the wagging tongues in every parish, that evil-speaking, lying, and slandering find a shining mark in the lapses and mistakes which are inevitable in our work. There is no reason for discord and disagreement, and the only way to avoid trouble is to have two plain rules. From the day you begin practice never under any circumstances listen to a tale told to the detriment of a brother practitioner. And when any dispute or trouble does arise, go frankly, ere sunset, and talk the matter over, in which way you may gain a brother and a friend. Very easy to carry out, you may think! Far from it; there is no harder battle to fight. Theoretically there seems to be no difficulty, but when the concrete wound is rankling, and after Mrs. Jones has rubbed in the cayenne pepper by declaring that Dr. J. told her in confidence of your shocking bungling, your attitude of mind is that you would rather see him in purgatory than make advances towards reconciliation. Wait until the day of your trial comes and then remember my words.

And in closing, may I say a few words to the younger practitioners in the audience whose activities will wax not wane with the growing years of the century which opens so auspiciously for this school, for this city, and for our country. You enter a noble heritage, made so by no efforts of your own, but by the generations of men who have unselfishly sought to do the best they could for suffering mankind. Much has been done, much remains to do; a way has been opened, and to the possibilities in the scientific development of medicine there

102. Laurence Sterne, *The Life and Opinions of Tristram Shandy* (1759–1767), book 1, chap. 21. Uncle Toby is Tristram Shandy's uncle.

103. Mark 12:30–31. Romans 13:8–10. 1. Corinthians 13:13. Galatians 5:14.

seems to be no limit. Except in its application, as general practitioners, you will not have much to do with this. Yours is a higher and more sacred duty. Think not to light a light to shine before men that they may see your good works;[104] contrariwise, you belong to the great army of quiet workers, physicians and priests, sisters and nurses, all over the world, the members of which strive not neither do they cry, nor are their voices heard in the streets,[105] but to them is given the ministry of consolation in sorrow, need, and sickness. Like the ideal wife of whom Plutarch speaks,[106] the best doctor is often the one of whom the public hears the least; but nowadays, in the fierce light that beats upon the hearth,[107] it is increasingly difficult to lead the secluded life in which our best work is done. To you the silent workers of the ranks, in villages and country districts, in the slums of our large cities, in the mining camps and factory towns, in the homes of the rich, and in the hovels of the poor, to you is given the harder task of illustrating with your lives the Hippocratic standards of Learning, of Sagacity, of Humanity, and of Probity.[108] Of learning, that you may apply in your practice the best that is known in our art, and that with the increase in your knowledge there may be an increase in that priceless endowment of sagacity, so that to all, everywhere, skilled succour may come in the hour of need. Of a humanity, that will show in your daily life tenderness and consideration to the weak, infinite pity to the suffering, and broad charity to all. Of a probity, that will make you under all circumstances true to yourselves, true to your high calling, and true to your fellow man.

104. *Think not to light a light to shine before men that they may see your good works:* Matthew 5:16. Osler has altered the quote slightly. The original reads: "Let your light so shine before men, that they may see your good works."

105. *strive not neither do they cry, nor are their voices heard in the streets:* Matthew 12:19. The original reads: "He shall not strive, nor cry; neither shall any man hear his voice in the streets."

106. According to Plutarch (c.46–c.120 A.D.), the ideal wife "ought to be modest and guarded about saying anything in the hearing of outsiders, since it is an exposure of herself; for in her talk can be seen her feelings, character, and disposition." "Advice to Bride and Groom," in *Plutarch's Moralia* 142d., trans. Frank Cole Babbitt (Cambridge, Mass: Harvard University Press, 1928), vol. 2, pp. 321–323.

107. Alfred Tennyson, "The Idylls of the King," dedication, line 26. The original line reads: "In that fierce light which beats upon a throne."

108. *Hippocrates* (c.460–c.375 B.C.): Greek physician and founder of scientific medicine, considered the father of medicine. The Hippocratic Oath continues to be the basis of medical ethics for present-day physicians. The text of the oath itself is divided into two major sections. "The first sets out the obligations of the physician to students of medicine and the duties of pupil to teacher. In the second section the physician pledges to prescribe only beneficial treatments, according to his abilities and judgment; to refrain from causing harm or hurt; and to live an exemplary personal and professional life" (*The New Encyclopædia Britannica*)

15

THE HOSPITAL AS

A COLLEGE

The Hospital is the only proper College in which to rear a true disciple of Æsculapius.
JOHN ABERNETHY, *source unknown*

The most essential part of a student's instruction is obtained, as I believe, not in the lecture room, but at the bedside. Nothing seen there is lost; the rhythms of disease are learned by frequent repetition; its unforeseen occurrences stamp themselves indelibly on the memory. Before the student is aware of what he has acquired he has learned the aspects and causes and probable issue of the diseases he has seen with his teacher, and the proper mode of dealing with them, so far as his master knows.
OLIVER WENDELL HOLMES, "Introductory Lecture," *Medical Essays*

OSLER ADVOCATES THAT the third and fourth years of medical training should be entirely clinical. For advanced students, there should be no teaching without "a patient for a text." Students should be placed in hospitals, not as observers but as practitioners. By 1903, when this talk was given to the New York Academy of Medicine, there had already been a revolution in medical education, including a longer period of study and stricter admission requirements. The most significant change had been the shift of emphasis from lectures to laboratory work, providing more practical knowledge, mental training, and exposure to the scientific habit of mind.

Osler recommends assigning third-year students to outpatient and surgical wards for long-term, routine patient checkups under skilled supervision. In the Johns Hopkins Medical School plan, the third year is spent in a systematic course of diagnosis in rooms adjacent to the outpatient department. Students take histories and report on their cases to teachers and fellow students. They study clinical microscopy in the hospital's teaching laboratory, working on their own cases under the direction of lab experts. The most interesting cases are shared in the amphitheatre.

The fourth year should be spent in ward *work,* not ward classes. Under supervision, students should be assigned four or five beds in a ward, with complete responsibility for the care of those patients, including the performance of lab work. They should also periodically help with rounds in all the wards.

These improvements would require changes in most hospitals. A system of clinical clerks and surgical dressers would be needed to give staff doctors more time to oversee students. Interaction with students would challenge doctors and keep them from becoming apathetic. Osler concludes with a reminder that students must always focus on the treatment of disease.

THE HOSPITAL AS
A COLLEGE

I

THE LAST QUARTER of the last century saw many remarkable changes and reformations, among which in far-reaching general importance not one is to be compared with the reform, or rather revolution, in the teaching of the science and art of medicine. Whether the conscience of the professors at last awoke, and felt the pricking of remorse, or whether the change, as is more likely, was only part of that larger movement toward larger events in the midst of which we are to-day, need not be here discussed. The improvement has been in three directions: in demanding of the student a better general education; in lengthening the period of professional study; and in substituting laboratories for lecture rooms—that is to say, in the replacement of theoretical by practical teaching. The problem before us as teachers may be very briefly stated: to give to our students an education of such a character that they can become sensible practitioners—the destiny of seven-eighths of them. Toward this end are all our endowments, our multiplying laboratories, our complicated curricula, our palatial buildings. In the four years' course a division is very properly made between the preparatory or scientific branches and the practical; the former are taught in the school or college, the latter in the hospital. Not that there is any essential difference; there may be as much science taught in a course of surgery as in a course of embryology. The special growth of the medical school[1] in the past twenty-five years has been in the direction of the

An address delivered at the Academy of Medicine, New York, in December 1903.
1. Regarding the situation of medical education, Henry E. Sigerist (1891–1957) later wrote: "The revo-

practical teaching of science. Everywhere the lectures have been supplemented or replaced by prolonged practical courses, and instead of a single laboratory devoted to anatomy, there are now laboratories of physiology, of physiological chemistry, of pathology, of pharmacology, and of hygiene. Apart from the more attractive mode of presentation and the more useful character of the knowledge obtained in this way, the student learns to use the instruments of precision, gets a mental training of incalculable value, and perhaps catches some measure of the scientific spirit. The main point is that he has no longer merely theoretical knowledge acquired in a lecture room, but a first-hand practical acquaintance with the things themselves. He not only has dissected the sympathetic system, but he has set up a kymograph and can take a blood pressure observation, he has personally studied the action of digitalis, of chloroform and of ether, he has made his own culture media and he has "plated" organisms. The young fellow who is sent on to us in his third year is nowadays a fairly well-trained man and in a position to begin his life's work in those larger laboratories, private and public, which nature fills with her mistakes and experiments.

How can we make the work of the student in the third and fourth year as practical as it is in his first and second? I take it for granted we all feel that it should be. The answer is, take him from the lecture-room, take him from the amphitheatre—put him in the out-patient department—put him in the wards. It is not the systematic lecture, not the amphitheatre clinic, not even the ward class—all of which have their value—in which the reformation is needed, but in the whole relationship of the senior student to the hospital. During the first two years, he is thoroughly at home in the laboratories, domiciled, we may say, with his place in each one, to which he can go and work quietly under a tutor's direction and guidance. To parallel this condition in the third and fourth years certain reforms are necessary. First, in the conception of how the art of medicine and surgery can be taught. My firm conviction is that we should start the third year student at once on his road of life. Ask any physician of twenty years' standing how he has become proficient in his art, and he will reply, by constant contact with disease; and he will add that the medicine he learned in the schools was totally different from the medicine he learned at the bedside. The graduate of a quarter of a century ago went out with little practical knowledge, which increased only as his practice increased. In what may be called the natural method of teaching the student begins with the patient, continues with the patient, and ends his studies with the patient, using books and lectures as tools, as means to an

lution in medical education began at Johns Hopkins, stressing that the teaching of medicine can never be an exclusively academic matter, that laboratories, dissection rooms, and clinics are indispensable for practical instruction." *American Medicine* (New York: W. W. Norton, 1934), p. 138.

end. The student starts, in fact, as a *practitioner,* as an observer of disordered machines, with the structure and orderly functions of which he is perfectly familiar. Teach him how to observe, give him plenty of facts to observe, and the lessons will come out of the facts themselves. For the junior student in medicine and surgery it is a safe rule to have no teaching without a patient for a text, and the best teaching is that taught by the patient himself. The whole art of medicine is in observation, as the old motto goes,[2] but to educate the eye to see, the ear to hear and the finger to feel takes time, and to make a beginning, to start a man on the right path, is all that we can do. We expect too much of the student and we try to teach him too much. Give him good methods and a proper point of view, and all other things will be added, as his experience grows.

The second, and what is the most important reform, is in the hospital itself. In the interests of the medical student, of the profession, and of the public at large we must ask from the hospital authorities much greater facilities than are at present enjoyed, at least by the students of a majority of the medical schools of this country. The work of the third and fourth year should be taken out of the medical school entirely and transferred to the hospital, which, as Abernethy[3] remarks, is the proper college for the medical student, in his last years at least. An extraordinary difficulty here presents itself. While there are institutions in which the students have all the privileges to be desired, there are others in which they are admitted by side entrances to the amphitheatre of the hospital, while from too many the students are barred as hurtful to the best interests of the patients. The work of an institution in which there is no teaching is rarely first class. There is not that keen interest, nor the thorough study of the cases, nor amid the exigencies of the busy life is the hospital physician able to escape clinical slovenliness unless he teaches and in turn is taught by assistants and students. It is, I think, safe to say that in a hospital with students in the wards the patients are more carefully looked after, their diseases are more fully studied and fewer mistakes made. The larger question, of the extended usefulness of the hospital in promoting the diffusion of medical and surgical knowledge, I cannot here consider.

I envy for our medical students the advantages enjoyed by the nurses, who live in daily contact with the sick, and who have, in this country at least, supplanted the former in the affections of the hospital trustees.[4]

2. In "Precepts" in the *Hippocratic Corpus* (Cambridge, Mass: Harvard University Press, 1957, p. 315) the unknown author writes: "For so I think the whole art has been set forth, by observing some part of the final end in each of many particulars, and then combining all into a single whole." Careful observation is also argued for by the unknown author of "Ancient Medicine" (also in the *Hippocratic Corpus*, pp. 12–63).

3. *Abernethy:* See p. 212, n. 37.

4. Osler probably had the situation of nurses at the Johns Hopkins Hospital in mind. Mary Adelaide Nut-

The objection often raised that patients do not like to have students in the wards is entirely fanciful. In my experience it is just the reverse. On this point I can claim to speak with some authority, having served as a hospital physician for more than twenty-five years, and having taught chiefly in the wards. With the exercise of ordinary discretion, and if one is actuated by kindly feelings towards the patients, there is rarely any difficulty. In the present state of medicine it is very difficult to carry on the work of a first-class hospital without the help of students. We ask far too much of the resident physicians, whose number has not increased in proportion to the enormous increase in the amount of work thrust upon them, and much of the routine work can be perfectly well done by senior students.

II

How, practically, can this be carried into effect? Let us take the third year students first. A class of one hundred students may be divided into ten sections, each of which may be called a clinical unit, which should be in charge of one instructor. Let us follow the course of such a unit through the day. On Mondays, Wednesdays, and Fridays at 9 A.M. elementary instruction in physical diagnosis. From 10 to 12 A.M. practical instruction in the out-patient department. This may consist in part in seeing the cases in a routine way, in receiving instruction on how to take histories, and in becoming familiar with the ordinary aspect of disease as seen in a medical outclinic. At 12 o'clock a senior teacher could meet four, or even five, of the units, dealing more systematically with special cases. The entire morning, or, where it is customary to have the hospital practice in the afternoon, a large part of the afternoon, two or three hours at least, should be spent in the out-patient department. No short six weeks' course, but each clinical unit throughout the session should as a routine see out-patient practice under skilled direction. Very soon these students are able to take histories, have learned how to examine the cases, and the out-patient records gradually become of some value. Of course all of this means abundance of clinical material, proper space in the out-patient department for teaching, sufficient apparatus and young men who are able and willing to undertake the work.

On the alternate days, Tuesdays, Thursdays and Saturdays, the clinical unit (which we are following) is in the surgical out-patient department, seeing minor surgery, learning how to bandage, to give ether, and helping in all the interesting

---

ting (1858–1948), as Superintendent of the Training School of Nurses, worked in close association with hospital administration and the leading minds in medical education, including Osler.

work of a surgical dispensary. Groups of three or four units should be in charge of a demonstrator of morbid anatomy, who would take them to postmortems, the individual men doing the work, and one day in the week all the units could attend the morbid anatomy demonstration of the professor of pathology. I take it for granted that the student has got so far that he has finished his pathological histology in his second year, which is the case in the more advanced schools.

Other hours of the day for the third year could be devoted to the teaching of obstetrics, materia medica, therapeutics, hygiene and clinical microscopy. At the end of the session in a well-conducted school the third-year student is really a very well-informed fellow. He knows the difference between Pott's disease and Pott's fracture; he can readily feel an enlarged spleen, and he knows the difference between Charcot's crystals and Charcot's joint.

In the fourth year I would still maintain the clinical unit of ten men, whose work would be transferred from the out-patient department to the wards. Each man should be allowed to serve in the medical, and, for as long a period as possible, in the surgical wards. He should be assigned four or five beds. He has had experience enough in his third year to enable him to take the history of the new cases, which would need, of course, supervision or correction by the senior house officer or attending physician. Under the supervision of the house physician he does all of the work connected with his own patients; analysis of the urine, etc., and takes the daily record as dictated by the attending physician. One or two of the clinical units are taken round the wards three or four times in the week by one of the teachers for a couple of hours, the cases commented upon, the students asked questions and the groups made familiar with the progress of the cases. In this way the student gets a familiarity with disease, a practical knowledge of clinical methods and a practical knowledge of how to treat disease. With equal advantage the same plan can be followed in the surgical wards and in the obstetrical and gynæcological departments.

An old method, it is the only method by which medicine and surgery can be taught properly, as it is the identical manner in which the physician is himself taught when he gets into practice. The radical reform needed is in the introduction into this country of the system of clinical clerks and surgical dressers, who should be just as much a part of the machinery of the wards as the nurses or the house physicians.

There is no scarcity of material; on the contrary, there is abundance. Think of the plethora of patients in this city, the large majority of whom are never seen, not to say touched, by a medical student! Think of the hundreds of typhoid fever patients, the daily course of whose disease is never watched or studied by our pupils! Think how few of the hundreds of cases of pneumonia which will enter the hospitals during the next three months, will be seen daily, hourly, in the wards by the fourth year men! And yet it is for this they are in the medical school, just as much as, more indeed, than they are in it to learn the physiology of the liver or the anatomy of the hip-joint.

But, you may ask, how does such a plan work in practice? From a long experience I can answer, admirably! It has been adopted in the Johns Hopkins Medical School, of which the hospital, by the terms of the founder's will, is an essential part.[5] There is nothing special in our material, our wards are not any better than those in other first-class hospitals, but a distinctive feature is that greater provision is made for teaching students and perhaps for the study of disease. Let me tell you in a few words just how the work is conducted. The third year students are taught medicine:

First, in a systematic course of physical diagnosis conducted by Drs. Thayer and Futcher,[6] the Associate Professors of Medicine, in the rooms adjacent to the out-patient department. In the second half of the year, after receiving instruction in history-taking, the students take notes and examine out-patients.

Secondly, three days in the week at the conclusion of the out-patient hours, the entire class meets the teacher in an adjacent room, and the students are taught how to examine and study patients. It is remarkable how many interesting cases can be shown in the course of a year in this way. Each student who takes a case is expected to report upon and "keep track" of it, and is questioned with reference to its progress. The opportunity is taken to teach the student how to look up questions in the literature by setting subjects upon which to report in connexion with the cases they have seen. A class of fifty can be dealt with very conveniently in this manner.

Thirdly, the clinical microscopy class. The clinical laboratory is part of the hospital equipment. It is in the charge of a senior assistant, who is one of the resident officers of the hospital. There is room in it for about one hundred students on two floors, each man having his own work-table and locker and a place in which he can have his own specimens and work at odd hours. The course is a systematic one, given throughout the session, from two hours to two hours and a half twice a week, and consists of routine instruction in the methods of exam-

---

5. The hospital and medical school were established with $7 million from the estate of Johns Hopkins (1795–1873), a wealthy, frugal businessman who was a bachelor. The London banker and philanthropist George Peabody convinced him that two things were sure to endure: "A university, for there will always be youth to train; and a hospital, for there will always be suffering to relieve" (Cushing, vol. 1, p. 311).

6. William Sydney *Thayer* (1864–1932): Professor of medicine at Johns Hopkins University. He was president of the American Medical Association (1928–1929).

Thomas Barnes *Futcher* (1871–1938): Professor of medicine at Johns Hopkins University.

ining the blood and secretions, the gastric contents, urine, etc. This can be made a most invaluable course, enabling the student to continue the microscopic work which he has had in his first and second years, and he familiarizes himself with the use of a valuable instrument, which becomes in this way a clinical tool and not a mere toy. The clinical laboratory in the medical school should be connected with the hospital, of which it is an essential part. Nowadays the microscopical, bacteriological and chemical work of the wards demands skilled labour, and the house physicians as well as the students need the help and supervision of experts in clinical chemistry and bacteriology, who should form part of the resident staff of the institution.

Fourthly, the general medical clinic. One day in the week, in the amphitheatre, a clinic is held for the third and fourth year students and the more interesting cases in the wards are brought before them. As far as possible we present the diseases of the seasons, and in the autumn special attention is given to malarial and typhoid fever, and later in the winter to pneumonia. Committees are appointed to report on every case of pneumonia and the complications of typhoid fever. There are no systematic lectures, but in the physical diagnosis classes there are set recitations, and in what I call the observation class in the dispensary held three times a week, general statements are often made concerning the diseases under consideration.

Fourth Year Ward Work.—The class is divided into three groups (one in medicine, one in surgery, and one in obstetrics and gynecology) which serve as clinical clerks and surgical dressers. In medicine each student has five or six beds. He takes notes of the new cases as they come in, does the urine and blood work and helps the house physician in the general care of the patients. From nine to eleven the visit is made with the clinical clerks, and systematic instruction is given. The interesting cases are seen and new cases are studied, and the students questioned with reference to the symptoms and nature of the disease and the course of treatment. What I wish to emphasize is that this method of teaching is not a ward-class in which a group of students is taken into the ward and a case or two demonstrated; it is *ward-work*, the students themselves taking their share in the work of the hospital, just as much as the attending physician, the interne, or the nurse. Moreover, it is not an occasional thing. His work in medicine for the three months is his major subject and the clinical clerks have from nine to twelve for their ward-work, and an hour in the afternoon in which some special questions are dealt with by the senior assistant or by the house physicians.

The Recitation Class.—As there are no regular lectures, to be certain that all of the subjects in medicine are brought before the students in a systematic manner, a recitation class is held once a week upon subjects set beforehand.

The Weekly Clinic in the amphitheatre, in which the clinical clerks take leading parts, as they report upon their cases and read the notes of their cases brought before the class for consideration. Certain important aspects of medicine are constantly kept before this class. Week after week the condition of the typhoid fever cases is discussed, the more interesting cases shown, the complications systematically placed upon the board. A pneumonia committee deals with all the clinical features of this common disease, and a list of the cases is kept on the blackboard, and during a session the students have reports upon fifty or sixty cases, a large majority of which are seen in the clinic by all of them, while the clinical clerks have in the wards an opportunity of studying them daily.

The general impression among the students and the junior teachers is that the system has worked well. There are faults, perhaps more than we see, but I am sure they are not in the system. Many of the students are doubtless not well informed theoretically on some subjects, as personally I have always been opposed to that base and most pernicious system of educating them with a view to examinations, but even the dullest learn how to examine patients, and get familiar with the changing aspects of the important acute diseases. The pupil handles a sufficient number of cases to get a certain measure of technical skill, and there is ever kept before him the idea that he is not in the hospital to learn everything that is known but to learn how to study disease and how to treat it, or rather, how to treat patients.

III

A third change is in reorganization of the medical school. This has been accomplished in the first two years by an extraordinary increase in the laboratory work, which has necessitated an increase in the teaching force, and indeed an entirely new conception of how such subjects as physiology, pharmacology and pathology should be taught. A corresponding reformation is needed in the third and fourth years. Control of ample clinical facilities is as essential to-day as large, well-endowed laboratories, and the absence of this causes the clinical to lag behind the scientific education. Speaking for the Departmnent of Medicine, I should say that three or four well-equipped medical clinics of fifty to seventy-five beds each, with out-patient departments under the control of the directors, are required for a school of maximum size, say eight hundred students. Within the next quarter of a century the larger universities of this country will have their own hospitals in which the problems of nature known as disease will be studied as thoroughly as are those of geology or Sanscrit. But even with present conditions much may be done. There are hundreds of earnest students, thousands of patients, and scores of well-equipped young men willing and anxious to do practical teaching. Too often, as you know full well, "the hungry sheep look up and are not fed;"[7] for the bread of the wards they are given the stones[8] of the lecture-room and amphitheatre. The dissociation of student and patient is a legacy of the pernicious system of theoretical teaching from which we have escaped in the first and second years.

For the third and fourth year students, the hospital is the college; for the juniors, the out-patient department and the clinics; for the seniors, the wards. They should be in the hospital as part of its equipment, as an essential part, without which the work cannot be of the best. They should be in it as the place in which alone they can learn the elements of their art and the lessons which will be of service to them when in practice for themselves. The hospital with students in its dispensaries and wards doubles its usefulness in a community. The stimulus of their presence neutralizes that clinical apathy certain, sooner or later, to beset the man who makes lonely "rounds" with his house-physician. Better work is done for the profession and for the public; the practical education of young men, who carry with them to all parts of the country good methods, extends enormously the work of an institution, and the profession is recruited by men who have been taught to think and to observe for themselves, and who become independent practitioners of the new school of scientific medicine—men whose faith in the possibilities of their art has been strengthened, not weakened, by a knowledge of its limitations. It is no new method which I advocate, but the old method of Boerhaave,[9] of the elder Rutherford of the Edinburgh school,[10] of the older men of this city, and of Boston and of Philadelphia—the men who had been pupils of John Hunter[11] and of Rutherford[12] and of Saunders.[13] It makes of the hospital a college in which, as clinical clerks and surgical dressers, the students slowly learn for themselves, under skilled direction, the phenomena of disease. It is the true method, because it is the natural one, the only one by which a physician grows in clinical wisdom after he begins practice for himself—all others are bastard substitutes.

7. John Milton, "Lycidas," line 125.

8. *bread and stones:* Matthew 7:9: "Or what man is there of you, whom if his son ask bread, will he give him a stone?" Also in Luke 11:11.

9. Hermann *Boerhaave* (1668–1738): Dutch physician who taught at Leyden (now Leiden) University, then the most famous medical institution in Europe. He was the first to teach by taking his students into a hospital.

10. John *Rutherford* (1695–1779): Scottish physician who introduced clinical teaching methods at the University of Edinburgh.

11. John *Hunter* (1728–1793): See "The Old Humanities and the New Science," p. 93, n. 214.

12. *Rutherford:* See p. 285, n. 10.

13. Richard Huck *Saunders* (1720–1785): Scottish physician. After a seventeen-year experience in the army he became physician at St. Thomas' Hospital in London until he retired in 1777.

16

THE FIXED PERIOD

Tho' much is taken, much abides.
ALFRED TENNYSON "Ulysses"

IN 1905, AFTER SIXTEEN YEARS, Osler left Johns Hopkins Medical School. On this occasion his speech, with praise for early retirement, caused much controversy. Osler was clearly surprised that this view had received so much negative attention.

This speech is an attempt to explain why one would retire before one is forced to, while still in good health and on good terms with congenial colleagues. Osler argues that individuals should not stay in one place too long and become stagnant. Furthermore, the university does not suffer from the loss of an individual. "A proper nomadic spirit" is desirable for an academic. Osler praises the English system of a "fixed period," with retirement either at a set age or after a fixed length of service. He maintains that one's most productive years are from ages twenty-five to forty; after that the role of older faculty should be to encourage and mentor younger ones.

He further argues that men over sixty should retire from commercial, political, and professional life. It is at this point that he mentions Trollope's thesis, adding that it does not seem so bad to one who has seen the problems that befall older people and some of the problems they cause (bad books, sermons, speeches, etc.)! Although urging early retirement (clearly in terms that were misunderstood) Osler emphasizes that one must live with the young and maintain a fresh outlook on the world's problems.

In what is meant to be the main point of this talk, Osler reviews the accomplishments of the Johns Hopkins Medical School. In sixteen years it had become one of the best schools in the world, demonstrating how medical students should be taught. Medical students at Johns Hopkins were integrated into the daily work of the hospital, giving them first-hand knowledge of diseases. Oster praises those who had connected the hospital with the university, required science courses for admission, and developed a curriculum emphasizing work in laboratory and clinic. He especially lauds the university's founder and president D. C. Gilman.

Osler notes that the United States no longer needs to depend on other countries for training and medical science. American scientific medicine had finally achieved a place in the world, including the establishment of prestigious journals. He notes there is still ample room for growth—for example, at the time of this address Germany had twenty-five times as many pathologists as did the United States. Osler concludes by suggesting future changes and developments.

THE FIXED PERIOD

I

As this is the last public function at which I shall appear as a member of the University, I very gladly embrace the opportunity which it offers to express the mingled feelings of gratitude and sorrow which are naturally in my mind—gratitude to you all for sixteen years of exceptionally happy life, sorrow that I am to belong to you no more. Neither stricken deeply in years, nor damaged seriously by illness, you may well wonder at the motives that have induced me to give up a position of such influence and importance, to part from colleagues so congenial, from associates and students so devoted, and to leave a country in which I have so many warm friends, and in which I have been appreciated at so much more than my real worth. It is best that you stay in the wonder-stage. Who can understand another man's motives? Does he always understand his own? This much I may say in explanation—not in palliation. After years of hard work, at the very time when a man's energies begin to flag, and when he feels the need of more leisure, the conditions and surroundings that have made him what he is and that have moulded his character and abilities into something useful in the community—these very circumstances ensure an ever increasing demand upon them; and when the call of the East comes,[1] which in one form or another is heard by all of us, and which

A farewell address delivered at the commencement exercises before the alumni, faculty, and students of Johns Hopkins University, February 22, 1905.

1. 1 Kings 17:2–3. The exact quotation is: "And the word of the Lord came unto him, saying, Get thee hence, and turn thee eastward, and hide thyself by the brook Cherith, that *is* before Jordan." Compare also Rudyard Kipling, stanza 4, line 4: "If you've 'eard the East a-callin,' you won't never 'eed naught else."

grows louder as we grow older, the call may come like the summons to Elijah,[2] and not alone the ploughing of the day, but the work of a life, friends, relatives, even father and mother, are left to take up new work in a new field. Or, happier far, if the call comes, as it did to Puran Das[3] in Kipling's story, not to new labours, but to a life "private, unactive, calm, contemplative."[4]

There are several problems in university life suggested by my departure. It may be asked in the first place, whether metabolism is sufficiently active in the professoriate body, is there change enough? May not the loss of a professor bring stimulating benefits to a university? We have not here lost very many—this is not a university that men care to leave—but in looking over its history I do not see that the departure of any one has proved a serious blow. It is strange of how slight value is the unit in a great system. A man may have built up a department and have gained a certain following, local or general; nay, more, he may have had a special value for his mental and moral qualities, and his fission may leave a scar, even an aching scar, but it is not for long. Those of us accustomed to the process know that the organism as a whole feels it about as much as a big polyzoon[5] when a colony breaks off, or a hive of bees after a swarm—'tis not indeed always a calamity, oftentimes it is a relief. Of course upon a few the sense of personal loss falls heavily; in a majority of us the faculty of getting attached to those with whom we work is strongly developed, and some will realize the bitterness of the lines:—

> Alas! that all we loved of him should be
> But for our grief as if it had not been.[6]

But to the professor himself these partings belong to the life he has chosen. Like the hero in one of Matthew Arnold's poems,[7] he knows that his heart was not framed to be 'long loved.'[8] Change is the very marrow of his existence—a

---

2. Osler, like many others, has confused Elijah with his disciple and successor Elisha. The passage he has in mind is 1 Kings 19:15–21. God orders Elijah to anoint Elisha to be prophet in his place after he is taken up to heaven. Elijah finds Elisha plowing and throws his cloak over him. Elisha asks to be allowed to say goodbye to his parents, and he sacrifices his oxen to God using the yokes and harness to feed the fire, then goes after Elijah.

3. *Puran Das* (also *Puran Dass*): A high-caste Brahmin, prime minister of an Indian state, who relinquished all and retired to the hills to live as a holy man. Rudyard Kipling, "The Miracle of Purun Bhagat," *The Second Jungle Book* (New York: Doubleday, Doran, 1929), pp. 35–60.

4. *private, unactive, calm, contemplative:* John Milton, *Paradise Regained*, book 2, line 81.

5. *polyzoon:* A small aquatic "colonial" animal.

6. Percy Bysshe Shelley, "Adonais: An Elegy on the Death of John Keats," stanza 21, lines 1–2.

7. This refers to Empedocles, Greek philosopher and statesman. Matthew Arnold, "Empedocles on Etna," Act II.

8. Matthew Arnold, "A Farewell," stanza 5, line 2. The exact quotation is:

new set of students every year, a new set of assistants, a new set of associates every few years to replace those called off to other fields; in any active department there is no constancy, no stability in the human surroundings. And in this there is an element of sadness. A man comes into one's life for a few years, and you become attached to him, interested in his work and in his welfare, and perhaps you grow to love him, as a son, and then off he goes!—leaving you with a bruised heart.

The question may be asked—whether as professors we do not stay too long in one place. It passes my persimmon [9] to tell how some good men—even lovable and righteous men in other respects—have the hardihood to stay in the same position for twenty-five years! To a man of active mind too long attachment to one college is apt to breed self-satisfaction, to narrow his outlook, to foster a local spirit, and to promote senility. Much of the phenomenal success of this institution has been due to the concentration of a group of light-horse intellectuals, without local ties, whose operations were not restricted, whose allegiance indeed was not always national, yet who were willing to serve faithfully in whatever field of action they were placed. And this should be the attitude of a vigilant professoriate. As St. Paul [10] preferred an evangelist without attachments, as more free for the work, so in the general interests of higher education a University President should cherish a proper nomadic spirit in the members of his faculties, even though it be on occasions a seeming detriment. A well-organized College Trust could arrange a rotation of teachers which would be most stimulating all along the line. We are apt to grow stale and thin mentally if kept too long in the same pasture. Transferred to fresh fields, amid new surroundings and other colleagues, a man gets a fillip which may last for several years. Interchange of teachers, national and international, will prove most helpful. How bracing the Turnbull lecturers [11] have been, for example. It would be an excellent work for

---

I blame thee not!—this heart, I know
To be long loved was never framed;
For something in its depths doth glow
Too strange, too restless, too untamed.

9. *It passes my persimmon:* (Archaic American colloquialism) the general meaning is "it is beyond my capacity to. . . ."

10. *St. Paul* (d. 67 A.D.): Apostle to the gentiles and writer of some of the epistles. In 1 Corinthians 7:29–35, St. Paul discusses marriage, and he says that the unmarried can more easily devote themselves wholeheartedly to God's service.

11. Percy Turnbull Memorial Lectureship on Poetry. A lectureship of poetry established at Johns Hopkins University by Frances L. Turnbull, an American novelist, and her husband Lawrence Turnbull in remembrance of their dead nine-year-old son, Percy Graeme Turnbull. Many distinguished scholars and poets have come to the University as Turnbull lecturers, among whom were T. S. Eliot, W. H. Auden, Archibald MacLeish, and Robert Frost.

the University Association which met here recently to arrange this interchange of instructors. Even to 'swap' College Presidents now and then might be good for the exchequer. We have an excellent illustration of the value of the plan in the transfer this year from Jena of Prof. Keutgen[12] to give the lectures on History. An international university clearing-house might be organized to facilitate the work. How delightful it would be to have a return to the mediaeval practice when the professor roamed Europe at his sweet will, or to the halcyon era of the old Greek teachers—of which Empedocles sings:—

> What days were those Parmenides!
> When we were young, when we could number friends
> In all the Italian cities like ourselves;
> When with elated hearts we joined your train
> Ye Sun-born Virgins on the road of truth.[13]

It is more particularly upon the younger men that I would urge the advantages of an early devotion to a peripatetic philosophy of life. Just so soon as you have your second teeth think of a change; get away from the nurse, cut the apron strings of your old teachers, seek new ties in a fresh environment, if possible where you can have a certain measure of freedom and independence. Only do not wait for a fully equipped billet almost as good as that of your master. A small one, poorly appointed, with many students and few opportunities for research, may be just what is needed to bring out the genius—latent and perhaps unrecognized—that will enable you in an unfavourable position to do well what another could not do at all, even in the most helpful surroundings. There are two appalling diseases which only a feline restlessness of mind and body may head off in young men in the academic career. There is a remarkable bodily condition, known as infantilism, in which adolescence does not come at the appointed time, or is deferred until the twentieth year or later, and is then incomplete, so that the childish mind and the childish form and features remain. The mental counterpart is even more common among us. Intellectual infantilism is a well recognized disease, and just as imperfect nutrition may cause failure of the marvellous changes which accompany puberty in the body, so the mind too long fed on the same diet in one place may be rendered rickety or even infantile. Worse than this may happen. A rare, but still more extraordinary, bodily state is that of progeria,[14] in which, as though touched with the wand of some malign fairy, the child does not remain

12. Friedrich Wilhelm Eduard *Keutgen* (1861–1936): German historian.

13. Matthew Arnold, "Empedocles on Etna," act 2, lines 235–239.

14. *progeria:* An abnormal state showing the symptoms both of infantilism and premature senility occurring in childhood.

infantile, but skips adolescence, maturity and manhood, and passes at once to senility, looking at eleven or twelve years like a miniature Tithonus [15] "marred and
wasted," [16] wrinkled and stunted, a little old man among his toys. It takes great
care on the part of any one to live the mental life corresponding to the phases
through which his body passes. How few minds reach puberty, how few come
to adolescence, how fewer attain maturity! It is really tragic—this wide-spread
prevalence of mental infantilism due to careless habits of intellectual feeding.
Progeria is an awful malady in a college. Few Faculties escape without an instance or two, and there are certain diets which cause it just as surely as there
are waters in some of the Swiss valleys that produce cretinism. I have known an
entire faculty attacked. The progeric himself is a nice enough fellow to look at
and to play with, but he is sterile, with the mental horizon narrowed, and quite
incapable of assimilating the new thoughts of his day and generation.

As in the case of many other diseases, it is more readily prevented than
cured, and, taken early, change of air and diet may do much to antagonize a tendency, inherited or acquired. Early stages may be relieved by a prolonged stay at
the University Baths [17] of Berlin or Leipzic, or if at the proper time a young man is
transferred from an American or Anglican to a Gallic or Teutonic diet. Through
no fault of the men, but of the system, due to the unfortunate idea on the part
of the denominations that in each one of the States they should have their own
educational institutions, collegiate infantilism is far too prevalent, against which
the freer air and better diet of the fully equipped State Universities is proving a
rapid, as it is the rational, antidote.

Nor would I limit this desire for change to the teachers. The student of the
technical school should begin his *wanderjahre* [18] early, not postponing them until
he has taken his M.D. or PH.D. A residence of four years in the one school is
apt to breed prejudice and to promote mental astigmatism which the after years
may never be able to correct. One great difficulty is the lack of harmony in the
curricula of the schools, but this time will correct and, once initiated and encouraged, the better students will take a year, or even two years, in schools other
than those at which they intend to graduate.

I am going to be very bold and touch upon another question of some deli-

15. In Greek mythology *Tithonus* was loved by Eos, who persuaded Zeus to give him the gift of immor-
tality. However, Eos forgot to ask for eternal youth for Tithonus, so he became old and infirm. In pity,
Eos turned him into a grasshopper. This is the subject of a dramatic monologue by Alfred Tennyson,
"Tithonus."

16. Alfred Tennyson, "Tithonus," line 19.

17. Osler is referring to places producing effects analogous to those of medical treatment by bathing. The
therapeutic use of baths is of ancient origin.

18. *wanderjahre:* (German) literally, wandering-years. Osler here means "journeyman's time of travel."

cacy, but of infinite importance in university life: one that has not been settled in this country. I refer to a fixed period for the teacher, either of time of service or of age. Except in some proprietary schools, I do not know of any institutions in which there is a time limit of, say, twenty years' service, as in some of the London hospitals, or in which a man is engaged for a term of years. Usually the appointment is *ad vitam aut culpam*,[19] as the old phrase reads. It is a very serious matter in our young universities to have all of the professors growing old at the same time. In some places, only an epidemic, a time limit, or an age limit can save the situation. I have two fixed ideas well known to my friends, harmless obsessions with which I sometimes bore them, but which have a direct bearing on this important problem. The first is the comparative uselessness of men above forty years of age.[20] This may seem shocking, and yet read aright the world's history bears out the statement. Take the sum of human achievement in action, in science, in art, in literature—subtract the work of the men above forty, and while we should miss great treasures, even priceless treasures, we would practically be where we are to-day. It is difficult to name a great and far-reaching conquest of the mind which has not been given to the world by a man on whose back the sun was still shining. The effective, moving, vitalizing work of the world is done between the ages of twenty-five and forty—these fifteen golden years of plenty, the anabolic or constructive period, in which there is always a balance in the mental bank and the credit is still good. In the science and art of medicine young or comparatively young men have made every advance of the first rank. Vesalius, Harvey, Hunter, Bichat, Laennec, Virchow, Lister, Koch[21]—the

19. *ad vitam aut culpam:* (Latin) for life or until a misdeed.

20. Osler may be misremembering and confusing two different passages in Plato's writings. In the *Republic* (book 5, 460e–461a) Socrates says that women are past their prime after forty, but men are not past theirs until fifty-five. In the *Laws* (book 6, 785b) Plato says that the limit for official posts shall be forty for a woman and thirty for a man.

Under his favorite phrase "la crise de quarante ans" (the crisis of forty years) he gave such examples as Locke, Milton, Darwin, and Goethe. Osler argued quite seriously for relatively early retirement, though not, of course, for euthanasia. This idea, however, led to the misunderstanding that he proposed early death, and to the coined verb "oslerize."

In the 1920s, every afternoon sightseeing buses used to go by Craigleigh, the house of his brother Sir Edmund Osler in Toronto, and the guide would shout through a megaphone from the open upper deck "This is the residence of Sir Edmund Osler, brother of Sir William Osler, the doctor who advocated euthanasia at sixty." Sir Edmund was very annoyed by this, and once said to his granddaughter "that is all they remember of a great man." (Anne) Wilkinson, *Lions in the Way* (Toronto: Macmillan, 1956), p. 236.

21. Andreas *Vesalius* (1514–1564): See "The Leaven of Science," p. 163, n. 62.

William *Harvey* (1578–1657): See "Teacher and Student," p. 116, n. 22.

John *Hunter* (1728–1793): See "The Master-Word in Medicine," p. 260, n. 36 and "The Old Humanities and the New Science," p. 93, n. 214.

green years were yet upon their heads when their epoch-making studies were made. To modify an old saying,[22] a man is sane morally at thirty, rich mentally at forty, wise spiritually at fifty—or never. The young men should be encouraged and afforded every possible chance to show what is in them. If there is one thing more than another upon which the professors of this university are to be congratulated it is this very sympathy and fellowship with their junior associates, upon whom really in many departments, in mine certainly, has fallen the brunt of the work. And herein lies the chief value of the teacher who has passed his climacteric and is no longer a productive factor, he can play the man midwife as Socrates did to Theaetetus,[23] and determine whether the thoughts which the young men are bringing to the light are false idols or true and noble births.

My second fixed idea is the uselessness of men above sixty years of age, and the incalculable benefit it would be in commercial, political and in professional life if, as a matter of course, men stopped work at this age. In his *Biathanatos* Donne tells us that by the laws of certain wise states sexagenarii were precipitated from a bridge,[24] and in Rome men of that age were not admitted to the suffrage and they were called *Depontani*[25] because the way to the senate was *per pontem*,[26] and they from age were not permitted to come thither. In that charming novel, *The Fixed Period*,[27] Anthony Trollope discusses the practical ad-

---

Marie François Xavier *Bichat* (1771–1802): See "Chauvinism in Medicine," p. 236, n. 34.

Théophile René Hyacinthe *Laënnec* (1781–1826): See "Chauvinism in Medicine," p. 236, n. 34.

Rudolf *Virchow* (1821–1902): See "The Old Humanities and the New Science," p. 75, n. 80.

Joseph *Lister* (1827–1912): English surgeon. He was deeply influenced by the discoveries of Pasteur and used carbolic acid to prevent septic infection. He founded antiseptic surgery.

Robert *Koch* (1843–1910): See "Books and Men," p. 222, n. 20.

22. "He that is not handsome at twenty, nor strong at thirty, nor rich at forty, nor wise at fifty, will never be handsome, strong, rich, or wise." This quotation was in a collection by George Herbert, *Outlandish Proverbs: The Works of George Herbert*, ed. F. E. Hutchinson (1639; Oxford: The Clarendon Press, 1941), p. 333.

23. Osler means here that the role of older teachers is to help give birth to "truth," Plato, *Theætetus*, 148e–151d. Osler quotes the passage in "Physic and Physicians as Depicted in Plato," pp. 141–144.

24. John Donne, *Biathanatos* (1646), a tract on suicide. The Greek word *biathanatos* could be applied to persons dying from any kind of violence but was most often applied to suicides. "To throw sixty-year-olds from the bridge" was an ancient proverb.

25. Pierio Valeriano, *Hieroglyphica* (1556), liber 17. The phrase *Depontani* properly means "put off the bridge."

26. John Donne, *Biathanatos*, part 1, dist. 4, sect. 2, lines 2328–2337. The phrase *per pontem* means "over the bridge." Men over sixty were indeed forbidden to vote in the *saepta*, the ancient Roman assembly held in the Campus Martius, and if any tried to go to it, they were thrust off the bridge that had to be crossed to reach the place; but that does not imply they were killed.

27. *The Fixed Period:* Anthony Trollope, *The Fixed Period* (1882). Trollope portrays a fictional state which has introduced compulsory euthanasia at the age of sixty-seven, not sixty as Osler maintains. David Skil-

vantages in modern life of a return to this ancient usage, and the plot hinges upon the admirable scheme of a college into which at sixty men retired for a year of contemplation before a peaceful departure by chloroform.[28] That incalculable benefits might follow such a scheme is apparent to any one who, like myself, is nearing the limit, and who has made a careful study of the calamities which may befall men during the seventh and eighth decades. Still more when he contemplates the many evils which they perpetuate unconsciously, and with impunity. As it can be maintained that all the great advances have come from men under forty, so the history of the world shows that a very large proportion of the evils may be traced to the sexagenarians—nearly all the great mistakes politically and socially, all of the worst poems, most of the bad pictures, a majority of the bad novels, not a few of the bad sermons and speeches. It is not to be denied that occasionally there is a sexagenarian whose mind, as Cicero remarks, stands out of reach of the body's decay.[29] Such a one has learned the secret of Hermippus,[30] that ancient Roman who feeling that the silver cord was loosening cut himself clear from all companions of his own age and betook himself to the company of young men, mingling with their games and studies, and so lived to the age of 153, *puerorum halitu refocillatus et educatus*.[31] And there is truth in

ton writes: "Although we find many points of interest in *The Fixed Period*, we must in the end rate it as a minor work, while still applauding Trollope's attempt. Of course, ironists are always liable to misinterpretation, and that most humane of physicians, Sir William Osler, in a retirement speech from Johns Hopkins University in 1905, drew a bitter stream of vilification down on himself from the press, by humorously approving Mr. Neverbend's scheme." David Skilton, "Introduction," *The Fixed Period* (1882 New York: Arno Press, 1981).

28. In Trollope's novel, after a year of retirement, death was not by chloroform as Osler said, but by "voluntary" suicide "by the traditional Roman method of immersing one's self in a warm bath opening a vein and bleeding to death." William Bennet Bean, "Osler, Trollope, and *The Fixed Period*," *Trans. Am. Clin. Climatol. Assoc.* 78:242–248, 1966.

29. *There is a sexagenarian whose mind, as Cicero remarks, stands out of reach of the body's decay:* Marcus Tullius *Cicero* (106–43 B.C.): Roman writer, statesman, and orator. Osler may have in mind *De Senectute*, where Cicero represents Cato the Elder, in his eighties, as recalling that at sixty-five he still "spoke publicly for the Voconian law, with loud voice and mighty lungs." *De Senectute*, trans. William Armistead Falconer (London: W. Heinemann, 1923), pp. 22–25.

30. *Hermippus:* Several medical writers of the seventeenth and eighteenth centuries quoted a supposed ancient Roman inscription, variously reported as commemorating Lucius Clodius Hermippus, who lived 115 years and 5 days on the breath of little girls, or Lucius Clodius Hirpanus, who lived 155 years on the breath of little boys. The inscription cannot now be traced and was probably either forged or misinterpreted. The versions are discussed in Sabine Baring-Gould, "Hermippus Redivivus," in *Curiosities of Olden Times*, rev. ed. (Edinburgh: John Grant, 1895), pp. 135–152. Osler may have read Johann Heinrich Cohausen, *Hermippus Redivivus: or, The Sage's Triumph over Old Age and the Grave* (London: J. Nourse, 1749).

31. *puerorum halitu refocillatus et educatus:* (Latin) revived and nourished by the breath of boys.

the story, since it is only those who live with the young who maintain a fresh outlook on the new problems of the world. The teacher's life should have three periods, study until twenty-five, investigation until forty, profession until sixty, at which age I would have him retired on a double allowance. Whether Anthony Trollope's suggestion of a college and chloroform should be carried out or not I have become a little dubious, as my own time is getting so short. (I may say for the benefit of the public that with a woman I would advise an entirely different plan, since, after sixty her influence on her sex may be most helpful, particularly if aided by those charming accessories, a cap and a fichu.) [32,33]

II

Such an occasion as the present affords an opportunity to say a few words on the work which the Johns Hopkins foundations have done and may do for medicine. The hospital was organized at a most favourable period, when the profession had at last awakened to its responsibilities, the leading universities had begun to take medical education seriously, and to the public at large had come a glimmering sense of the importance of the scientific investigation of disease and of the advantages of well trained doctors in a community. It would have been an easy matter to have made colossal mistakes with these great organizations. There are instances in which larger bequests have been sterile from the start; but in the history of educational institutions it is hard to name one more prolific than the Johns Hopkins University. Not simply a seed farm, it has been a veritable nursery from which the whole country has been furnished with cuttings, grafts, slips, seedlings, etc. It would be superfluous in this audience to refer to the great work which the Trustees and Mr. Gilman [34] did in twenty-five years—their praise is in all the colleges. But I must pay a tribute to the wise men who planned the hospital, who refused to establish an institution on the old lines—a great city charity for the sick poor, but gave it vital organic connexion with a University. I do not know who was directly responsible for the provision in Mr. Hopkins' will [35] that the hospital should form part of the Medical School, and that it should be an institution for the study as well as for the cure of disease. Perhaps the founder himself may be credited with the idea, but I have always felt that Francis T. King [36]

32. *fichu:* A woman's triangular scarf of light weight fabric, worn over the shoulders.

33. This passage about women reminds us that Osler was a Victorian.

34. Daniel Coit *Gilman* (1831–1908): American educator and first president of Johns Hopkins University.

35. Johns *Hopkins* (1795–1873): Baltimore businessman. He founded Johns Hopkins University.

36. Francis T. *King* (1819–1891): Baltimore businessman. First president of the Johns Hopkins Hospital Board and also a trustee of the university.

was largely responsible, as he had strong and sensible convictions on the subject, and devoted the last years of his useful life putting them into execution. As first President of the Hospital Board he naturally did much to shape the policy of the institution, and it is a pleasure to recall the zeal and sympathy with which he was always ready to co-operate. It is sad that in so few years all of the members of the original Board have passed away, the last, Mr. Corner[37]—faithful and interested to the end—only a few weeks ago. They did a great work for this city, and their names should be held in everlasting remembrance. Judge Dobbin and James Carey Thomas,[38] in particular, the members of the staff in the early days remember with gratitude for their untiring devotion to the medical school side of the problems which confronted us. To John S. Billings,[39] so long the skilled adviser of the Board, we all turned for advice and counsel, and his influence was deeper and stronger than was always apparent. For the admirable plan of preliminary medical study, and for the shaping of the scientific work before the hospital was opened for patients, we are indebted to Newell Martin, Ira Remsen and W. H. Welch.[40] The present excellent plan of study leading to medicine, in which the classics, science and literature are fully represented, is the outcome of their labours.

About this time sixteen years ago Mr. King, Dr. Billings, Dr. Welch and myself had many conferences with reference to the opening of the hospital. I had been appointed January 1, but had not yet left Philadelphia. As so often happens the last steps in a great organization are the most troublesome, and after some delay the whole matter was intrusted to Mr. Gilman, who became acting director, and in a few months everything was ready, and on May 7 the hospital was opened. I look back with peculiar pleasure to my association with Mr. Gilman. It was both an education and a revelation. I had never before been brought into

37. George W. *Corner* (d.1905): Baltimore businessman and one of the early members of the Hospital Board of Trustees.

38. George W. *Dobbin* (1809–1891): Baltimore judge, one of the early members of both the hospital and university boards.

   James Carey *Thomas* (1833–1897): Baltimore physician in practice, a member of the University Board of Trustees.

39. John Shaw *Billings* (1838–1913): See "Books and Men," p. 222, n. 18.

40. Henry Newell *Martin* (1848–1896): American biologist and physiologist. Professor and colleague of Osler at Johns Hopkins University. He introduced the evolutionary approach to zoology in the United States.

   Ira *Remsen* (1846–1927): American chemist who introduced German methods of advanced laboratory instruction at Johns Hopkins University, and in 1901 became the university's second president. One of the buildings is still called Remsen Hall.

   William Henry *Welch* (1850–1934): See "Physic and Physicians as Depicted in Plato," p. 127, n. 2.

close contact with a man who loved difficulties just for the pleasure of making them disappear. But I am not going to speak of those happy days lest it should forestall the story I have written of the inner history of the first period of the hospital.

At the date of the organization of the hospital the two great problems before the profession of this country were, how to give to students a proper education, in other words how to give them the culture, the science and the art commensurate with the dignity of a learned profession; and, secondly, how to make this great and rich country a contributor to the science of medicine.

The conditions under which the medical school opened in 1893 were unique in the history of American medicine. It would have been an easy matter, following the lead of the better schools, to have an entrance examination which guaranteed that a man had an ordinary education, but Miss Garett's[41] splendid gift enabled us to say, no! we do not want a large number of half-educated students; we prefer a select group trained in the sciences preliminary to medicine, and in the languages which will be most useful for a modern physician. It was an experiment, and we did not expect more than twenty five or thirty students each year for eight or ten years at least. As is so often the case, the country was better prepared than we thought to meet our conditions, and the number of admissions to the school has risen until we have about reached our capacity. Our example in demanding the preliminary arts or science course for admission to the school has been followed by Harvard, and is to be adopted at Columbia. It is not a necessary measure in all the schools, but there has been everywhere a very salutary increase in the stringency of the entrance examinations. Before we took up the work great reforms in the scientific teaching in medicine had already begun in this country. Everywhere laboratory work had replaced to some extent the lecture, and practical courses in physiology, pathology and pharmacology had been organized. We must not forget however that to Newell Martin,[42] the first professor of physiology in this university, is due the introduction of practical classes in biology and physiology. The rapid growth of the school necessitated the erection of a separate building for physiology, pharmacology and physiological chemistry, and in these departments and in anatomy the equipment is as complete as is required. Of the needs in pathology, hygiene and experimental pathology this is not the occasion to speak. It is sufficient to say that for instruc-

41. Mary Elizabeth *Garett* (1854–1915): Baltimore resident and active feminist. She gave the $300,000 necessary to complete the $500,000 endowment to start the medical school. To her gift she attached the conditions that women should be accepted as students and that one of the buildings should bear the inscribed name of the "Women's Memorial Fund Building" (Cushing, vol. 1, pp. 373–374)

42. *Martin:* See p. 298, n. 40.

tion in the sciences, upon which the practice of the art is based, the school is in first class condition.

Indeed the rapidity with which the scientific instruction in our medical schools has been brought to a high level is one of the most remarkable educational features of the past twenty years. Even in small unendowed colleges admirable courses are given in bacteriology and pathology, and sometimes in the more difficult subject of practical physiology. But the demand and the necessity for these special courses has taxed to the utmost the resources of the private schools. The expense of the new method of teaching is so great that the entire class fees are absorbed by the laboratories. The consequence is that the old proprietary colleges are no longer profitable ventures, certainly not in the north, and fortunately they are being forced into closer affiliation with the universities, as it is not an easy matter to get proper endowments for private corporations.

The great difficulty is in the third part of the education of the student: viz., his art. In the old days when a lad was apprenticed to a general practitioner, he had good opportunities to pick up the essentials of a rough and ready art, and the system produced many self-reliant, resourceful men. Then with the multiplication of the medical schools and increasing rivalry between them came the two year course, which for half a century lay like a blight on the medical profession, retarding its progress, filling its ranks with half-educated men, and pandering directly to all sorts of quackery, humbuggery and fraud among the public. The awakening came about thirty years ago, and now there is scarcely a school in the country which has not a four years course, and all are trying to get clear of the old shackles and teach rational medicine in a rational way. But there are extraordinary difficulties in teaching the medical student his Art. It is not hard, for example, to teach him all about the disease pneumonia, how it prevails in the winter and spring, how fatal it always has been, all about the germ, all about the change which the disease causes in the lungs and in the heart—he may become learned, deeply learned, on the subject—but put him beside a case, and he may not know which lung is involved, and he does not know how to find out, and if he did find out, he might be in doubt whether to put an ice-bag or a poultice on the affected side, whether to bleed or to give opium, whether to give a dose of medicine every hour or none at all, and he may not have the faintest notion whether the signs look ominous or favourable. So also with other aspects of the art of the general practitioner. A student may know all about the bones of the wrist, in fact he may carry a set in his pocket and know every facet and knob and nodule on them, he may have dissected a score of arms, and yet when he is called to see Mrs. Jones who has fallen on the ice and broken her wrist, he may not know a Colles' from a Pott's fracture, and as for setting it *secundum artem*,[43] he may not have the faintest notion, never having seen a case. Or he may be called to preside at one of those awful domestic tragedies—the sudden emergency, some terrible accident of birth or of childhood, that requires skill, technical skill, courage—the courage of full knowledge, and if he has not been in the obstetrical wards, if he has not been trained practically, if he has not had the opportunities that are the rights of every medical student, he may fail at the critical moment, a life, two lives, may be lost, sacrificed to ignorance, often to helpless, involuntary ignorance. By far the greatest work of the Johns Hopkins Hospital has been the demonstration to the profession of the United States and to the public of this country of how medical students should be instructed in their art. I place it first because it was the most needed lesson, I place it first because it has done the most good as a stimulating example, and I place it first because never before in the history of this country have medical students lived and worked in a hospital as part of its machinery, as an essential part of the work of the wards. In saying this, Heaven forbid that I should obliquely disparage the good and faithful work of my colleagues elsewhere. But the amphitheatre clinic, the ward and dispensary classes, are but bastard substitutes for a system which makes the medical student himself help in the work of the hospital as part of its human machinery. He does not see the pneumonia case in the amphitheatre from the benches, but he follows it day by day, hour by hour; he has his time so arranged that he can follow it; he sees and studies similar cases and the disease itself becomes his chief teacher, and he knows its phases and variations as depicted in the living; he learns under skilled direction when to act and when to refrain, he learns insensibly principles of practice and he possibly escapes a "nickel-in-the-slot" attitude of mind [44] which has been the curse of the physician in the treatment of disease. And the same with the other branches of his art; he gets a first hand knowledge which, if he has any sense, may make him wise unto the salvation of his fellows. And all this has come about through the wise provision that the hospital was to be part of the medical school, and it has become for the senior students, as it should be, their college. Moreover they are not in it upon sufferance and admitted through side-doors, but they are welcomed as important aids without which the work could not be done efficiently. The whole question of the practical education of the medical student is one in which the public is vitally interested. Sane, intelligent physicians and surgeons with culture, science, and art, are worth much in a community, and they are worth paying for in rich endowments of our medical schools and hospitals. Personally, there

43. *secundum artem:* (Latin) "according to the established method."

44. The point is either taking whatever comes up (with gambling machines) or being satisfied with cheap, ordinary things (dispensed by vending machines).

is nothing in life in which I take greater pride than in my connexion with the organization of the medical clinic of the Johns Hopkins Hospital and with the introduction of the old-fashioned methods of practical instruction. I desire no other epitaph—no hurry about it, I may say—than the statement that I taught medical students in the wards,[45] as I regard this as by far the most useful and important work I have been called upon to do.

The second great problem is a much more difficult one, surrounded as it is with obstacles inextricably connected with the growth and expansion of a comparatively new country. For years the United States had been the largest borrower in the scientific market of the world, and more particularly in the sciences relating to medicine. To get the best that the world offered, our young men had to go abroad; only here and there was a laboratory of physiology or pathology, and then equipped as a rule for teaching. The change in twenty years has been remarkable. There is scarcely to-day a department of scientific medicine which is not represented in our larger cities by men who are working as investigators, and American scientific medicine is taking its rightful place in the world's work. Nothing shows this more plainly than the establishment within a few years of journals devoted to scientific subjects; and the active participation of this school as a leader is well illustrated by the important publications which have been started by its members. The Hospital Trustees early appreciated the value of these scientific publications, and the Bulletin and the Reports have done much to spread the reputation of the Hospital as a medical centre throughout the world. But let us understand clearly that only a beginning has been made. For one worker in pathology—a man, I mean, who is devoting his life to the study of the causes of disease—there are twenty-five at least in Germany, and for one in this country there are a dozen laboratories of the first class in any one of the more important sciences cognate to medicine. It is not alone that the money is lacking; the men are not always at hand. When the right man is available he quickly puts American science into the forefront. Let me give you an illustration. Anatomy is a fundamental branch in medicine. There is no school, even amid sylvan glades,[46] without its dissecting room; but it has been a great difficulty to get the higher anatomy represented in American universities. Plenty of men have always been available to teach the subject to medical students, but when it came to questions of morphology and embryology and the really scientific study

45. Presidential Art Medals, Inc., Vandalia, Ohio, issued an Osler Medal as one of its "Great Men of Medicine" series. The obverse shows a frontal bust of Osler, and the reverse shows Osler at the bedside with a patient and his students. Above them Osler's own chosen epitaph is inscribed: HE TAUGHT MEDICAL STUDENTS IN THE WARDS.
46. Woodland regions.

of the innumerable problems connected with them, it was only here and there and not in a thorough manner that the subjects were approached. And the young men had to go abroad to see a completely equipped, modern working anatomical institute. There is to-day connected with this university a school of anatomy of which any land might be proud, and the work of Dr. Mall[47] demonstrates what can be done when the man fits his environment.

It is a hopeful sign to see special schools established for the study of disease such as the Rockefeller Institute in New York, the McCormick Institute in Chicago and the Phipps Institute in Philadelphia. They will give a great impetus in the higher lines of work in which the country has heretofore been so weak. But it makes one green with envy to see how much our German brethren are able to do. Take, for example, the saddest chapter in the history of disease—insanity, the greatest curse of civilized life. Much has been done in the United States for the care of the insane, much in places for the study of the disease, and I may say that the good work which has been inaugurated in this line at the Sheppard Hospital[48] is attracting attention everywhere; but what a bagatelle it seems in comparison with the modern development of the subject in Germany, with its great psychopathic clinics connected with each university, where early and doubtful cases are skilfully studied and skilfully treated. The new department for insanity connected with the University of Munich has cost nearly half a million dollars! Of the four new departments for which one side of the hospital grounds lies vacant, and which will be built within the next twenty-five years, one should be a model psychopathic clinic to which the acute and curable cases may be sent. The second, a clinic for the diseases of children. Much has been done with our out-patient department under Dr. Booker,[49] who has helped to clarify one of the dark problems in infant mortality, but we need a building with fine wards and laboratories in which may be done work of a character as notable and worldwide as that done in Dr. Kelly's[50] division for the diseases of women.[51] The third great

47. Franklin Paine *Mall* (1862–1917): American anatomist and professor at Johns Hopkins University. Also director of the embryology department of the Carnegie Institution in Washington.

48. Sheppard Insane Asylum, founded in 1853.

49. William David *Booker* (1844–1921): American pediatrician and professor at Johns Hopkins University. He was one of the founders of the American Pediatric Society, of which he became president in 1901.

50. Howard Atwood *Kelly* (1858–1943): American surgeon and professor of gynecology at Johns Hopkins University. He was one of the first to use radium in cancer treatment and also to use cocaine as a local anesthetic.

51. Osler's original note reads: "It is most gratifying to know that the Harriet Lane Johnston Hospital for children will be associated with the Johns Hopkins Hospital, and will meet the requirements of which I have spoken." The Harriet Lane Home, one of the first pediatric hospitals in the country, opened in 1912, with the university supplying medical staff and the hospital giving nursing and other staff.

department for which a separate building must be provided is that of Syphilis and Dermatology. Already no small share of the reputation of this hospital has come from the good work in these specialities by the late Dr. Brown, by Dr. Gilchrist, and by Dr. Hugh Young;[52] and lastly, for diseases of the eye, ear, and throat, a large separate clinic is needed, which will give to these all-important subjects the equipment they deserve.

For how much to be thankful have we who have shared in the initiation of the work of these two great institutions. We have been blessed with two remarkable Presidents, whose active sympathies have been a stimulus in every department, and whose good sense has minimized the loss of energy through friction between the various parts of the machine—a loss from which colleges are very prone to suffer. A noteworthy feature is that in so motley a collection from all parts of the country the men should have fitted into each other's lives so smoothly and peacefully, so that the good fellowship and harmony in the faculties has been delightful. And we have been singularly blessed in our relationship with the citizens, who have not only learned to appreciate the enormous benefits which these great trusts confer upon the city and the state, but they have come forward in a noble way to make possible a new era in the life of the university. And we of the medical faculty have to feel very grateful to the profession, to whose influence and support much of the success of the hospital and the medical school is due; and not only to the physicians of the city and of the state, who have dealt so truly with us, but to the profession of the entire country, and more particularly to that of the Southern States, whose confidence we have enjoyed in such a practical way. Upon a maintenance of this confidence the future rests. The character of the work of the past sixteen years is the best guarantee of its permanence.

What has been accomplished is only an earnest of what shall be done in the future. Upon our heels a fresh perfection must tread, born of us, fated to excel us.[53] We have but served and have but seen a beginning. Personally I feel deeply grateful to have been permitted to join in this noble work and to have been united in it with men of such high and human ideals.

---

52. Thomas Richardson *Brown* (1845–1879): American specialist in gastroenterology and professor of clinical medicine at Johns Hopkins University.

   Thomas Caspar *Gilchrist* (1862–1927): Dermatologist from England and professor of dermatology at Johns Hopkins University.

   Hugh Hampton *Young* (1879–1945): American surgeon and clinical professor of urology at Johns Hopkins University.

53. John Keats, "Hyperion," book 2, lines 212–214.

17

THE STUDENT LIFE

"Take therefore no thought for the morrow:
for the morrow shall take thought for
the things of itself."
MATTHEW 6:34, Sermon on the Mount

THIS IS A FAREWELL ADDRESS to American and Canadian medical students in 1905. Osler discusses the fragmentary nature of discovered truth and urges the students to pursue it with receptive minds and open, honest hearts. Medicine deals with "man and his mental and bodily anomalies and diseases." Hence, medicine requires special traits—a sense of humor and a balance between knowledge from books and that acquired by travel and close observation of others. Success depends both on early training and on persistence. Osler urges concentration and the thorough study of subjects, always keeping a sense of proportion. Being a student, particularly of medicine, implies belonging to a fraternity in which the faculty are brothers, not masters.

Education must be a lifelong course, for which the few years at school are just a preparation. Systematic learning and observation must continue after graduation. Osler offers advice for lifelong success and serenity:

1. Take notes on all cases systematically, then honestly categorize your diagnoses as clear, doubtful, or mistaken—in order to profit from your experience. This will help you develop wisdom, defined as "knowledge ready for use."

2. Be prepared to gather new information and to learn how to apply it to your own cases. Also, do reading that is not related to your profession.

3. Although difficult for practicing physicians, it is important to get away every five years, back to a hospital or laboratory for a rejuvenation or "brain-dusting."

Osler warns physicians of the various dangers encountered in prosperity, politics, and moving to a larger place. He also cautions against pitfalls such as entering a specialty presuming it will be easier than general practice. He warns about the loss of perspective due to narrow focus on a specialty, which can be avoided by keeping a strong contact with workers in other areas. Those who will teach, especially at small schools, need to avoid stagnation due to the routine and to the isolation from others working in the same subject. To teach with fresh enthusiasm and devotion requires a sense of responsibility and proportion. He remembers his mentor, Dr. Palmer Howard, as an ideal teacher. The noble calling of medicine requires humility, confidence, pride in the medical heritage, and hope for the future.

THE STUDENT LIFE

I

EXCEPT IT BE A LOVER, no one is more interesting as an object of study than a student. Shakespeare might have made him a fourth in his immortal group.[1] The lunatic with his fixed idea, the poet with his fine frenzy, the lover with his frantic idolatry, and the student aflame with the desire for knowledge are of "imagination all compact."[2] To an absorbing passion, a whole-souled devotion, must be joined an enduring energy, if the student is to become a devotee of the grey-eyed goddess[3] to whose law his services are bound. Like the quest of the Holy Grail,[4] the quest of Minerva is not for

A farewell address to American and Canadian medical students, delivered at McGill University, April 14, 1905, and later the same month at the University of Pennsylvania.

1. William Shakespeare, *A Midsummer Night's Dream*, V, i, 7–8.

2. Ibid. The exact quotation is:

> The lunatic, the lover, and the poet
> Are of imagination all compact.

3. Minerva, the Roman goddess of wisdom, arts, and war (identified with the Greek Athena). She was born from Zeus' head, representing the idea of conception on the intellectual level as opposed to merely in the generative sense, and symbolic of a whole new level in human consciousness. Alexander Eliot, *Myths* (New York: McGraw-Hill, c.1976), p. 196.

4. *Holy Grail:* According to legend, the cup used by Jesus at the Last Supper and in which his blood was caught as he hung on the cross. It was supposed to have been brought to Britain by Joseph of Arimathea, and miraculously appeared to King Arthur and his knights as they sat at dinner at the Round Table. The knights then all vowed to go on quest for it; but only three who were morally pure—Galahad, Percival, and Bors—ever achieved more than a glimpse. Hence it became a symbol for any goal whose attainment requires perfection and steadfast dedication.

all. For the one, the pure life; for the other, what Milton calls "a strong propensity of nature."[5] Here again the student often resembles the poet—he is born, not made.[6] While the resultant of two moulding forces, the accidental, external conditions, and the hidden germinal energies, which produce in each one of us national, family, and individual traits, the true student possesses in some measure a divine spark which sets at naught their laws. Like the Snark,[7] he defies definition, but there are three unmistakable signs by which you may recognize the genuine article from a Boojum[8]—an absorbing desire to know the truth, an unswerving steadfastness in its pursuit, and an open, honest heart, free from suspicion, guile, and jealousy.

At the outset do not be worried about this big question—Truth. It is a very simple matter if each one of you starts with the desire to get as much as possible. No human being is constituted to know the truth, the whole truth, and nothing but the truth;[9] and even the best of men must be content with fragments, with partial glimpses, never the full fruition. In this unsatisfied quest the attitude of mind, the desire, the thirst—a thirst that from the soul must rise![10]—the fervent longing, are the be-all and the end-all.[11] What is the student but a lover courting a fickle mistress[12] who ever eludes his grasp? In this very elusiveness is brought out his second great characteristic—steadfastness of purpose. Unless from the start the limitations incident to our frail human faculties are frankly accepted, nothing but disappointment awaits you. The truth is the best you can get with your best endeavour, the best that the best men accept—with this you must learn to be satisfied, retaining at the same time with due humility an earnest desire for an ever larger portion. Only by keeping the mind plastic and receptive does the student escape perdition. It is not, as Charles Lamb[13] remarks, that some people do not know what to do with truth when it is offered to them, but the tragic fate is to reach, after years of patient search, a condition of mind-blindness in which the truth is not recognized, though it stares you in the face. This can never

5. John Milton, "Introduction" *The Reason of Church-government Urg'd against Prelaty*, book 2, ed. Harry Morgan Ayres, *The Works of John Milton* (New York: Columbia University Press, 1931), vol. 3, p. 236.

6. *Poets are born, not made:* A common Latin maxim.

7. *Snark:* An imaginary, elusive monster in *The Hunting of the Snark* (1876) by Lewis Carroll.

8. *Boojum:* A very dangerous variety of Snark.

9. Before testifying in court, one places a hand on the Bible and swears "to tell the truth, the whole truth, and nothing but the truth."

10. Ben Jonson, "The Forest: To Celia," stanza 1.

11. *the be-all and the end-all:* William Shakespeare, *Macbeth*, I, vii, 5.

12. The "fickle mistress" whom the student pursues is Truth or Knowledge personified.

13. Charles *Lamb* (1775–1834): English author and essayist. Osler paraphrased this more briefly in his memo book. We could not find this quote in Lamb's writings.

happen to a man who has followed step by step the growth of a truth, and who knows the painful phases of its evolution. It is one of the great tragedies of life that every truth has to struggle to acceptance against honest but mind-blind students. Harvey knew his contemporaries well,[14] and for twelve successive years demonstrated the circulation of the blood before daring to publish the facts on which the truth was based.[15] Only steadfastness of purpose and humility enable the student to shift his position to meet the new conditions in which new truths are born, or old ones modified beyond recognition. And, thirdly, the honest heart will keep him in touch with his fellow students, and furnish that sense of comradeship without which he travels an arid waste alone. I say advisedly an honest *heart*—the honest head is prone to be cold and stern, given to judgment, not mercy, and not always able to entertain that true charity which, while it thinketh no evil,[16] is anxious to put the best possible interpretation upon the motives of a fellow worker. It will foster, too, an attitude of generous, friendly rivalry untinged by the green peril, jealousy, that is the best preventive of the growth of a bastard[17] scientific spirit, loving seclusion and working in a lock-and-key laboratory, as timorous of light as is a thief.

You have all become brothers in a great society, not apprentices, since that implies a master, and nothing should be further from the attitude of the teacher than much that is meant in that word, used though it be in another sense, particularly by our French brethren in a most delightful way, signifying a bond of intellectual filiation. A fraternal attitude is not easy to cultivate—the chasm between the chair and the bench is difficult to bridge. Two things have helped to put up a cantilever[18] across the gulf. The successful teacher is no longer on a height, pumping knowledge at high pressure into passive receptacles. The new methods have changed all this. He is no longer *Sir Oracle*,[19] perhaps unconsciously by his very manner antagonizing minds to whose level he cannot possibly descend, but he is a senior student anxious to help his juniors. When a simple, earnest

14. William Harvey (1578–1657): See "Teacher and Student," p. 116, n. 22.

15. Osler's original note reads: " 'These views, as usual, pleased some more, others less; some chid and calumniated me, and laid it to me as a crime that I had dared to depart from the precepts and opinions of all Anatomists.'—*De Motu Cordis*, chap. i." Osler is quoting from the English version of *De Motu Cordis, Anatomical Dissertation upon the Movement of the Heart and Blood in Animals* (Canterbury: G. Moreton, 1894), p. 20. The translator's name is not given.

16. *that true charity which, while it thinketh no evil:* 1 Corinthians 13:5.

17. *bastard:* Spurious; not genuine; corrupt.

18. *cantilever:* A bracket-like arm projecting from a bank or pier which supports the span of a bridge. Osler implies by it cooperation between teachers and students.

19. *Sir Oracle:* One who thinks he is well-informed and delivers pompous pronouncements. He is not a character in the play, but a mocking nickname bestowed by Graziano on people who want an undeserved reputation for wisdom. William Shakespeare, *The Merchant of Venice*, I, i, 93.

spirit animates a college, there is no appreciable interval between the teacher and the taught—both are in the same class, the one a little more advanced than the other. So animated, the student feels that he has joined a family whose honour is his honour, whose welfare is his own, and whose interests should be his first consideration.

The hardest conviction to get into the mind of a beginner is that the education upon which he is engaged is not a college course, not a medical course, but a life course, for which the work of a few years under teachers is but a preparation. Whether you will falter and fail in the race or whether you will be faithful to the end depends on the training before the start, and on your staying powers, points upon which I need not enlarge. You can all become good students, a few may become great students, and now and again one of you will be found who does easily and well what others cannot do at all, or very badly, which is John Ferriar's excellent definition of a genius.[20]

In the hurry and bustle of a business world, which is the life of this continent, it is not easy to train first-class students. Under present conditions it is hard to get the needful seclusion, on which account it is that our educational market is so full of wayside fruit. I have always been much impressed by the advice of St. Chrysostom: "Depart from the highway and transplant thyself in some enclosed ground, for it is hard for a tree which stands by the wayside to keep her fruit till it be ripe."[21] The dilettante is abroad in the land, the man who is always venturing on tasks for which he is imperfectly equipped, a habit of mind fostered by the multiplicity of subjects of the curriculum; and while many things are studied, few are studied thoroughly. Men will not take time to get to the heart of a matter. After all, concentration is the price the modern student pays for success. Thoroughness is the most difficult habit to acquire, but it is the pearl of great price, worth all the worry and trouble of the search. The dilettante lives an easy, butterfly life, knowing nothing of the toil and labour with which the treasures of knowledge are dug out of the past, or wrung by patient research in the laboratories. Take, for example, the early history of this country—how easy for the student of the one type to get a smattering, even a fairly full acquaintance with the events of the French and Spanish settlements. Put an original document before him, and it might as well be Arabic.[22] What we need is the other

20. John *Ferriar* (1761–1815): Scottish physician. He writes: "In a word, that genius consists in the power of doing best, what many endeavour to do well." "Of Genius," in *Illustrations of Sterne* (1798; London: Cadell and Davies, 1812), vol. 1, p. 180.

21. Regarding St. John *Chrysostom* (347–407) and this metaphor: See "The Master-Word in Medicine," p. 267, n. 69.

22. *and it might as well be Arabic:* Arabic is written with a completely different alphabet from the languages of Europe.

type, the man who knows the records, who, with a broad outlook and drilled in what may be called the embryology of history, has yet a powerful vision for the minutiae of life. It is these kitchen and backstair men who are to be encouraged, the men who know the subject in hand in all possible relationships. Concentration has its drawbacks. It is possible to become so absorbed in the problem of the "enclitic $\delta\epsilon$,"[23] or the structure of the flagella of the Trichomonas, or of the toes of the prehistoric horse, that the student loses the sense of proportion in his work, and even wastes a lifetime in researches which are valueless because not in touch with current knowledge. You remember poor Casaubon, in *Middlemarch*,[24] whose painful scholarship was lost on this account. The best preventive to this is to get denationalized early. The true student is a citizen of the world, the allegiance of whose soul, at any rate, is too precious to be restricted to a single country. The great minds, the great works transcend all limitations of time, of language, and of race, and the scholar can never feel initiated into the company of the elect until he can approach all of life's problems from the cosmopolitan standpoint. I care not in what subject he may work, the full knowledge cannot be reached without drawing on supplies from lands other than his own—French, English, German, American, Japanese, Russian, Italian—there must be no discrimination by the loyal student, who should willingly draw from any and every source with an open mind and a stern resolve to render unto all their dues. I care not on what stream of knowledge he may embark, follow up its course, and the rivulets that feed it flow from many lands. If the work is to be effective he must keep in touch with scholars in other countries. How often has it happened that years of precious time have been given to a problem already solved or shown to be insoluble, because of the ignorance of what had been done elsewhere. And it is not only book knowledge and journal knowledge, but a knowledge of men that is needed. The student will, if possible, see the men in other lands. Travel not only widens the vision and gives certainties in place of vague surmises, but the personal contact with foreign workers enables him to appreciate better the failings or successes in his own line of work, perhaps to look with more charitable eyes on the work of some brother whose limitations and opportunities have been more restricted than his own. Or, in contact with a mastermind, he may take

23. enclitic $\delta\epsilon$: (Greek) an unaccented word that becomes attached in speech to the word that comes before it. Osler's point seems to be that enclitic $\delta\epsilon$ is a colorless word, used merely to connect sentences in continuous prose and often not worth translating, and yet whole studies have been written on its correct use.

24. Rev. Edward *Casaubon:* A dreary scholar who married Dorothea. He intended to show, in his life's project, that all mythologies (e.g., Greek mythology, South Sea island creation stories, and African tribal theophanies) were corruption of the narratives of the Bible, but his ardent labor was all in vain because he was ignorant of the new discoveries of his time. George Eliot, *Middlemarch* (1871–1872).

fire, and the glow of the enthusiasm may be the inspiration of his life. Concentration must then be associated with large views on the relation of the problem, and a knowledge of its status elsewhere; otherwise it may land him in the slough of a specialism so narrow that it has depth and no breadth, or he may be led to make what he believes to be important discoveries, but which have long been current coin in other lands. It is sad to think that the day of the great polymathic student is at an end; that we may, perhaps, never again see a Scaliger, a Haller, or a Humboldt[25]—men who took the whole field of knowledge for their domain and viewed it as from a pinnacle. And yet a great specializing generalist may arise, who can tell? Some twentieth-century Aristotle may be now tugging at his bottle, as little dreaming as are his parents or his friends of a conquest of the mind, beside which the wonderful victories of the Stagirite[26] will look pale. The value of a really great student to the country is equal to half a dozen grain elevators or a new transcontinental railway. He is a commodity singularly fickle and variable, and not to be grown to order. So far as his advent is concerned there is no telling when or where he may arise. The conditions seem to be present even under the most unlikely externals. Some of the greatest students this country has produced have come from small villages and country places. It is impossible to predict from a study of the environment, which a "strong propensity of nature,"[27] to quote Milton's phrase again, will easily bend or break.

The student must be allowed full freedom in his work, undisturbed by the utilitarian spirit of the Philistine,[28] who cries, *Cui bono?*[29] and distrusts pure science. The present remarkable position in applied science and in industrial trades

25. The following three figures are Osler's examples of men having very versatile talents:

Julius Caesar *Scaliger* (1484–1558): Italian physician and scholar. His writings included Latin verse, Latin grammar on scientific principles, and commentaries on works of Aristotle, Hippocrates, etc.

Albrecht von *Haller* (1708–1777): Swiss anatomist who traveled to France, England, and Germany to study. See "The Leaven of Science," p. 163, n. 63.

Alexander von *Humboldt* (1769–1859): German naturalist, geographer, and traveler, who explored and mapped Mexico, Central and South America, and later Central Asia. His five-volume *Cosmos* (1845–1858) tried to describe the physical universe. It was considered to be the most valuable contribution to natural science of its time.

26. *the Stagirite:* Aristotle, who was born in Stagira, a city of ancient Macedonia.

27. See p. 308, n. 5.

28. *the Philistine:* A prosaic, materialistic person who scorns intellectual and artistic values. This is a term used in contempt to signify people who are contentedly commonplace in ideas and tastes. "Philister" is a derogatory nickname applied by students at the German universities to hostile townsfolk (*OED*). Carlyle seems to have been the first to use the term this way in English, but it was popularized by Matthew Arnold's use of it in *Culture and Anarchy* (1869).

29. *Cui bono:* (Latin) Osler, like many, seems to have misunderstood it as "whom is it of use to?" rather than "who stands to gain from it?" See "The Leaven of Science," p. 170, n. 91.

of all sorts has been made possible by men who did pioneer work in chemistry, in physics, in biology, and in physiology, without a thought in their researches of any practical application. The members of this higher group of productive students are rarely understood by the common spirits, who appreciate as little their unselfish devotion as their unworldly neglect of the practical side of the problems.

Everywhere now the medical student is welcomed as an honoured member of the guild. There was a time, I confess, and it is within the memory of some of us, when, like Falstaff,[30] he was given to "taverns and sack and wine and metheglins,[31] and to drinkings and swearings and starings, pribbles and prabbles";[32] but all that has changed with the curriculum, and the "Meds" now roar you as gently as the "Theologs."[33] On account of the peculiar character of the subject-matter of your studies, what I have said upon the general life and mental attitude of the student applies with tenfold force to you. Man, with all his mental and bodily anomalies and diseases—the machine in order, the machine in disorder, and the business yours to put it to rights. Through all the phases of its career this most complicated mechanism of this wonderful world will be the subject of our study and of your care—the naked, new-born infant, the artless child, the lad and the lassie just aware of the tree of knowledge overhead, the strong man in the pride of life, the woman with the benediction of maternity on her brow, and the aged, peaceful in the contemplation of the past. Almost everything has been renewed in the science and in the art of medicine, but all through the long centuries there has been no variableness or shadow of change in the essential features of the life which is our contemplation and our care. The sick lovechild of Israel's sweet singer,[34] the plague-stricken hopes of the great Athenian statesman,[35] Elpenor, bereft of his beloved Artemidora,[36] and "Tully's

---

30. *Falstaff:* Jovial fat knight in William Shakespeare's *Henry IV*, parts 1 and 2, and *The Merry Wives of Windsor*, V, v, 168.

31. *metheglins:* Spiced or medicated liquor made by fermenting honey and water.

32. *pribbles and prabbles:* This means "vain chatter" and seems intended as Welsh dialect, because Shakespeare puts it in the mouth of Sir Hugh, the Welsh parson. William Shakespeare, *The Merry Wives of Windsor*, V, v, 156–158.

33. The medical students now are no more rowdy and noisy than the theological students.

34. *Israel's sweet singer:* A reminiscence of 2 Samuel 23:1, where David is called "the sweet psalmist of Israel." He had an illegitimate child with Uriah's wife. The exact quotation is: "And the Lord struck the child that Uriah's wife bare unto David, and it was very sick. David therefore besought God for the child; and David fasted, and went in, and lay all night upon the earth" (2 Samuel 12:15–23).

35. *Pericles* (c.493–429 B.C.): Leader of Athens for thirty years at the peak of its power, prosperity, and cultural achievement. The period of his ascendancy is known as the Golden Age of Athens. Pericles made many reforms that allowed commoners to be elected to high office, and he devoted a great deal of attention to the cultural life of Athens. His policy of foreign conquest led to the Peloponnesian War between

daughter mourned so tenderly,"[37] are not of any age or any race—they are here with us to-day, with the Hamlets, the Ophelias, and the Lears. Amid an eternal heritage of sorrow and suffering our work is laid, and this eternal note of sadness would be insupportable if the daily tragedies were not relieved by the spectacle of the heroism and devotion displayed by the actors.[38] Nothing will sustain you more potently than the power to recognize in your humdrum routine, as perhaps it may be thought, the true poetry of life—the poetry of the commonplace, of the ordinary man, of the plain, toil-worn woman, with their loves and their joys, their sorrows and their griefs. The comedy, too, of life will be spread before you, and nobody laughs more often than the doctor at the pranks Puck plays upon the Titanias and the Bottoms[39] among his patients. The humorous side is really almost as frequently turned towards him as the tragic. Lift up one hand to heaven and thank your stars if they have given you the proper sense to enable you to appreciate the inconceivably droll situations in which we catch our fellow creatures. Unhappily, this is one of the free gifts of the gods, unevenly distributed, not bestowed on all, or on all in equal portions. In undue measure it is not without risk, and in any case in the doctor it is better appreciated by the eye than expressed on the tongue. Hilarity and good humour, a breezy cheerfulness, a nature "sloping toward the southern side,"[40] as Lowell has it, help enormously both in the study and in the practice of medicine. To many of a sombre and sour disposition it is hard to maintain good spirits amid the trials and tribulations of the day, and yet it is an unpardonable mistake to go about among patients with a long face.

Divide your attentions equally between books and men. The strength of the student of books is to sit still—two or three hours at a stretch—eating the heart out of a subject with pencil and notebook in hand, determined to master the details and intricacies, focussing all your energies on its difficulties. Get ac-

---

Athens and Sparta from 431 to 404 B.C., which resulted in the transfer of power in Greece from Athens to Sparta. Pericles died of the plague during this war. Osler's point is that the plague gravely weakened the population and thereby the war effort.

36. *Elpenor:* A companion of Odysseus who died from accidentally falling off the roof of Circe's house. He had been the youngest member of Odysseus' crew. Homer, *Odyssey,* book 10, lines 550–560.

37. Marcus Tullius Cicero: (also Tully) (106–43 B.C.). Roman statesman and writer, had a daughter, Tullia (c.76–45 B.C.), to whom he was devoted. She died in 45 B.C.—the hardest blow he suffered in his private life. Cicero wrote his *Consolatio* (on the deaths of great men) to console himself after Tullia's death.

38. Osler is eased by the knowledge that others have borne similar griefs well and still achieved greatness.

39. Puck is a mischievous fairy who plays tricks on Titania, queen of the fairies, on Bottom, a weaver, and on others in William Shakespeare's *A Midsummer Night's Dream.*

40. The phrase means a sunny disposition. James Russell Lowell, "An Epistle to George William Curtis," postscript, line 54.

customed to test all sorts of book problems and statements for yourself, and take as little as possible on trust. The Hunterian "Do not think, but try" attitude of mind[41] is the important one to cultivate. The question came up one day, when discussing the grooves left on the nails after fever, how long it took for the nail to grow out, from root to edge. A majority of the class had no further interest; a few looked it up in books; two men marked their nails at the root with nitrate of silver, and a few months later had positive knowledge on the subject. They showed the proper spirit. The little points that come up in your reading try to test for yourselves. With one fundamental difficulty many of you will have to contend from the outset—a lack of proper preparation for really hard study. No one can have watched successive groups of young men pass through the special schools without profoundly regretting the haphazard, fragmentary character of their preliminary education. It does seem too bad that we cannot have a student in his eighteenth year sufficiently grounded in the humanities and in the sciences preliminary to medicine—but this is an educational problem upon which only a Milton or a Locke could discourse with profit.[42] With pertinacity you can overcome the preliminary defects and once thoroughly interested, the work in books becomes a pastime. A serious drawback in the student life is the selfconsciousness, bred of too close devotion to books. A man gets shy, "dysopic,"[43] as old Timothy Bright[44] calls it, and shuns the looks of men, and blushes like a girl.

The strength of a student of men is to travel—to study men, their habits, character, mode of life, their behaviour under varied conditions, their vices, virtues, and peculiarities. Begin with a careful observation of your fellow stu-

41. Hunter's approach to physiology and pathology was practical, based on experiment and observations rather than on theory. He said, "Don't think: try; be patient; be accurate." Quoted in James Paget, "Hunterian Oration" (February 13, 1877), in *Selected Essays and Addresses* (London: Longmans, Green, 1902), p. 192. For biographical information, see "The Old Humanities and the New Science," p. 93, n. 214.

42. Both men worked as tutors and wrote on the problems of education.

John *Milton* (1608–1674) was tutor to his nephews Edward and John Phillips. While tutoring he developed and practiced his educational theories later outlined in *Of Education* (1644).

John *Locke* (1632–1704) was tutor to Anthony Ashley Cooper (later earl of Shaftesbury). In the "Epistle Dedicatory" to his book *Some Thoughts Concerning Education*, addressed to Edward Clarke, he wrote that "I my self have been consulted of late by so many, who profess themselves at a loss how to breed their Children." John Locke, *Some Thoughts Concerning Education*, ed. John W. Yolton and Jean S. Yolton (Oxford: Clarendon Press, 1989), p. 79.

43. *dysopic*: (Greek) shy. Timothy Bright cited *dysopia* as a Greek word meaning "confusion of face, shamefacedness" in *A Treatise of Melancholie* (1586; New York: Da Capo Press, 1969), p. 166.

44. Timothy *Bright* (c.1551–1615): English inventor of shorthand. He abandoned the medical profession to take holy orders in 1590.

dents and of your teachers; then, every patient you see is a lesson in much more than the malady from which he suffers. Mix as much as you possibly can with the outside world, and learn its ways. Cultivated systematically, the student societies, the students' union, the gymnasium, and the outside social circle will enable you to conquer the diffidence so apt to go with bookishness and which may prove a very serious drawback in after-life. I cannot too strongly impress upon the earnest and attentive men among you the necessity of overcoming this unfortunate failing in your student days. It is not easy for every one to reach a happy medium, and the distinction between a proper self-confidence and "cheek,"[45] particularly in junior students, is not always to be made. The latter is met with chiefly among the student pilgrims who, in travelling down the Delectable Mountains, have gone astray and have passed to the left hand, where lieth the country of Conceit, the country in which you remember the brisk lad Ignorance met Christian.[46]

I wish we could encourage on this continent among our best students the habit of wandering. I do not know that we are quite prepared for it, as there is still great diversity in the curricula, even among the leading schools, but it is undoubtedly a great advantage to study under different teachers, as the mental horizon is widened and the sympathies enlarged. The practice would do much to lessen that narrow "I am of Paul and I am of Apollos"[47] spirit which is hostile to the best interests of the profession.

There is much that I would like to say on the question of work, but I can spare only a few moments for a word or two. Who will venture to settle upon so simple a matter as the best time for work? One will tell us there is no best time; all are equally good; and truly, all times are the same to a man whose soul is absorbed in some great problem. The other day I asked Edward Martin,[48] the well-known story-writer, what time he found best for work. "Not in the evening, and never between meals!" was his answer, which may appeal to some of my hearers. One works best at night; another, in the morning; a majority of the students of the past favour the latter. Erasmus,[49] the great exemplar, says, "Never work at night; it dulls the brain and hurts the

45. *cheek*: (Colloq.) impudence, or insolent boldness.

46. John Bunyan, *The Pilgrim's Progress* (1678; London: George Routledge and Son, n.d.).

47. The actual quote is: "I am a disciple of Paul and I am a disciple of Apollos." Each man or "I" proclaims himself to be strictly of one school or another, while Osler favors a more open attitude (1 Corinthians 1:10–17).

48. Edward S. *Martin* (1856–1939): American journalist. Author of *A Little Brother of the Rich, and Other Verses* (1890), *What's Ahead and Meanwhile* (1927), and many other works.

49. Desiderius *Erasmus* (c.1466–1536): See "The Old Humanities and the New Science," p. 66, n. 11.

health."[50] One day, going with George Ross[51] through Bedlam,[52] Dr. Savage,[53] at that time the physician in charge, remarked upon two great groups of patients—those who were depressed in the morning and those who were cheerful, and he suggested that the spirits rose and fell with the bodily temperature—those with very low morning temperatures were depressed, and vice versa. This, I believe, expresses a truth which may explain the extraordinary difference in the habits of students in this matter of the time at which the best work can be done. Outside of the asylum there are also the two great types, the student-lark[54] who loves to see the sun rise, who comes to breakfast with a cheerful morning face, never so "fit" as at 6 a.m. We all know the type. What a contrast to the student-owl[55] with his saturnine[56] morning face, thoroughly unhappy, cheated by the wretched breakfast bell of the two best hours of the day for sleep, no appetite, and permeated with an unspeakable hostility to his *vis-à-vis*,[57] whose morning garrulity and good humour are equally offensive. Only gradually, as the day wears on and his temperature rises, does he become endurable to himself and to others. But see him really awake at 10 p. m. while our blithe lark is in hopeless coma over his books, from which it is hard to rouse him sufficiently to get his boots off for bed, our lean owl-friend, Saturn no longer in the ascendant,[58] with bright eyes and cheery face, is ready for four hours of anything you wish—deep study, or

Heart-affluence in discursive talk,[59]

and by 2 a.m. he will undertake to unsphere the spirit of Plato.[60] In neither a virtue, in neither a fault we must recognize these two types of students, differently constituted, owing possibly—though I have but little evidence for the belief—to thermal peculiarities.

THE STUDENT
LIFE

50. The passage is from Erasmus' letter 79. Osler made a note of it when reading J. A. Froude's *Life and Letters of Erasmus* (New York: Charles Scribner's Sons, 1894), p. 65 (Cushing, vol. 1, p. 534).

51. George *Ross* (1845–1892): See "After Twenty-Five Years," p. 206, n. 18.

52. *Bedlam:* Popular name for the hospital of St. Mary of Bethlehem, an insane asylum in south London.

53. Probably George Henry *Savage* (1842–1921): Physician at London's Bethlehem Hospital and later at St. Thomas' Hospital. Author of *Dreams: Normal and Morbid* (1908).

54. With allusion to the lark's habit of singing at dawn.

55. With allusion to the owl's nocturnal habit.

56. *saturnine:* Gloomy; sluggish.

57. *vis-à-vis:* (French) this is used in the sense of "the person sitting across the table."

58. In astrology Saturn was thought to produce melancholy, and its influence was believed to be greatest when it was in the ascendant; that is, above the eastern horizon and proceeding toward its zenith.

59. Alfred Tennyson, "In Memoriam A.H.H.," stanza 109, line 1.

60. *unsphere the spirit of Plato:* John Milton, "Il Penseroso," lines 88–89.

II

In the days of probation the student's life may be lived by each one of you in its fullness and in its joys, but the difficulties arise in the break which follows departure from college and the entrance upon new duties. Much will now depend on the attitude of mind which has been encouraged. If the work has been for your degree, if the diploma has been its sole aim and object, you will rejoice in a freedom from exacting and possibly unpleasant studies, and with your books you will throw away all thoughts of further systematic work. On the other hand, with good habits of observation you may have got deep enough into the subject to feel that there is still much to be learned, and if you have had ground into you the lesson that the collegiate period is only the beginning of the student life, there is a hope that you may enter upon the useful career of the *student-practitioner.* Five years, at least, of trial await the man after parting from his teachers, and entering upon an independent course—years upon which his future depends, and from which his horoscope may be cast with certainty. It is all the same whether he settles in a country village or goes on with hospital and laboratory work; whether he takes a prolonged trip abroad; or whether he settles down in practice with a father or a friend—these five waiting years fix his fate so far as the student life is concerned. Without any strong natural propensity to study,[61] he may feel such a relief after graduation that the effort to take to books is beyond his mental strength, and a weekly journal with an occasional textbook furnish pabulum[62] enough, at least to keep his mind hibernating. But ten years later he is dead mentally, past any possible hope of galvanizing into life as a student, fit to do a routine practice, often a capable, resourceful man, but without any deep convictions, and probably more interested in stocks or in horses than in diagnosis or therapeutics. But this is not always the fate of the student who finishes his work on Commencement Day.[63] There are men full of zeal in practice who give good service to their fellow creatures, who have not the capacity or the energy to keep up with the times. While they have lost interest in science, they are loyal members of the profession, and appreciate their responsibilities as such. That fateful first lustrum[64] ruins some of our most likely material. Nothing is more trying to the soldier than inaction, to

61. See p. 308, n. 5. Osler changed the phrasing slightly.

62. *pabulum:* Blended food, such as baby food, easily digested for nourishment; also, material for intellectual nourishment.

63. *Commencement Day:* The day when candidates formally take their degrees, and so "commence" to be bachelors of arts, masters of science, and the like.

64. *lustrum:* A period of five years.

mark time while the battle is raging all about him; and waiting for practice is a serious strain under which many yield. In the cities it is not so hard to keep up: there is work in the dispensaries and colleges, and the stimulus of the medical societies; but in smaller towns and in the country it takes a strong man to live through the years of waiting without some deterioration. I wish the custom of taking junior men as partners and assistants would grow on this continent. It has become a necessity, and no man in large general practice can do his work efficiently without skilled help. How incalculably better for the seniors, how beneficial to the patients, how helpful in every way if each one of you, for the first five or ten years, was associated with an older practitioner, doing his night work, his laboratory work, his chores of all sorts. You would, in this way, escape the chilling and killing isolation of the early years, and amid congenial surroundings you could, in time, develop into that flower of our calling—the cultivated general practitioner. May this be the destiny of a large majority of you! Have no higher ambition! You cannot reach any better position in a community; the family doctor is the man behind the gun, who does our effective work. That his life is hard and exacting; that he is underpaid and overworked; that he has but little time for study and less for recreation—these are the blows that may give finer temper to his steel, and bring out the nobler elements in his character. What lot or portion has the general practitioner in the student life? Not, perhaps, the fruitful heritage of Judah or Benjamin[65] but he may make of it the goodly portion of Ephraim.[66] A man with powers of observation, well trained in the wards, and with the strong natural propensity[67] to which I have so often referred, may live the ideal student life, and even reach the higher levels of scholarship. Adams,[68] of Banchory (a little Aberdeenshire village), was not only a good practitioner and a skilful operator, but he was an excellent naturalist. This is by no means an unusual or remarkable combination, but Adams became, in addition, one of the great scholars of the profession. He had a perfect passion for the classics, and amid a very exacting practice found time to read "almost

THE STUDENT LIFE

65. *Judah:* The fourth son of Jacob and Leah. *Benjamin:* The youngest and favorite son of Jacob and Rachel, and brother of Joseph. This is from Jacob's prophecy concerning his sons. The exact quotations are: "Judah, thou *art he* whom thy brethren shall praise: . . . Judah *is* a lion's whelp: from thy prey, my son, thou art gone up" (Genesis 49:8–12), and "Benjamin shall ravin *as* a wolf: in the morning he shall devour the prey, and at night he shall divide the spoil" (Genesis 49:27).

66. *Ephraim:* The younger son of Joseph. He was chosen over his older brother Manasseh by his dying grandfather, Jacob, to receive a greater inheritance in Israel. The exact quotation is: "But truly his younger brother shall be greater than he, and his seed shall become a multitude of nations" (Genesis 48:17–22).

67. See p. 308, n. 5.

68. Francis *Adams* (1796–1861): Scottish physician and outstanding scholar of Greek medicine.

every Greek work which has come down to us from antiquity, except the ecclesiastical writers."[69] He translated the works of Paulus Aegineta,[70] the works of Hippocrates,[71] and the works of Aretaeus,[72] all of which are in the Sydenham Society's publications,[73] monuments of the patient skill and erudition of a Scottish village doctor, an incentive to every one of us to make better use of our precious time.

Given the sacred hunger and proper preliminary training, the student-practitioner requires at least three things with which to stimulate and maintain his education, a notebook, a library, and a quinquennial braindusting. I wish I had time to speak of the value of note-taking. You can do nothing as a student in practice without it. Carry a small notebook which will fit into your waistcoat pocket, and never ask a new patient a question without notebook and pencil in hand. After the examination of a pneumonia case two minutes will suffice to record the essentials in the daily progress. Routine and system when once made a habit, facilitate work, and the busier you are the more time you will have to make observations after examining a patient. Jot a comment at the end of the notes: "clear case," "case illustrating obscurity of symptoms," "error in diagnosis," etc. The making of observations, may become the exercise of a jackdaw trick,[74] like the craze which so many of us have to collect articles of all sorts. The study of the cases, the relation they bear to each other and to the cases in literature—here comes in the difficulty. Begin early to make a threefold category—clear cases, doubtful cases, mistakes. And learn to play the game fair, no self-deception, no shrinking from the truth; mercy and consideration for the other man, but none for yourself, upon whom you have to keep an incessant watch. You remember Lincoln's famous *mot*[75] about the impossibility of fooling all of the people all the time. It does not hold good for the individual who can fool himself to his heart's

---

69. The quote comes from J. F. Payne's article on Francis Adams in *The Dictionary of National Biography*.

70. Paulus *Aegineta* (fl. *ante* 700): Greek medical writer. He was the last major ancient Greek encyclopaedist, whose *Epitomae medicae libri septem* (Abridgement of Medicine in Seven Books) contained almost all the knowledge concerning medical arts at the time.

71. *Hippocrates* (c.460–c.375 B.C.): See "The Master-Word in Medicine," p. 274, n. 108.

72. *Aretaeus* of Cappadocia (c.1st to 2nd cent. A.D.): See "Chauvinism in Medicine," p. 231, n. 10.

73. Society named after Thomas Sydenham (1624–1689), the "English Hippocrates," who is considered the founder of modern clinical medicine and epidemiology.

74. *jackdaw:* A crow-like bird, which is said to collect all sorts of things. Osler might have been thinking of "The Jackdaw of Rheims" in *The Ingoldsby Legends* (1840) by Richard Harris Barham. In this poem a jackdaw carries off a cardinal's ring.

75. Attributed words in a speech at Charleston, the fourth of the Lincoln-Douglas debates, September 8, 1858, during his campaign for a Senate seat.

content all of the time. If necessary, be cruel; use the knife and the cautery to cure the intumescence[76] and moral necrosis which you will feel in the posterior parietal region, in Gall and Spurzheim's[77] centre of self-esteem, where you will find a sore spot after you have made a mistake in diagnosis. It is only by getting your cases grouped in this way that you can make any real progress in your post-collegiate education; only in this way can you gain wisdom with experience. It is a common error to think that the more a doctor sees the greater his experience and the more he knows. No one ever drew a more skilful distinction than Cowper in his oft-quoted lines, which I am never tired of repeating in a medical audience:

> Knowledge and wisdom, far from being one,
> Have oft-times no connexion. Knowledge dwells
> In heads replete with thoughts of other men;
> Wisdom in minds attentive to their own.
> Knowledge is proud that he has learned so much;
> Wisdom is humble that he knows no more.[78]

What we call sense or wisdom is knowledge, ready for use, made effective, and bears the same relation to knowledge itself that bread does to wheat. The full knowledge of the parts of a steam engine and the theory of its action may be possessed by a man who could not be trusted to pull the lever to its throttle. It is only by collecting data and using them that you can get sense. One of the most delightful sayings of antiquity is the remark of Heraclitus upon his predecessors[79]—that they had much knowledge but no sense—which indicates that the noble old Ephesian[80] had a keen appreciation of their difference; and the distinction, too, is well drawn by Tennyson in the oft-quoted line:

---

76. *intumescence:* A swelling of the tissue.

77. Franz Joseph *Gall* (1758–1828): See "The Leaven of Science," p. 165, n. 70.

   Johann Kaspar *Spurzheim* (1776–1832): See "The Leaven of Science," p. 165, n. 70.

78. William Cowper, *The Task* (1784), book 6, "The Winter Walk at Noon," lines 89–97. Osler omitted the following four lines:

> Knowledge, a rude unprofitable mass,
> The mere materials with which wisdom builds,
> Till smooth'd and squar'd and fitted to its place,
> Does but encumber whom it seems t' enrich.

79. *Heraclitus* (c.540–c.470 B.C.): Greek philosopher and early metaphysician. He is known as "the Weeping Philosopher" because of his gloomy view of life. His phrase *panta rhei* (all things are in a state of flux) is well known. The writings of Heraclitus are lost except for fragments preserved as quotations by other ancient writers. This idea is referred to by Aristotle in *De Caelo*, book 3, chap. 1, sect. 298b.

80. Heraclitus was born in Ephesus, an ancient city in West Asia Minor, south of Smyrna.

Knowledge comes but wisdom lingers.[81]

Of the three well-stocked rooms which it should be the ambition of every young doctor to have in his house, the library, the laboratory, and the nursery—books, balances, and bairns [82]—as he may not achieve all three, I would urge him to start at any rate with the books and the balances. A good weekly and a good monthly journal to begin with, and read them. Then, for a systematic course of study, supplement your college textbooks with the larger systems—Allbutt or Nothnagel [83]—a system of surgery, and, as your practice increases, make a habit of buying a few special monographs every year. Read with two objects: first, to acquaint yourself with the current knowledge on the subject and the steps by which it has been reached; and secondly, and more important, read to understand and analyse your cases. To this line of work we should direct the attention of the student before he leaves the medical school, pointing in specific cases just where the best articles are to be found, sending him to the Index Catalogue—that marvellous storehouse, every page of which is interesting and the very titles instructive. Early learn to appreciate the differences between the descriptions of disease and the manifestations of that disease in an individual—the difference between the composite portrait and one of the component pictures. By exercise of a little judgment you can collect at moderate cost a good working library. Try, in the waiting years, to get a clear idea of the history of medicine. Read Foster's *Lectures on the History of Physiology* [84] and Baas's *History of Medicine*.[85] Get the "Masters of Medicine" Series,[86] and subscribe to the *Library and Historical Journal*.[87]

Every day do some reading or work apart from your profession. I fully realize, no one more so, how absorbing is the profession of medicine; how applicable

81. Alfred Tennyson, "Locksley Hall," line 141.

82. *bairn:* (Scottish) A child.

83. Thomas Clifford *Allbutt* (1836–1925): English medical writer and physician. He invented the short clinical thermometer (1866) and wrote *Systems of Medicine* (1896–1899).

Carl W. H. *Nothnagel* (1841–1905): German physician. He studied the physiology and pathology of the nervous system and edited *Spezielle Pathologie und Therapie* in 24 volumes (1894–1908), trans. Alfred Stengel, *Nothnagel's Encyclopedia of Practical Medicine* (Philadelphia: W.B. Saunders, 1904).

84. Michael *Foster* (1836–1907): English physiologist and professor at Cambridge. Author of *Lectures on the History of Physiology during the 16th, 17th and 18th Centuries* (1901). He was a medical historian who introduced modern methods of teaching biology, physiology, and embryology with an emphasis on laboratory training.

85. Johann Herman *Baas* (1838–1909): German physician and author of *History of Medicine* (1876).

86. *Masters of Medicine Series:* (New York: Longman, Green, 1897–1899). The series includes Hunter, Harvey, Helmholtz, Sydenham, Vesalius, and others.

87. Osler's original note reads: "Brooklyn. Price $2 per annum."

to it is what Michelangelo says: "There are sciences which demand the whole of a man, without leaving the least portion of his spirit free for other distractions";[88] but you will be a better man and not a worse practitioner for an avocation. I care not what it may be; gardening or farming, literature or history or bibliography, any one of which will bring you into contact with books. (I wish that time permitted me to speak of the other two rooms which are really of equal importance with the library, but which are more difficult to equip, though of co-ordinate value in the education of the head, the heart, and the hand.) The third essential for the practitioner as a student is the quinquennial brain-dusting, and this will often seem to him the hardest task to carry out. Every fifth year, back to the hospital, back to the laboratory, for renovation, rehabilitation, rejuvenation, re-integration, resuscitation, etc. Do not forget to take the notebooks with you, or the sheets, in three separate bundles, to work over. From the very start begin to save for the trip. Deny yourself all luxuries for it; shut up the room you meant for the nursery—have the definite determination to get your education thoroughly well started; if you are successful you may, perhaps, have enough saved at the end of three years to spend six weeks in special study; or in five years you may be able to spend six months. Hearken not to the voice of old "Dr. Hayseed,"[89] who tells you it will ruin your prospects, and that he "never heard of such a thing" as a young man, not yet five years in practice, taking three months' holiday. To him it seems preposterous. Watch him wince when you say it is a speculation in the only gold mine which the physician should invest—*Grey Cortex:*[90] What about the wife and babies, if you have them? Leave them! Heavy as are your responsibilities to those nearest and dearest, they are outweighed by the responsibilities to yourself, to the profession, and to the public. Like Isaphaena, the story of whose husband—ardent, earnest soul, peace to his ashes![91]—I have told in the little sketch of *An Alabama Student*, your wife will be glad to bear her share in the sacrifice you make.

88. *Michelangelo* Buonarroti (1475–1564): Italian sculptor, painter, and poet of the High Renaissance. He drew anatomical sketches that Osler admired.

  Michelangelo here discusses the art of painting with Hollanda (1517–1584) a young Portuguese artist. Francisco de Hollanda, *Four Dialogues on Painting*, trans. Aubrey F. G. Bell (Westport, Conn.: Hyperion Press, 1979), p. 13.

89. The word "hayseed" means a countryman, rustic, or "yokel" or "hick" in U.S. slang. Osler refers to a rustic doctor as someone who does not understand the necessity of study.

90. *The layer of grey matter:* Nervous tissue that covers the cerebral hemispheres and the cerebellum. Here Osler uses the term to refer to brains or intellect.

91. William Osler, *An Alabama Student and Other Biographical Essays* (London: Chiswick Press, 1906). The Alabama student refers to Dr. John Y. Bassett (1805–1851) of Huntsville, Alabama. He left his wife Isaphaena and two children in Alabama to study in Paris.

With good health and good habits the end of the second lustrum should find you thoroughly established—all three rooms well furnished, a good stable, a good garden, no mining stock, but a life insurance, and, perhaps, a mortgage or two on neighbouring farms. Year by year you have dealt honestly with yourself; you have put faithfully the notes of each case into their proper places, and you will be gratified to find that, though the doubtful cases and mistakes still make a rather formidable pile, it has grown relatively smaller. You literally "own" the countryside, as the expression is. All the serious and dubious cases come to you, and you have been so honest in the frank acknowledgment of your own mistakes, and so charitable in the contemplation of theirs, that neighbouring doctors, old and young, are glad to seek your advice. The work, which has been very heavy, is now lightened by a good assistant, one of your own students, who becomes in a year or so your partner. This is not an overdrawn picture, and it is one which may be seen in many places except, I am sorry to say, in the particular as to the partner. This is the type of man we need in the country districts and the smaller towns. He is not a whit too good to look after the sick, not a whit too highly educated—impossible! And with an optimistic temperament and a good digestion he is the very best product of our profession, and may do more to stop quackery and humbuggery, inside and outside of the ranks, than could a dozen prosecuting county attorneys. Nay, more! such a doctor may be a daily benediction in the community—a strong, sensible, whole-souled man, often living a life of great self-denial, and always of tender sympathy, worried neither by the vagaries[92] of the well nor by the testy waywardness of the sick, and to him, if to any, may come (even when he knows it not) the true spiritual blessing—that "blessing which maketh rich and addeth no sorrow."[93]

The danger in such a man's life comes with prosperity. He is safe in the hard-working day, when he is climbing the hill, but once success is reached, with it come the temptations to which many succumb. Politics has been the ruin of many country doctors, and often of the very best, of just such a good fellow as he of whom I have been speaking. He is popular; he has a little money; and he, if anybody, can save the seat for the party! When the committee leaves you, take the offer under consideration, and if in the ten or twelve years you have kept on intimate terms with those friends of your student days, Montaigne and Plutarch,[94] you will know what answer to return. If you live in a large town, resist the temptation to open a sanatorium. It is not the work for a general prac-

92. *vagaries:* Capricious or eccentric acts.

93. Proverbs 10:22.

94. Michel Eyquem de *Montaigne* (1533–1592): See "Sir Thomas Browne," p. 57, n. 179.

Plutarch (c.46–c.125 A.D.): See "The Old Humanities and the New Science," p. 73, n. 62.

titioner, and there are risks that you may sacrifice your independence and much else besides. And, thirdly, resist the temptation to move into a larger place. In a good agricultural district, or in a small town, if you handle your resources aright, taking good care of your education, of your habits, and of your money, and devoting part of your energies to the support of the societies, etc., you may reach a position in the community of which any man may be proud. There are country practitioners among my friends with whom I would rather change places than with any in our ranks, men whose stability of character and devotion to duty make one proud of the profession.

Curiously enough, the student-practitioner may find studiousness to be a stumbling-block[95] in his career. A bookish man may never succeed; deep-versed in books, he may not be able to use his knowledge to practical effect; or, more likely, his failure is not because he has studied books much, but because he has not studied men more. He has never got over that shyness, that diffidence, against which I have warned you. I have known instances in which this malady was incurable; in others I have known a cure effected not by the public, but by the man's professional brethren, who, appreciating his work, have insisted upon utilizing his mental treasures. It is very hard to carry student habits into a large city practice; only zeal, a fiery passion, keeps the flame alive, smothered as it is so apt to be by the dust and ashes of the daily routine. A man may be a good student who reads only the book of nature. Such a one I remember[96] in the early days of my residence in Montreal—a man whose devotion to patients and whose kindness and skill quickly brought him an enormous practice. Reading in his carriage and by lamplight at Lucina's bedside,[97] he was able to keep well informed; but he had an insatiable desire to know the true inwardness of a disease, and it was in this way I came into contact with him. Hard pushed day and night, yet he was never too busy to spend a couple of hours with me searching for data which had not been forthcoming during life, or helping to unravel the mysteries of a new disease, such as pernicious anaemia.

III

The *student-specialist* has to walk warily, as with two advantages there are two great dangers against which he has constantly to be on guard. In the bewilder-

95. Isaiah 8:14 and Romans 9:33. The phrase means "an obstacle to one's progress or anything that causes people to offend." See also "After Twenty-Five Years," p. 212, n. 35.

96. Osler's original note reads: "The late John Bell." John *Bell* (1852–1897): Canadian surgeon at the Montreal General Hospital and professor of clinical surgery at McGill University.

97. *Lucina:* Roman goddess presiding over childbirth.

ing complexity of modern medicine it is a relief to limit the work of a life to a comparatively narrow field which can be thoroughly tilled. To many men there is a feeling of great satisfaction in the mastery of a small department, particularly one in which technical skill is required. How much we have benefited from this concentration of effort in dermatology, laryngology, ophthalmology, and in gynecology! Then, as a rule, the specialist is a free man, with leisure or, at any rate, with some leisure; not the slave of the public, with the incessant demands upon him of the general practitioner. He may live a more rational life, and has time to cultivate his mind, and he is able to devote himself to public interests and to the welfare of his professional brethren, on whose suffrage he so largely depends. How much we are indebted in the larger cities to the disinterested labours of this favoured class the records of our libraries and medical societies bear witness. The dangers do not come to the strong man in a speciality, but to the weak brother who seeks in it an easier field in which specious garrulity and mechanical dexterity may take the place of solid knowledge. All goes well when the man is larger than his speciality and controls it, but when the speciality runs away with the man there is disaster, and a topsy-turvy condition which, in every branch, has done incalculable injury. Next to the danger from small men is the serious risk of the loss of perspective in prolonged and concentrated effort in a narrow field. Against this there is but one safeguard—the cultivation of the sciences upon which the speciality is based. The student-specialist may have a wide vision—no student wider—if he gets away from the mechanical side of the art, and keeps in touch with the physiology and pathology upon which his art depends. More than any other of us, he needs the lessons of the laboratory, and wide contact with men in other departments may serve to correct the inevitable tendency to a narrow and perverted vision, in which the life of the ant-hill is mistaken for the world at large.

Of the *student-teacher* every faculty affords examples in varying degrees. It goes without saying that no man can teach successfully who is not at the same time a student. Routine, killing routine, saps the vitality of many who start with high aims, and who, for years, strive with all their energies against the degeneration which it is so prone to entail. In the smaller schools isolation, the absence of congenial spirits working at the same subject, favours stagnation, and after a few years the fires of early enthusiasm no longer glow in the perfunctory lectures. In many teachers the ever-increasing demands of practice leave less and less time for study, and a first-class man may lose touch with his subject through no fault of his own, but through an entanglement in outside affairs which he deeply regrets yet cannot control. To his five natural senses the student-teacher must add two more—the sense of responsibility and the sense of proportion. Most of us start with a highly developed sense of the importance of the work, and with a desire to live up to the responsibilities entrusted to us. Punctuality, the class first, always and at all times; the best that a man has in him, nothing less; the best the profession has on the subject, nothing less; fresh energies and enthusiasm in dealing with dry details; animated, unselfish devotion to all alike; tender consideration for his assistants—these are some of the fruits of a keen sense of responsibility in a good teacher. The sense of proportion is not so easy to acquire, and much depends on the training and on the natural disposition. There are men who never possess it; to others it seems to come naturally. In the most careful ones it needs constant cultivation—*nothing over-much*[98] should be the motto of every teacher. In my early days I came under the influence of an ideal student-teacher, the late Palmer Howard,[99] of Montreal. If you ask what manner of man he was, read Matthew Arnold's noble tribute to his father in his well-known poem, *Rugby Chapel.*[100] When young, Dr. Howard had chosen a path— "path to a clear-purposed goal,"[101] and he pursued it with unswerving devotion. With him the study and the teaching of medicine were an absorbing passion, the ardour of which neither the incessant and ever-increasing demands upon his time nor the growing years could quench. When I first, as a senior student, came into intimate contact with him in the summer of 1871, the problem of tuberculosis was under discussion, stirred up by the epoch-making work of Villemin[102] and the radical views of Niemeyer.[103] Every lung lesion at the Montreal General Hospital had to be shown to him, and I got my first-hand introduction to Laënnec, to Graves, and to Stokes,[104] and became familiar with their works. No matter what the hour, and it usually was after 10 p. m., I was welcome with my bag, and if Wilks and Moxon, Virchow, or Rokitanski[105] gave us no help, there

98. This phrase derives from the Latin expression *ne quid nimis* (nothing in excess), advocating the middle ground in all things. The Latin, in turn, derives from the Greek quoted in Plato's *Protagoras*, 343b.

99. Robert Palmer *Howard* (1823–1889): Osler's teacher and mentor at McGill University. For further information, see "Aequanimitas," p. 28, n. 42.

100. Matthew Arnold (1822–1888): English poet, whose father, Dr. Thomas Arnold, a distinguished headmaster of Rugby, was buried in the school chapel in 1842.

101. Matthew Arnold, "Rugby Chapel," line 85.

102. Jean Antoine *Villemin* (1827–1892): French bacteriologist whose studies on tuberculosis led Pasteur to believe that a microscopic germ was the transmissible aetiological agent of the disease.

103. Felix von *Niemeyer* (1820–1871): German physician. Author of the much-translated *Lehrbuch der Speziellen Pathologie und Therapie* (1858–1861).

104. Théophile René Hyacinthe *Laënnec* (1781–1826): See "Chauvinism in Medicine," p. 236, n. 34.
Robert James *Graves* (1796–1853): See "The Master-Word in Medicine," p. 260, n. 34.
William *Stokes* (1804–1878): See "The Master-Word in Medicine," p. 260, n. 34.

105. Samuel *Wilks* (1824–1911): English physician at Guy's Hospital and the Royal Hospital for Children, London. Author of the eight-volume *Lectures on the Specific Fevers and Diseases of the Chest* (1875).
Walter *Moxon* (1836–1886): English physician and lecturer at Guy's Hospital.
Rudolf *Virchow* (1821–1902): See "The Old Humanities and the New Science," p. 75, n. 80.

were the Transactions of the Pathological Society[106] and the big *Dictionnaire* of Dechambre.[107] An ideal teacher because a student, ever alert to the new problems, an indomitable energy enabled him in the midst of an exacting practice to maintain an ardent enthusiasm, still to keep bright the fires which he had lighted in his youth. Since those days I have seen many teachers, and I have had many colleagues, but I have never known one in whom were more happily combined a stern sense of duty with the mental freshness of youth.

But as I speak, from out of the memory of the past there rises before me a shadowy group, a long line of students whom I have taught and loved, and who have died prematurely—mentally, morally, or bodily. To the successful we are willing and anxious to bring the tribute of praise, but none so poor to give recognition to the failures. From one cause or another, perhaps because when not absorbed in the present, my thoughts are chiefly in the past, I have cherished the memory of many young men whom I have loved and lost. *Io victis:*[108] let us sometimes sing of the vanquished. Let us sometimes think of those who have fallen in the battle of life, who have striven and failed, who have failed even without the strife. How many have I lost from the student band by mental death, and from so many causes—some stillborn from college, others dead within the first year of infantile marasmus,[109] while mental rickets, teething, tabes,[110] and fits have carried off many of the most promising minds! Due to improper feeding within the first five fateful years, scurvy and rickets head the mental mortality bills of students. To the teacher-nurse it is a sore disappointment to find at the end of ten years so few minds with the full stature, of which the early days gave promise. Still, so widespread is mental death that we scarcely comment upon it in our friends. The real tragedy is the moral death which, in different forms, overtakes so many good fellows who fall away from the pure, honourable, and righteous service of Minerva[111] into the idolatry of Bacchus, of

---

Karl von *Rokitanski* (1804–1878): Austrian physician and one of the founders of modern pathological anatomy. Author of *Handbuch der Pathologischen Anatomie* (1842–1846).

106. The transactions published in London 1847–1893.

107. *Dictionnaire Encyclopédique des Sciences Médicales: A one-hundred-volume work* (1864–1889) compiled by the French physician Amédée Dechambre (1812–1886).

108. *Io victis:* (Latin) Osler coined this. The usual expression is *Vae victis,* Latin for "Woe to the vanquished!" spoken by Brennus the Gaul when he conquered Rome, according to Livy (59 B.C.–17 A.D.) in his *History of Rome,* book 5, chap. 48, the last sentence. Osler has changed this to "Hail to the vanquished," *Io* in Latin being an interjection to express joy.

109. *infantile marasmus:* Emaciation and wasting in an infant, as from malnutrition rather than from actual disease.

110. *tabes:* Gradual, progressive emaciation in any chronic disease

111. *Minerva:* Roman goddess of wisdom and the arts, identified with the Greek Athena.

Venus, or of Circe.[112] Against the background of the past these tragedies stand out, lurid and dark, and as the names and faces of my old boys recur (some of them my special pride), I shudder to think of the blighted hopes and wrecked lives, and I force my memory back to those happy days when they were as you are now, joyous and free from care, and I think of them on the benches, in the laboratories, and in the wards—and there I leave them. Less painful to dwell upon, though associated with a more poignant grief, is the fate of those whom physical death has snatched away in the bud or blossom of the student life. These are among the tender memories of the teacher's life, of which he does not often care to speak, feeling with Longfellow that the surest pledge of their remembrance is "the silent homage of thoughts unspoken."[113] As I look back it seems now as if the best of us had died, that the brightest and the keenest had been taken and the more commonplace among us had been spared. An old mother, a devoted sister, a loving brother, in some cases a broken-hearted wife, still pay the tribute of tears for the untimely ending of their high hopes, and in loving remembrance I would mingle mine with theirs. What a loss to our profession have been the deaths of such true disciples as Zimmerman, of Toronto; of Jack Cline and of R. L. MacDonnell, of Montreal; of Fred Packard and of Kirkbride, of Philadelphia; of Livingood, of Lazear, of Oppenheimer, and of Oechsner, in Baltimore[114]—cut off with their leaves still in the green, to the inconsolable grief of their friends!

112. *Bacchus:* God of wine and revelry.

Venus: Roman goddess of sexual desire identified with the Greek Aphrodite.

Circe: An enchantress who turned the companions of Odysseus into swine with a magical drink. Homer, *Odyssey,* book 10.

113. Henry Wadsworth Longfellow, "The Herons of Elmwood," line 36.

114. Richard *Zimmerman* (1851–1888): See "The Master-Word in Medicine," p. 261, n. 40.

Jack *Cline* (1852–1877): One of Osler's friends at McGill and a member of Osler's Journal Club for the circulation of French and German journals. He died of diphtheria at age twenty-five.

Richard Lee *MacDonnel* (1853–1891): A colleague of Osler at McGill. He died untimely from tuberculosis in 1891. For further information, see "Teaching and Thinking," p. 182, n. 30.

Frederick A. *Packard* (1862–1902): Physician of the Children's Hospital and the Pennsylvania Hospital who died of typhoid in 1902.

Thomas Story *Kirkbride* (1809–1883): Physician-in-chief of the Pennsylvania Hospital for the Insane.

Louis Eugene *Livingood* (1860–1898): One of those who helped Osler to revise the textbook. At the end of the preface to the text, Osler "spoke of his obligations to Livingood, a victim of the Bourgogne disaster, who had been on his way for a year's study abroad." The *Bourgogne* was an ocean liner that sank in the North Atlantic in 1898.

Jesse W. *Lazear* (1866–1900): One of Osler's assistants and one of the doctors who allowed themselves to be bitten by mosquitoes to prove that they transmitted the germ of yellow fever. He died of it in 1900.

To each one of you the practice of medicine will be very much as you make it—to one a worry, a care, a perpetual annoyance; to another, a daily joy and a life of as much happiness and usefulness as can well fall to the lot of man. In the student spirit you can best fulfil the high mission of our noble calling—in his *humility*, conscious of weakness, while seeking strength; in his *confidence*, knowing the power, while recognizing the limitations of his art; in his *pride* in the glorious heritage from which the greatest gifts to man have been derived; and in his sure and certain hope that the future holds for us richer blessings than the past.

Arthur *Oppenheim* (also *Oppenheimer*) (d.c.1895): One of Osler's assistant residents at Johns Hopkins who died of typhoid.

Henry William *Oechsner* (date unknown): One of Osler's interns at Johns Hopkins who also died of typhoid. Osler noted how deeply moved he was by his death.

18

UNITY, PEACE, AND CONCORD

"In necessariis unitas, in non-necessariis libertas, in omnibus caritas." (In essentials, unity; in non-essentials, liberty; in all things charity [love])
ST. AUGUSTINE, *Confessions*

> Life is too short to waste,
> In critic peep or cynic bark,
> Quarrel or reprimand:
> 'Twill soon be dark;
> Up! Mind thine own aim, and
> God speed the mark!
> RALPH WALDO EMERSON, "To J.W."

OSLER RETIRED IN 1905 from Johns Hopkins Medical School in order "to work in another part of the same vineyard" on more literary pursuits in England. His farewell to the medical profession of the United States expresses his gratitude to his professional colleagues, especially those idealists who generated the reforms of the preceding years: specifically the scientific advances in medicine, in medical education, and in medical humanism. Such idealism is exemplified by the traditional prayer for the nations to attain unity, peace, and concord.

Unity: Physicians have been united by the increased international exchange of information and by recent advances in disease prevention (vaccination, sanitation, etc.) and cures (anaesthesia, antiseptic surgery, etc.). For further fostering the unity of the profession, Osler suggests reciprocity of licensing between states (and eventually between nations), consolidation of medical schools to meet the demands for laboratory science and clinical facilities, and reconciliation with homoeopathic physicians.

Peace: To achieve peace, physicians need to fight three great foes: (1) ignorance, which leads to quackery; (2) apathy and the needless deaths it causes; and (3) vice and personal impurity.

Concord: Osler stresses the great need for professional harmony, especially between medical schools. Increasingly, national and specialized societies promote this. Osler gives specific suggestions to doctors on avoiding quarrels: cultivate friendly social relationships with rival schools, mentor younger doctors—treating them as sons, not rivals—and seek the advice of older doctors. He urges doctors to avoid gossip, strife, and uncharitable judgements.

UNITY, PEACE,
& CONCORD

O N THIS OCCASION I have had no difficulty in selecting a subject
on which to address you. Surely the hour is not for the head but
for the heart, out of the abundance of which I may be able to express,[1] however feebly, my gratitude for the many kindnesses I
have received from the profession of this country during the past twenty-one
years, and from you, my dear colleagues of this state and city, during the sixteen
years I have dwelt among you. Truly I can say that I have lived my life in our beloved profession—perhaps too much! but whatever success I have had has come
directly through it, and my devotion is only natural. Few men have had more
from their colleagues than has fallen to my lot. As an untried young man my
appointment at McGill College came directly through friends in the faculty who
had confidence in me as a student. In the ten happy years I lived in Montreal I
saw little of any save physicians and students, among whom I was satisfied to
work—and to play. In Philadelphia the hospitals and the societies absorbed the
greater part of my time, and I lived the peaceful life of a student with students.
An ever-widening circle of friends in the profession brought me into closer contact with the public, but I have never departed from my ambition to be first of
all a servant of my brethren, willing and anxious to do anything in my power to
help them. Of my life here you all know. I have studied to be quiet and to do my

A farewell address to the Medical Profession of the United States, delivered at the annual meeting of the
Medical and Chirurgical Faculty of the State of Maryland, April 26, 1905. The title comes from the Litany
in the *Book of Common Prayer*. See p. 335, n. 7.

1. *the heart, out of the abundance of which I may be able to express:* This is an echo of Matthew 12:34:
"for out of the abundance of the heart the mouth speaketh."

own business and to walk honestly toward them that are without;[2] and one of my chief pleasures has been to work among you as a friend, sharing actively in your manifold labours. But when to the sessions of sweet, silent thought I summon up the past,[3] not what I have done but the many things I have left undone,[4] the opportunities I have neglected, the battles I have shirked, the precious hours I have wasted—these rise up in judgment.

A notable period it has been in our history through which we have lived, a period of reconstruction and renovation, a true renaissance, not only an extraordinary revival of learning, but a complete transformation in our educational methods; and I take pride in the thought that, in Philadelphia and in Baltimore, I have had the good fortune to be closely associated with men who have been zealous in the promotion of great reforms, the full value of which we are too close to the events to appreciate. On the far-reaching influence of these changes time will not permit us to dwell. I propose to consider another aspect of our work of equal importance, neither scientific nor educational, but what may be called humanistic, as it deals with our mutual relations and with the public.

Nothing in life is more glaring than the contrast between possibilities and actualities, between the ideal and the real. By the ordinary mortal, idealists are regarded as vague dreamers, striving after the impossible; but in the history of the world how often have they gradually moulded to their will conditions the most adverse and hopeless! They alone furnish the *Geist*[5] that finally animates the entire body and makes possible reforms and even revolutions. Imponderable, impalpable, more often part of the moral than of the intellectual equipment, are the subtle qualities so hard to define, yet so potent in everyday life, by which these fervent souls keep alive in us the reality of the ideal. Even in a lost cause, with aspirations utterly futile, they refuse to acknowledge defeat, and, still nursing an unconquerable hope,[6] send up the prayer of faith in face of a scoffing

2. *I have studied to be quiet and to do my own business and to walk honestly toward them that are without:* This is an echo of 1 Thessalonians 4:11–12: "And that ye study to be quiet, and to do your own business . . . that ye may walk honestly toward them that are without." "Without" here means "outside." St. Paul is thinking of those outside the fold of the Christian church; Osler of those outside the medical profession.

3. *when to the sessions of sweet, silent thought I summon up the past:* This is an echo of William Shakespeare, "Sonnet 30," lines 1–2: "When to the sessions of sweet silent thought I summon up remembrance of things past."

4. *not what I have done but the many things I have left undone:* The *Book of Common Prayer*. The General Confession, from which these words come, is appointed in the Prayerbook at both Morning and Evening Prayer. The exact quotation is: "We have left undone those things which we ought to have done; And we have done those things which we ought not to have done."

5. *Geist:* (German) mind or spirit.

6. *still nursing an unconquerable hope:* Matthew Arnold, "The Scholar-Gipsy," line 211. Arnold actually wrote "the unconquerable hope."

world. Most characteristic of aspirations of this class is the petition of the Litany in which we pray that to the nations may be given 'unity, peace, and concord.'[7] Century after century from the altars of Christendom this most beautiful of all prayers has risen from lips of men and women, from the loyal souls who have refused to recognize its hopelessness, with the war-drums ever sounding in their ears. The desire for unity, the wish for peace, the longing for concord, deeply implanted in the human heart, have stirred the most powerful emotions of the race, and have been responsible for some of its noblest actions. It is but a senti-ment, you may say: but is not the world ruled by feeling and by passion? What but a strong sentiment baptized this nation in blood;[8] and what but sentiment, the deep-rooted affection for country which is so firmly implanted in the hearts of all Americans, gives to these states to-day unity, peace, and concord? As with the nations at large, so with the nation in particular; as with people, so with indi-viduals; and as with our profession, so with its members, this fine old prayer for unity, peace, and concord, if in our hearts as well as on our lips, may help us to realize its aspirations. What some of its lessons may be to us will be the subject of my address.

Unity

Medicine is the only world-wide profession, following everywhere the same methods, actuated by the same ambitions, and pursuing the same ends. This homogeneity, its most characteristic feature, is not shared by the law, and not by the Church, certainly not in the same degree. While in antiquity the law rivals medicine, there is not in it that extraordinary solidarity which makes the physi-cian at home in any country, in any place where two or three sons of men are gathered together.[9] Similar in its high aims and in the devotion of its officers, the Christian Church, widespread as it is, and saturated with the humanitarian instincts of its Founder, yet lacks that catholicity — *urbi et orbi*[10] — which enables the physician to practise the same art amid the same surroundings in every coun-try of the earth. There is a unity, too, in its aims — the prevention of diseases by discovering their causes, and the cure and relief of sickness and suffering. In a

7. From the Litany in the *Book of Common Prayer.* The exact quotation is: "That it may please thee to give to all nations unity, peace, and concord; We beseech thee to hear us, good Lord."

8. *baptized this nation in blood:* This refers to the American Civil War (1860–1865), which was fought to preserve the union of the states.

9. *where two or three sons of men are gathered together:* This is an echo of Matthew 18:20: "For where two or three are gathered together in my name, there am I in the midst of them."

10. *urbi et orbi:* (Latin) literally, "to the city (Rome) and to the world." This is the phrase used particularly for the blessing that the Pope occasionally gives from the balcony of one of the basilicas of Rome.

little more than a century a united profession, working in many lands, has done more for the race than has ever before been accomplished by any other body of men. So great have been these gifts that we have almost lost our appreciation of them. Vaccination, sanitation, anaesthesia, antiseptic surgery, the new science of bacteriology, and the new art in therapeutics have effected a revolution in our civilization to which can be compared only the extraordinary progress in the mechanical arts. Over the latter there is this supreme advantage, it is domestic [11]—a bedroom revolution which sooner or later touches each one of us, if not in person, in those near and dear—a revolution which for the first time in the history of poor, suffering humanity brings us appreciably closer to that promised day when the former things should pass away, when there should be no more unnecessary death, when sorrow and crying should be no more, and there should not be any more pain.[12]

One often hears as a reproach that more has been done in the prevention than in the cure of disease. It is true; but this second part of our labours has also made enormous progress. We recognize to-day the limitations of the art; we know better the diseases curable by medicine, and those which yield to exercise and fresh air; we have learned to realize the intricacy of the processes of disease, and have refused to deceive ourselves with half-knowledge, preferring to wait for the day instead of groping blindly in the dark or losing our way in the twilight. The list of diseases which we can positively cure is an ever-increasing one, the number of diseases the course of which we can modify favourably is a growing one, the number of incurable diseases (which is large and which will probably always be large) is diminishing—so that in this second point we may feel that not only is the work already done of the greatest importance, but that we are on the right path, and year by year as we know disease better we shall be able to treat it more successfully. The united efforts of countless workers in many lands have won these greatest victories of science. Only by ceaseless co-operation and the intelligent appreciation by all of the results obtained in each department has the present remarkable position been reached. Within a week or ten days a great discovery in any part of the world is known everywhere, and, while in a certain sense we speak of German, French, English, and American medicine, the differences are trifling in comparison with the general similarity. The special workers know each other and are familiar with each other's studies in a way that is truly

---

11. *domestic:* Refers here to the sense that vaccination, sanitation, anesthesia, etc. affect us in our daily life.

12. *when there should be more unnecessary death, when sorrow and crying should be no more, and there should not be any more pain:* Revelation 21:4. The exact quotation is: "And God shall wipe away all tears from their eyes; and there shall be no more death, neither sorrow, nor crying, neither shall there be any more pain: for the former things are passed away."

remarkable. And the knowledge gained by the one, or the special technic he may devise, or the instrument he may invent is at the immediate disposal of all. A new lifesaving operation of the first class devised by a surgeon in Breslau[13] would be performed here the following week. A discovery in practical medicine is common property with the next issue of the weekly journals.

A powerful stimulus in promoting this wide organic unity is our great international gatherings—not so much the International Congress of the profession, which has proved rather an unwieldy body, but of the special societies which are rapidly denationalizing science. In nearly every civilized country medical men have united in great associations which look after their interests and promote scientific work. It should be a source of special pride to American physicians to feel that the national association of this country—the American Medical Association—has become one of the largest and most influential bodies of the kind in the world. We cannot be too grateful to men who have controlled its course during the past ten years. The reorganization so efficiently carried out has necessitated a readjustment of the machinery of the state societies, and it is satisfactory to know that this meeting of our state society, the first held under the new conditions, has proved so satisfactory. But in the whole scheme of readjustment nothing commands our sympathy and co-operation more than the making of the county societies the materials out of which the state and national associations are built. It is not easy at first to work out such a scheme in full detail, and I would ask of the members of this body not only their co-operation, but an expectant consideration, if the plan at first does not work as smoothly as could be desired. On the county members I would urge the support of a plan conceived on broad national lines—on you its success depends, and to you its benefits will chiefly come.

Linked together by the strong bonds of community of interests, the profession of medicine forms a remarkable world-unit in the progressive evolution of which there is a fuller hope for humanity than in any other direction.

Concentration, fusion, and consolidation are welding together various subunits in each nation. Much has been done, much remains to do; and to three desiderata I may refer briefly.

In this country reciprocity between the state licensing boards remains one of the most urgent local needs. Given similar requirements, and examinations practically of the same character, with evidence of good character, the state board should be given power to register a man on payment of the usual fee. It is preposterous to restrict in his own country, as is now done, a physician's liberty. Take a

13. A city then in southeastern Germany; now in southwestern Poland and called Wrocław.

case in point: A few months ago a man who is registered in three states, an able, capable practitioner of twenty years' standing, a hard student in his profession, a physician who has had charge of some of the most important lives of this country, had to undergo another examination for licence. What an anomaly! What a reflection on a united profession! I would urge you all most strongly to support the movement now in progress to place reciprocity on a proper basis. International reciprocity is another question of equal importance, but surrounded with greater difficulties; and, though a long way off, it will come within this century.

The second urgent need is a consolidation of many of our medical schools. Within the past twenty-five years conditions have so changed that the tax on the men in charge of the unendowed schools has become ever more burdensome.

In the old days of a faculty with seven professors, a school with three hundred students was a good property, paying large salaries, but the introduction of laboratory and practical teaching has so increased the expenses that very little is now left for distribution at the end of the year. The students' fees have not increased proportionately, and only the self-sacrifice and devotion of men who ungrudgingly give their time, and often their means, save a hopeless situation. A fusion of the schools is the natural solution of the problem. Take a concrete example: A union of three of the medical schools of this city would enable the scientific departments to be consolidated at an enormous saving of expense and with a corresponding increase in efficiency. Anatomy, physiology, pathology, physiological chemistry, bacteriology, and pharmacology could be taught in separately organized departments which the funds of the united school could support liberally. Such a school could appeal to the public for aid to build and endow suitable laboratories. The clinical work could be carried on at the separate hospitals, which would afford unequalled facilities for the scientific study of disease. Not only in this city, but in Richmond, in Nashville, in Columbus, in Indianapolis, and in many cities a "merger" is needed. Even the larger schools of the larger cities could "pool" their scientific interests to the great advantage of the profession.

And the third desideratum is the recognition by our homoeopathic brethren that the door is open. It is too late in this day of scientific medicine to prattle of such antique nonsense as is indicated in the "pathies."[14] We have long got past the stage when any "system" can satisfy a rational practitioner, long past the time

14. *pathies:* Osler means homoeopathy and allopathy, which were rival systems of medicine in vogue in the first half of the nineteenth century. "Allopathy" was the name given by homoeopaths to traditional medicine, implying that it sought to cure diseases by producing contrary effects—that is, by merely repressing the symptoms. Homoeopathy sought to cure diseases by augmenting the symptoms, on the theory that they represented the body's way of fighting the disease. Osler is saying that both theories have some merit but neither can be made the sole basis of scientific medicine.

when a difference of belief in the action of drugs—the most uncertain element in our art!—should be allowed to separate men with the same noble traditions, the same hopes, the same aims and ambitions. It is not as if our homoeopathic brothers are asleep; far from it, they are awake—many of them at any rate—to the importance of the scientific study of disease, and all of them must realize the anomaly of their position. It is distressing to think that so many good men live isolated, in a measure, from the great body of the profession. The original grievous mistake was ours—to quarrel with our brothers over infinitesimals was a most unwise and stupid thing to do. That we quarrel with them now is solely on account of the old Shibboleth [15] under which they practise. Homoeopathy [16] is as inconsistent with the new medicine as is the old-fashioned polypharmacy, to destruction of which it contributed so much. The rent in the robe of Æsculapius,[17] wider in this country than elsewhere, could be repaired by mutual concessions— on the one hand by the abandonment of special designations,[18] and on the other by an intelligent toleration of therapeutic vagaries [19] which in all ages have beset the profession, but which have been mere flies on the wheels [20] of progress.

Peace

Many seek peace, few ensue it actively, and among these few we, alas! are not often to be found. In one sense every one of us may be asked the question which Jehu returned to Joram: "What hast thou to do with peace?" [21] since our life must be a perpetual warfare, dominated by the fighting spirit. The physician, like the Christian, has three great foes [22]—ignorance, which is sin; apathy, which is the

15. *Shibboleth:* A password. See "Teacher and Student," p. 112, n. 11.

16. A treatment started by a German physician, Samuel Hahnemann (1755–1843), in which diseases are treated by giving minute doses of drugs that would produce in a healthy person symptoms similar to those of the disease.

17. *Æsculapius:* Greek god of medicine. See "Physic and Physicians as Depicted in Plato," p. 128, n. 8.

18. *special designations:* This refers to the controversy over homoeopathy versus allopathy as explained above.

19. Wild, capricious treatment.

20. The phrase, "flies on the wheel," is derived from Aesop's fable, which is as follows: "What a dust do I raise, said the fly upon the chariot wheel." Although the fly is boasting, it is the chariot, not the fly, that raises the dust.

21. 2 Kings 9:17–19. The exact quotation is: "Then he sent out a second on horseback, which came to them, and said, Thus saith the king, *Is it* peace? And Jehu answered, What hast thou to do with peace? turn thee behind me." Jehu was an army captain who raised a rebellion against King Joram of Israel. Jehu's answer to the king's messenger means that it is no time for peace and that he ought to join the rebellion.

22. Osler is thinking of the service of Baptism in the *Book of Common Prayer* where the priest marks the newly baptized Christian with the sign of the cross "in token that hereafter he shall not be ashamed to

world; and vice, which is the devil. There is a delightful Arabian proverb two lines of which run: "He that knows not, and knows not that he knows not, is a fool. Shun him. He that knows not, and knows that he knows not, is simple. Teach him." To a large extent these two classes represent the people with whom we have to deal. Teaching the simple and suffering the fools gladly, we must fight the wilful ignorance of the one and the helpless ignorance of the other, not with the sword of righteous indignation, but with the skilful weapon of the tongue. On this ignorance the charlatan and the quack live, and it is by no means an easy matter to decide how best to conduct a warfare against these wily foes, the oldest and most formidable with whom we have to deal. As the incomparable Fuller[23] remarks: "Well did the poets feign Æsculapius[24] and Circe[25] brother and sister, . . . for in all times (in the opinion of the multitude) witches, old women, and impostors have had a competition with doctors."[26] Education of the public of a much more systematic and active kind is needed. The congress on quackery which is announced to take place in Paris, with some twenty-five subjects for discussion, indicates one important method of dealing with the problem. The remarkable exhibit held last year in Germany of everything relating to quacks and charlatans did an immense good in calling attention to the colossal nature of the evil. A permanent museum of this sort might well be organized in Washington in connexion with the Department of Hygiene. It might be worth while to imitate our German brethren in a special national exhibit, though I dare say many of the most notorious sinners would apply for large space, not willing to miss the opportunity for a free advertisement! One effective measure is enforced in Germany: any proprietary medicine sold to the public must be submitted to a government analyst, who prepares a statement (as to its composition, the price of its ingredients, etc.), which is published at the cost of the owner of the supposed remedy in a certain number of the daily and weekly papers.

By far the most dangerous foe we have to fight is apathy—indifference from whatever cause, not from a lack of knowledge, but from carelessness, from absorption in other pursuits, from a contempt bred of self-satisfaction. Fully 25 percent of the deaths in the community are due to this accursed apathy, fos-

confess the faith of Christ crucified, and manfully to fight under his banner against sin, the world, and the devil." Hence, the Christian's great foes are "sin, the world, and the devil."

23. Thomas *Fuller* (1608–1661): See "Sir Thomas Browne," p. 57, n. 178.

24. *Æsculapius:* See "Physic and Physicians as Depicted in Plato," p. 128, n. 8.

25. *Circe:* An enchantress in the *Odyssey* by Homer as well as in Greek mythology. See "The Student Life," p. 329, n. 112.

26. Fuller is saying that true doctors (like Æsculapius) and false ones (like Circe) are close relations, in competition. Thomas Fuller, "The Good Physician," in *The Holy State and the Profane State,* ed. James Nichols (1642; London: Thomas Tegg, 1841), book 2, chap. 2, maxime 8, line 53.

tering a human inefficiency, and going far to counterbalance the extraordinary achievements of the past century. Why should we take pride in the wonderful railway system with which enterprise and energy have traversed the land, when the supreme law, the public health,[27] is neglected? What comfort in the thought of a people enjoying great material prosperity when we know that the primary elements of life (on which even the old Romans were our masters) are denied to them? What consolation does the 'little red school-house'[28] afford when we know that a Lethean apathy[29] allows toll to be taken of every class, from the little tots to the youths and maidens? Western civilization has been born of knowledge, of knowledge won by hard, honest sweat of body and brain, but in many of the most important relations of life we have failed to make that knowledge effective. And, strange irony of life, the lesson of human efficiency is being taught us by one of the little nations of the earth,[30] which has so far bettered our instruction that we must again turn eastward for wisdom. Perhaps in a few years our civilization may be put on trial,[31] and it will not be without benefit if it arouses the individual from apathy and makes him conscious of the great truth that only by earnest individual human effort can knowledge be made effective, and if it arouses communities from an apathy which permits mediaeval conditions to prevail without a protest.

Against our third great foe—vice in all its forms—we have to wage an incessant warfare, which is not less vigorous because of the quiet, silent kind. Better than any one else the physician can say the word in season[32] to the immoral, to the intemperate, to the uncharitable in word and deed. Personal impurity is the

27. *the supreme law, the public health:* This is an echo of the Latin maxim *salus populi suprema est lex,* which is usually translated "the safety (or welfare) of the people is the supreme law," but *salus* can be understood, as it is by Osler, as "health."

28. The "little red school-house" refers to the typical local rural elementary school. They were often painted red or built of red brick. To Osler they were the physical testimonial to universal, compulsory, free elementary education; and he is saying that the establishment of that system throughout the United States and Canada is one of the great achievements of his lifetime, but much of its benefit is lost because so many pupils still die young needlessly, owing to ignorance or lack of effort at preventing and treating diseases.

29. The river Lethe in Hades caused forgetfulness of the past. The souls of the dead drink from its water and forget their past life before being reborn back into the world. Plato, *Republic,* book 10, 614–621.

30. Osler probably refers to Japan. He wrote an editorial "Progress Made by the Japanese in Modern Medical Methods . . ." (*Medical News,* Philadelphia, 1887). When he says "we must again turn eastward for wisdom," he is probably thinking of the Wise Men from the east (Matthew 2).

31. What soon afterward put on trial Osler's civilization was the Great War that broke out between European nations in 1914. In the light of history, his words here seem prophetic.

32. *say the word in season:* means "give advice when the recipient is willing to hear it." This is a vague echo of 2 Timothy 4:2: "Preach the word; be instant in season, out of season," where "instant" means "insistent."

evil against which we can do most good, particularly to the young, by showing the possibility of the pure life and the dangers of immorality. Had I time, and were this the proper occasion, I would like to rouse the profession to a sense of its responsibility toward the social evil—the black plague[33] which devastates the land. I can but call your attention to an important society, of which Dr. Prince Morrow,[34] of New York, is the organizer, which has for one of its objects the education of the public on this important question. I would urge you to join in a crusade quite as important as that in which we are engaged against tuberculosis.

Concord

Unity promotes concord—community of interests, the same aims, the same objects give, if anything can, a feeling of comradeship, and the active co-operation of many men, while it favours friction, lessens the chances of misunderstanding and ill will. One of the most gratifying features of our professional life is the good feeling which prevails between the various sections of the country. I do not see how it could be otherwise. One has only to visit different parts and mingle with the men to appreciate that everywhere good work is being done, everywhere an earnest desire to elevate the standard of education, and everywhere the same self-sacrificing devotion on the part of the general practitioner. Men will tell you that commercialism is rife, that the charlatan and the humbug were never so much in evidence, and that in our ethical standards there has been a steady declension. These are the Elijahs[35] who are always ready to pour out their complaints, mourning that they are not better than their fathers. Few men have had more favourable opportunities than I have had to gauge the actual conditions in professional private life, in the schools, and in the medical societies, and as I have seen them in the past twenty years I am filled with thankfulness for the present and with hope for the future. The little rift within the lute is the absence in many places of that cordial professional harmony which should exist among us. In the larger cities professional jealousies are dying out. Read Charles Caldwell's *Autobiography*[36] if you wish for spicy details of the quarrels of the

33. *the social evil—the black plague:* Osler here means venereal diseases, especially syphilis. "Black plague" (or, more usually, "black death") is the bubonic plague, with particular reference to the successive epidemics that more than halved the population of Europe in the fourteenth century.

34. *Prince Morrow* (1846–1913): American physician who specialized in venereal and genito-urinary diseases and who pioneered public education on sex hygiene.

35. *Elijah:* (9th cent. B.C.) Hebrew prophet (1 Kings 19:4). The exact quotation is: "But he himself went a day's journey into the wilderness, and came and sat down under a juniper tree: and he requested for himself that he might die; and said, It is enough; now, O Lord, take away my life; for I *am* not better than my fathers."

36. Charles *Caldwell, Autobiography* (1855; New York: Da Capo Press, 1968), pp. 407–411.

doctors in this country during the first half of the last century. I am sorry to say the professors have often been the worst offenders, and the rivalry between medical schools has not always been friendly and courteous. That it still prevails to some extent must be acknowledged, but it is dying out, though not so rapidly as we could wish. It makes a very bad impression on the public, and is often a serious stumbling-block [37] in the way of progress. Only the other day I had a letter from an intelligent and appreciative layman who is interested in a large hospital scheme about which I had been consulted. I quote this sentence from it in sorrow, and I do so because it is written by a strong personal friend of the profession, a man who has had long and varied experience with us: "I may say to you that one of the distressing bewilderments of the layman who only desires the working out of a broad plan is the extraordinary bitterness of professional jealousy between not only schoolmen and non-schoolmen, but between school-men themselves, and the reflections which are cast on one another as belonging to that clique, which makes it exceedingly difficult for the layman to understand what way there is out of these squabbles."

The national and special societies, and particularly the American Medical Association, have brought men together and have taught them to know each other and to appreciate the good points which at home may have been over-looked. As Dr. Brush [38] said yesterday in his address, it is in the smaller towns and country districts that the conditions are most favourable for mutual misunder-standings. Only those of us who have been brought up in such surroundings can appreciate how hard it is for physicians to keep on good terms with each other. The practice of medicine calls equally for the exercise of the heart and the head; and when a man has done his best, to have his motives misunderstood and his conduct of a case harshly criticized not only by the family, but by a colleague who has been called in, small wonder, when the opportunity arises, if the old Adam [39] prevails and he pays in kind. So far as my observation goes there are three chief causes for the quarrels of doctors. The first is lack of proper friendly intercourse, by which alone we can know each other. It is the duty of the older man to look on the younger one who settles near him not as a rival, but as a son. He will do to you just what you did to the old practitioner, when, as a young man, you started—get a good many of your cases; but if you have the sense to realize that this is inevitable, unavoidable, and the way of the world, and if you have the sense to talk over, in a friendly way, the first delicate situation that arises, the difficulties will disappear and recurrences may be made impossible.

37. *stumbling-block:* an obstacle. See "After Twenty-Five Years," p. 212, n. 35.

38. Edward Nathaniel *Brush* (1852–1933): Professor of psychiatry at the University of Maryland and the College of Physicians and Surgeons in Baltimore, Maryland.

39. The evil inherent in man.

The young men should be tender with the sensibilities of their seniors, deferring to their judgment and taking counsel with them. If young graduates could be taken more frequently as assistants or partners, the work of the profession would be much lightened, and it would promote amity and good fellowship. A man of whom you may have heard as the incarnation of unprofessional conduct, and who has been held up as an example of all that is pernicious, may be, in reality, a very good fellow, the victim of petty jealousies, the mark of the arrows of a rival faction; and you may, on acquaintance, find that he loves his wife and is devoted to his children, and that there are people who respect and esteem him. After all, the attitude of mind is the all-important factor in the promotion of concord. When a man is praised, or when a young man has done a good bit of work in your special branch, be thankful—it is for the common good. Envy, that pain of the soul, as Plato calls it,[40] should never for a moment afflict a man of generous instincts who has a sane outlook in life. The men of rival schools should deliberately cultivate the acquaintance of each other and encourage their students and the junior teachers to fraternize. If you hear that a young fellow just starting has made mistakes or is a little "off colour,"[41] go out of your way to say a good word to him, or for him. It is the only cure; any other treatment only aggravates the malady.

The second great cause is one over which we have direct control. The most widespread, the most pernicious of all vices, equal in its disastrous effects to impurity, much more disastrous often than intemperance, because destructive of all mental and moral nobility as are the others of bodily health, is uncharitableness—the most prevalent of modern sins, peculiarly apt to beset all of us, and the chief enemy to concord in our ranks. Oftentimes it is a thoughtless evil, a sort of tic or trick, an unconscious habit of mind and tongue which gradually takes possession of us. No sooner is a man's name mentioned than something slighting is said of him, or a story is repeated which is to his disadvantage, or the involuntary plight of a brother is ridiculed, or even his character is traduced.[42] In chronic and malign offenders literally "with every word a reputation dies."[43] The work of a school is disparaged, or the character of the work in a laboratory is belittled; or it may be only the faint praise that damns, not the generous meed from a full and thankful heart. We have lost our fine sense of the tragic element in this vice, and of its debasing influence on the character. It is interesting that

40. Plato, *Philebus*, 47e.

41. *off colour:* Slightly odd, or seeming to act strangely and improperly.

42. *traduced:* Slandered.

43. Alexander Pope, "The Rape of the Lock," canto 3, line 16. The exact quotation is: "At every word a reputation dies."

Christ and the Apostles lashed it more unsparingly than any other. Who is there among us who does not require every day to lay to heart that counsel of perfection: "Judge not according to the appearance, but judge righteous judgment?"[44] One of the apostles of our profession, Sir Thomas Browne, has a great thought on the question:

> While thou so hotly disclaimest the devil, be not guilty of diabolism. Fall not into one name with that unclean spirit, nor act his nature whom thou so much abhorrest—that is, to accuse, calumniate, backbite, whisper, detract, or sinistrously interpret others. Degenerous depravities, and narrow-minded vices! not only below St. Paul's noble Christian, but Aristotle's true gentleman.[45] Trust not with some that the Epistle of St. James[46] is apocryphal, and so read with less fear that stabbing truth, that in company with this vice thy religion is in vain. Moses broke the tables without breaking the law;[47] but where charity is broke the law itself is shattered, which cannot be whole without love, which is the fulfilling of it. Look humbly upon thy virtues; and though thou art rich in some, yet think thyself poor and naked without that crowning grace, which thinketh no evil, which envieth not, which beareth, hopeth, believeth, endureth all things.[48] With these sure graces, while busy tongues are crying out for a drop of cold water, mutes may be in happiness, and sing the Trisagion[49] in heaven.[50]

44. John 7:24.

45. St. Paul's noble Christian refers to Philippians 4:8. The whole of the *Nicomachean Ethics* by Aristotle (384–322 B.C.) is about the nature of the good man.

46. The authenticity of this book was questioned by some scholars in Browne's time.

47. Moses had gone up on Mount Sinai and communed with God, who gave him two stone tables (tablets) inscribed with the Ten Commandments. On coming back down, Moses found that the Israelites had turned away from his teaching to worship the Golden Calf, and in his shock and anger he threw down the stone tablets and broke them. After he had destroyed the calf and brought the people to repent, God told him to make two new tablets. On these tablets he wrote the Commandments again, to show that his covenant with Israel still stood (Exodus 31:18, 32:19, and 34:1).

48. *which thinketh no evil, which envieth not, which beareth, hopeth, believeth, endureth all things:* 1 Corinthians 13:5–7, part of St. Paul's hymn to charity.

49. "Trisagion" strictly is the hymn "Holy God, Holy Mighty (One), Holy Immortal (One), have mercy upon us", which is used in the Greek eucharistic Liturgy and in the Roman Catholic Church in the Good Friday rites. But English writers as old as Trevisa (1387) have applied the Greek name to the Western hymn "Tersanctus" in both its Latin and its English version, and that is clearly what Browne had in mind. Hence Browne here means the hymn sung in the Communion service of the *Book of Common Prayer*, as "Holy, Holy, Holy, Lord God of Hosts, heaven and earth are full of thy glory."

50. Thomas Browne, "A Letter to a Friend, Upon the Occasion of the Death of His Intimate Friend" in *The Works of Sir Thomas Browne*, ed. Geoffrey Keynes (London: Faber and Faber, 1964), pp. 116–117; also *Christian Morals* (1716), part I, sect. 16, p. 248.

And the third cause is the wagging tongue of others[51] who are too often ready to tell tales and make trouble between physicians. There is only one safe rule—never listen to a patient who begins with a story about the carelessness and inefficiency of Dr. Blank. Shut him or her up with a snap, knowing full well that the same tale may be told of you a few months later. Fully half of the quarrels of physicians are fomented by the tittle-tattle[52] of patients, and the only safeguard is not to listen. Sometimes it is impossible to check the flow of imprecation and slander; and then apply the other rule—perfectly safe, and one which may be commended as a good practice—never believe what a patient tells you to the detriment of a brother physician, even though you may think it to be true.

To part from the profession of this country and from this old Faculty, which I have learned to love so dearly, is a great wrench, one which I would feel more deeply were it not for the nearness of England, and for the confidence I feel that I am but going to work in another part of the same vineyard,[53] and were it not for the hope that I shall continue to take interest in your affairs and in the welfare of the medical school to which I owe so much. It may be that in the hurry and bustle of a busy life I have given offence to some—who can avoid it? Unwittingly I may have shot an arrow o'er the house and hurt a brother[54]—if so, I am sorry, and I ask his pardon. So far as I can read my heart I leave you in charity with all. I have striven with none, not, as Walter Savage Landor says, because none was worth the strife,[55] but because I have had a deep conviction of the hatefulness of strife, of its uselessness, of its disastrous effects, and a still deeper conviction of the blessings that come with unity, peace, and concord. And I would give to each of you, my brothers—you who hear me now, and to you who may elsewhere read my words—to you who do our greatest work labouring incessantly for small rewards in towns and country places—to you the more favoured ones

51. People talking about others, gossipping.

52. Encouraged by the trivial complaining or criticizing.

53. *work in another part of the vineyard:* This is a metaphor for going to another place while continuing to work at the same profession. It is derived from the parables of Isaiah (Isaiah 5) and Jesus (Matthew 20–21). Osler compares the field of his activity, the medical profession, to a vineyard.

54. *I may have shot an arrow o'er the house and hurt a brother:* William Shakespeare, *Hamlet,* V, ii, 254. The original reads: "And hurt my brother."

55. Walter Savage Landor (1775–1864): English poet and prose writer. He had a problem with his temper, quarreling with his wife, family, neighbors, tenants, and many others. The exact quotation is:

> I strove with none, for none was worth my strife:
>
> Nature I loved, and next to Nature Art:
>
> I warm'd both hands before the fire of Life;
>
> It sinks; and I am ready to depart.

"Dying Speech of an Old Philosopher," in *Poems by Walter Savage Landor* (London: Centaur Press, 1964), p. 172.

who have special fields of work—to you teachers and professors and scientific workers—to one and all, through the length and breadth of the land—I give a single word as my parting commandment:

"It is not hidden from thee, neither is it far off. It is not in heaven, that thou shouldest say, 'Who shall go up for us to heaven, and bring it unto us, that we may hear it, and do it?' Neither is it beyond the sea, that thou shouldest say, 'Who shall go over the sea for us, and bring it unto us, that we may hear it, and do it?' But the word is very nigh unto thee, in thy mouth and in thy heart, that thou mayest do it"—CHARITY.[56]

56. Deuteronomy 30:11–14. However, it should be noted that Osler added the eotf "charity" at the end of this quotation.

19

L'ENVOI

"I am a part of all that I have met."
ALFRED TENNYSON, "Ulysses"

THIS IS AN EMOTIONAL after-dinner speech at a farewell dinner in New York in 1905. It marks Osler's retirement from Johns Hopkins and his impending departure for England. Osler credits his happiness to the friendship and esteem of his colleagues, his family, his patients, and the public.

He jokes about coming to the United States from Canada years before. He had assumed the invitation to apply for a position at the University of Pennsylvania was a hoax because it had been forwarded to him by a friend on whom he had played many pranks. The job interview meal had also tested his finesse: the cherries in the pie had not been pitted. His years at Pennsylvania and at Johns Hopkins were very happy due to cordial colleagues. Osler discusses his two long-term professional ambitions: to be a good clinical physician and to build a scientifically based clinic patterned after those in Germany. He gives thanks for the opportunities to be able to accomplish as much at Johns Hopkins.

In this speech he also shares his personal ideals: to focus on doing the day's work well without worrying about tomorrow; to act according to the Golden Rule; and to cultivate equanimity, a spiritual calmness. He concludes that he does not care what the future holds because the memories of his past cannot be taken away. He quotes Matthew Arnold:

> I have loved no darkness,
> Sophisticated no truth,
> Nursed no delusion,
> Allowed no fear.

L'ENVOI

I AM SURE YOU ALL sympathize with me in the feelings which naturally almost overpower me on such an occasion. Many testimonials you have already given me of your affection and of your regard, but this far exceeds them all, and I am deeply touched that so many of you have come long distances,[1] and at great inconvenience, to bid me Godspeed in the new venture I am about to undertake. Pardon me, if I speak of myself, in spite of Montaigne's warning that one seldom speaks of oneself without some detriment to the person spoken of.[2] Happiness comes to many of us and in many ways, but I can truly say that to few men has happiness come in so many forms as it has come to me. Why I know not, but this I do know, that I have not deserved more than others, and yet, a very rich abundance of it has been vouchsafed to me. I have been singularly happy in my friends, and for that I say "God be praised." I have had exceptional happiness in the profession of my choice, and I owe all of this to you. I have sought success in life, and if, as some one has said, this consists in getting what you want and being satisfied with it, I have found what I sought in the estimation, in the fellowship and friendship of the members of my profession.

I have been happy too in the public among whom I have worked—happy

Speech at a farewell dinner in New York, delivered before the leaders of the medical profession of the United States and Canada, May 2, 1905. *L'envoi* "is French for "the sendoff" or "the dispatch." This word is the traditional heading for the last stanza of a ballade or certain other complexly rhyming poems. Such poems were originally in fashion late in the Middle Ages, but they were revived in Osler's lifetime. *L'envoi* is often used as the title of poems by James Russell Lowell (1819–1891), Alfred Tennyson (1809–1892), and Rudyard Kipling (1865–1936), Osler's favorite authors.
1. There were some five hundred participants from all over the continent (Cushing, vol. 1, p. 681).
2. Michel de Montaigne, *Essais,* book 1, chap. 21. Osler has quoted this in his memo book.

in my own land in Canada, happy here among you in the country of my adoption, from which I cannot part without bearing testimony to the nobility and the grace of character which I have found here in my colleagues. It fills me with joy to think that I have had not only the consideration and that ease of fellowship which means so much in life, but the warmest devotion on the part of my patients and their friends.

Of the greatest of all happiness I cannot speak—of my home. Many of you know it, and that is enough.

I would like to tell you how I came to this country. The men responsible for my arrival were Samuel W. Gross and Minis Hays[3] of Philadelphia, who concocted the scheme in the *Medical News* office and asked James Tyson[4] to write a letter asking if I would be a candidate for the professorship of Clinical Medicine in the University of Pennsylvania. That letter reached me at Leipsic,[5] having been forwarded to me from Montreal by my friend Shepherd.[6] So many pranks had I played on my friends there that, when the letter came, I felt sure it was a joke, so little did I think that I was one to be asked to succeed Dr. Pepper.[7] It was several weeks before I ventured to answer that letter, fearing that Dr. Shepherd had perhaps surreptitiously taken a sheet of University of Pennsylvania notepaper on purpose to make the joke more certain. Dr. Mitchell[8] cabled me to meet him in London, as he and his good wife were commissioned to "look me over," particularly with reference to personal conditions. Dr. Mitchell said there was only one way in which the breeding of a man suitable for such a position, in such a city as Philadelphia, could be tested:—give him cherry pie and see how he disposed of the stones. I had read of the trick before and disposed of them genteelly in my spoon—and got the Chair!

My affiliations with the profession in this country have been wide and to

3. Samuel Weissel *Gross* (1837–1889): Professor of surgery at Jefferson Medical College. For further information, see "Aequanimitas," p. 28, n. 41.

Isaac Minis *Hays* (1847–1925): American ophthalmologist. He was coeditor of *The American Journal of the Medical Sciences* and *The Medical News*. While serving as secretary and librarian of the American Philosophical Society he collected and catalogued the great mass of Benjamin Franklin's papers and manuscripts.

4. James *Tyson* (1841–1919): American physician. Professor at the University of Pennsylvania and later dean of the medical faculty.

5. Osler was then (1884) studying in Cohnheim's pathological institute in Leipzig (Leipsic), Germany.

6. Francis John *Shepherd* (1851–1929): Canadian anatomist and surgeon and Osler's colleague at McGill.

7. William *Pepper* Jr. (1843–1898): American physician. As provost of the University of Pennsylvania and professor of medicine, he significantly enlarged its educational opportunities. Osler was his biographer.

8. Silas Weir *Mitchell* (1829–1914): American neurologist, poet, and novelist, and a trustee of the University of Pennsylvania. He was responsible for developing the "rest cure," or Weir Mitchell treatment, for nervous disorders.

me most gratifying. At the University of Pennsylvania I found men whom I soon learned to love and esteem, and when I think of the good men who have gone—of Pepper, of Leidy, of Wormley, of Agnew, of Ashhurst[9]—I am full of thankfulness to have known them before they were called to their long rest. I am glad to think that my dear friends Tyson and Wood[10] are here still to join in a demonstration to me.

At Johns Hopkins University I found the same kindly feeling of friendship and my association with my colleagues there has been, as you all know, singularly happy and delightful.

With my fellow workers in the medical societies—in the American Medical Association, in the Association of American Physicians, in the Pediatric, Neurological and Physiological Societies—my relations have been most cordial and I would extend to them my heartfelt thanks for the kindness and consideration shown me during the past twenty years.

With the general practitioners throughout the country my relations have been of a peculiarly intimate character. Few men present, perhaps very few men in this country, have wandered so far and have seen in so many different sections the doctor at work. To all of these good friends who have given me their suffrage I express my appreciation and heartfelt thanks for their encouragement and support.

And lastly, my relations with my students—so many of whom I see here—have been of a close and most friendly character. They have been the inspiration of my work, and I may say truly, the inspiration of my life.

I have had but two ambitions in the profession: first, to make of myself a good clinical physician, to be ranked with the men who have done so much for the profession of this country—to rank in the class with Nathan Smith, Bartlett, James Jackson, Bigelow, Alonzo Clark, Metcalfe, W. W. Gerhard, Draper, Pepper, DaCosta and others.[11] The chief desire of my life has been to become a

9. Professors at the University of Pennsylvania. *Pepper:* See p. 351, n. 7. Joseph *Leidy* (1823–1891): American anatomist. For further information, see "The Leaven of Science," pp. 160–162. Theodore George *Wormley* (1826–1897): American toxicologist who also taught chemistry. David Hayes *Agnew* (1818–1892): American surgeon and anatomist. John *Ashhurst* Jr. (1839–1900): American surgeon and Dr. Agnew's successor in 1888.

10. *Tyson:* See p. 351, n. 4. Horatio Charles *Wood* (1841–1920): American clinical professor of nervous diseases and later professor of materia medica and therapeutics at Pennsylvania. Before Osler's appointment, Dr. Wood went to Montreal to inquire about Osler and returned home with the conviction that Osler was the right man for the job.

11. Nathan Ryno *Smith* (1797–1877): See "Books and Men," p. 224, n. 30. Elisha *Bartlett* (1804–1855): See "Books and Men," p. 224, n. 30. James *Jackson* (1777–1867): American physician and influential educator. American medical education was influenced by his reorganization of Harvard Medical School (1810) and

clinician of the same stamp with these great men, whose names we all revere and who did so much good work for clinical medicine.

My second ambition has been to build up a great clinic on Teutonic lines, not on those previously followed here and in England, but on lines which have proved so successful on the Continent, and which have placed the scientific medicine of Germany in the forefront of the world. And if I have done anything to promote the growth of clinical medicine it has been in this direction, in the formation of a large clinic with a well organized series of assistants and house physicians and with proper laboratories in which to work at the intricate problems that confront us in internal medicine. For the opportunities which I have had at Johns Hopkins Hospital to carry out these ideas, I am truly thankful. How far I have been successful, or not, remains to be seen. But of this I am certain:—If there is one thing above another which needs a change in this country, it is the present hospital system in relation to the medical school. It has been spoken of by Dr. Jacobi [12] but cannot be referred to too often. In every town of fifty thousand inhabitants a good model clinic could be built up, just as good as in smaller German cities,[13] if only a self-denying ordinance were observed on the part of the profession and only one or two men given the control of the hospital service, not half a dozen. With proper assistants and equipment, with good clinical and pathological laboratories there would be as much clinical work done in this country as in Germany.

I have had three personal ideals. One to do the day's work well and not to bother about to-morrow. It has been urged that this is not a satisfactory ideal. It is; and there is not one which the student can carry with him into practice with greater effect. To it, more than to anything else, I owe whatever success I have had—to this power of settling down to the day's work and trying to do it well to the best of one's ability, and letting the future take care of itself.[14]

---

by the foundation of the Massachusetts General Hospital. Henry Jacob *Bigelow* (1818–1890): American surgeon and professor of surgery at Harvard. He published the first account of the use of ether in surgery. Alonzo *Clark* (1807–1887): See "Books and Men," p. 224, n. 30. Samuel Lyther *Metcalfe* (1798–1856): American physician and chemist. He practiced medicine in Indiana, Mississippi, and New York and wrote articles and books on science. William Wood *Gerhard* (1809–1872): American pathologist who published a series of articles on the pathology of smallpox, pneumonia in children, tuberculous meningitis, and typhus. William H. *Draper* (1809–1872): American dermatologist. Professor of dermatology and later of clinical medicine at Columbia. *Pepper:* See p. 351, n. 7. Jacob Mendez *Dacosta* (1833–1900): American physician and professor of medicine at Jefferson, noted for his use of newer methods in physical diagnosis.

12. Abraham *Jacobi* (1830–1919): American pediatrician who taught at the College of Physicians and Surgeons.

13. Osler refers to Munich and other German cities in Bavaria. See "Teacher and Student," p. 213.

14. This philosophy is often repeated in other writings by Osler. See "A Way of Life," pp. 5–6.

The second ideal has been to act the Golden Rule,[15] as far as in me lay, towards my professional brethren and towards the patients committed to my care.

And the third has been to cultivate such a measure of equanimity as would enable me to bear success with humility, the affection of my friends without pride and to be ready when the day of sorrow and grief came to meet it with the courage befitting a man.

What the future has in store for me, I cannot tell—you cannot tell. Nor do I care much, so long as I carry with me, as I shall, the memory of the past you have given me. Nothing can take that away.

I have made mistakes, but they have been mistakes of the head not of the heart. I can truly say, and I take upon myself to witness, that in my sojourn among you:—

> I have loved no darkness,
> Sophisticated no truth,
> Nursed no delusion,
> Allowed no fear.[16]

15. *The Golden Rule* is a precept of Jesus in the Sermon on the Mount and a central teaching of Christianity. "Therefore all things whatsoever ye would that men should do to you, do ye even so to them" (Matthew 7:12 and Luke 6:31). This philosophy is also found in other religions or teachings; for example, "What I do not wish others to do unto me I also wish not to do unto others," Confucius, *Analects*, book 5, chap. 11 and book 12, chap. 2.

16. Matthew Arnold, *Empedocles on Etna*, act 2, lines 400–403.

20

MAN'S REDEMPTION OF MAN

And a man shall be as an hiding-place from the wind,
and a covert from the tempest; as rivers of water in a dry place;
as the shadow of a great rock in a weary land.
And the voice of weeping shall be no more heard in her,
nor the voice of crying. There shall be no more thence an infant
of days, nor an old man that has not filled his days.

ISAIAH, 32:2, 65:19–20

THIS IS A LAY SERMON given in Edinburgh, Scotland, in 1910 for students in connection with a meeting on tuberculosis.

In the past, suffering from tuberculosis was often so great that death seemed preferable. Although the book of Psalms in the Bible says no man may redeem his brother, Osler propounds that redemption of man has come, due to the reduction of pain and suffering from scientific advances in medicine. This great triumph has its roots in Greek medical thought, which sought ways to improve life and to balance the body and soul. The Greeks initiated careful observation of nature, coupled with making generalizations and seeking principles. Galen carried this forward to include experimentation. Unfortunately, the Dark Ages then eclipsed this brilliant progress for many centuries until the renaissance of learning later transformed the world at an accelerating pace. In the sixty years before this talk, in addition to Darwin's theory of evolution, great strides were made in healing and in harnessing nature through advances in chemistry and physics.

Truly the best measure of this progress is the decrease in suffering. It is hard even to imagine the horrors of surgery before the development of anesthesia. Its introduction in 1846 at Massachusetts General in Boston was "the greatest single gift ever made to suffering humanity." Equally important was the widespread effect of modern ideas in sanitation. Lister's treatment of wounds made surgery much safer, and recovery less painful, than when dressings had to be changed daily. As causes of epidemics were researched, infectious diseases such as smallpox, typhus, and malaria could be prevented. Osler challenges those who oppose vaccination to volunteer to work in the next epidemic, promising them suitable funerals.

These advances resulted in unparalleled decreases in deaths and indicate the enormous strides being made in progress toward man's redemption of man. In spite of these advances, however, tuberculosis is still a common worldwide cause of death from disease, even though its causes have been determined and its mortality rate reduced by 40 percent. Osler urges a crusade to improve the prevention and treatment of tuberculosis. Since the factors that stand in the way of implementing the needed measures are social rather than medical, education of the public becomes paramount.

Although human nature has not changed, this increased scientific knowledge has broken forever the medieval linkage of disease with sin. It has given a whole new value to human life. Even the glories of Greece and the Biblical promises were dulled by the extent of suffering and the resultant fear and anxiety. The increasing well-being gives a hopeful outlook for the future. Osler quotes the Greek philosopher Prodicus, who said, "That which benefits human life is God."

MAN'S REDEMPTION OF MAN

T O MAN THERE HAS BEEN published a triple gospel—of his soul, of his goods, of his body.[1] Growing with his growth, preached and professed in a hundred different ways in various ages of the world, these gospels represent the unceasing purpose of his widening thoughts.

The gospel of his relation to the powers unseen has brought sometimes hope, too often despair. In a wide outlook on the immediate and remote effects of the attempts to establish this relation, one event[2] discredits the great counsel of Confucius[3] (who realized what a heavy yoke religion might be) to keep aloof from spiritual beings. Surviving the accretions of twenty centuries, the life and immortality brought to light by the gospel of Christ, remain the earnest desire of the best portion of the race.

The gospel of his goods—of man's relation to his fellow men, is written in blood on every page of history. Quietly and slowly the righteousness that exalt-

This address was delivered at a service held for the students of the University of Edinburgh in connection with the Edinburgh meeting of the National Association for the Prevention of Tuberculosis, July 3, 1910.

1. Osler explains each one as follows: *the gospel of his soul:* man's relation to the powers unseen, the gospel of Christ; *the gospel of his goods:* man's relation to his fellow men; *the gospel of his body:* man's relation with nature.

2. Probably the resurrection, as in the poem by Alfred Tennyson, "In Memoriam A.H.H.," epilogue, stanza 36, lines 143–144. The exact quotation is:

> And one far-off divine event,
>
> To which the whole creation moves.

3. The Doctrine of the Mean. Confucius (552–479 B.C.), the great Chinese philosopher concerned primarily with morality and social order. He had a humanistic tendency in that he talked about men rather than spiritual things (*Analects,* book 5, sect. 12.

eth a nation,[4] the principles of eternal justice, have won acquiescence, at any rate in theory, though as nations and individuals we are still far from carrying them into practice.

And the third gospel, the gospel of his body, which brings man into relation with nature,—a true *evangelion*, the glad tidings of a conquest beside which all others sink into insignificance—is the final conquest of nature, out of which has come man's redemption of man, the subject to which I am desirous of directing your attention.

In the struggle for existence in which all life is engaged, disease and pain loom large as fundamental facts. The whole creation groaneth and travaileth,[5] and so red in tooth and claw with ravin is Nature,[6] that, it is said, no animal in a wild state dies a natural death. The history of man is the story of a great martyrdom—plague, pestilence and famine, battle and murder,[7] crimes unspeakable, tortures inconceivable, and the inhumanity of man to man[8] has even outdone what appear to be atrocities in nature. In the *Grammar of Assent*[9] (chap. x) Cardinal Newman has an interesting paragraph on this great mystery of the physical world. Speaking of the amount of suffering bodily and mental which is our lot and heritage, he says: "Not only is the Creator far off, but some being of malignant nature seems to have got hold of us, and to be making us his sport. Let us say that there are a thousand millions of men on the earth at this time; who can weigh and measure the aggregate of pain which this one generation has endured, and will endure from birth to death? Then add to this all the pain which has fallen and will fall upon our race through generations past and to come. Is there not then some great gulf fixed between us and the good God?"[10]

Dwelling too exclusively on this aspect of life, who does not echo the wish of Euripides:[11] "Not to be born is the best, and next to die as soon as possible."[12]

4. *righteousness that exalteth a nation:* Proverbs 14:34.

5. *The whole creation groaneth and travaileth:* Romans 8:22.

6. *so red in tooth and claw with ravin is Nature:* This phrase is a reminiscence of Tennyson's "In Memoriam A.H.H.," part 56, stanza 4, lines 15–16. The original quotation is:

> Tho' Nature, red in tooth and claw
>
> With ravine, shriek'd against his creed.

7. *plague, pestilence and famine, battle and murder:* This phrase echoes the Litany in the *Book of Common Prayer:* "From lightning and tempest; from plague, pestilence, and famine; from battle and murder, and from sudden death, Good Lord, deliver us."

8. *the inhumanity of man to man:* Robert Burns, "Man Was Made to Mourn," lines 55–56.

9. John Henry *Newman* (1801–1890): See "Teacher and Student," p. 112, n. 8.

10. John Henry *Newman, The Grammar of Assent* (on the philosophy of faith) (1870), chap. 10, sect. 1. Toward the end of the quote Newman is recalling Luke 16:26, "And beside all this, between us and you there is a great gulf fixed."

11. *Euripides* (480–406 B.C.): One of the three great tragic poets of Greece; he was a friend of Socrates.

Some of you may remember Edwin Markham's poem, "The Man with the Hoe," based on Millet's famous picture.

> Bowed by the weight of centuries he leans
> Upon his hoe and gazes on the ground,
> The emptiness of ages in his face,
> And on his back the burden of the world.
> Who made him dead to rapture and despair,
> A thing that grieves not and that never hopes,
> Stolid and stunned, a brother to the ox?[13]

It is a world-old tale, this of the trembling heart, the failing eyes, the desponding mind of the natural man. "And thy life shall hang in doubt before thee; and thou shalt fear day and night, and shalt have none assurance of thy life: In the morning thou shalt say, Would God it were even! and at even thou shalt say, Would God it were morning! for the fear of thine heart wherewith thou shalt fear, and for the sight of thine eyes which thou shalt see" (Deut. xxviii.).[14]

The condition of Hopeful and Christian put by Giant Despair[15] into "a very dark dungeon, nasty and stinking to their spirits,"[16] and beaten with stripes, and made to feel that the bitterness of death was as nothing to the bitterness of life, illustrates in allegory the state of man for countless centuries. In darkness and in the shadow of death he lay helpless, singing like the prisoners vain hymns of hope, and praying vain prayers of patience, yet having all the while in his bosom, like Christian, a key called Promise, capable of unlocking the doors of his dungeon. Groping between what Sir Thomas Browne so finely calls "the night of our fore-being"[17] and the unknown future, the dark before and after, he at last came to himself, and with the help of this key unlocked the mysteries of Nature, and found a way of physical salvation.

Man's redemption of man is the great triumph of Greek thought. The taproot of modern science sinks deep in Greek soil, the astounding fertility of which

12. This bitter saying exhibits the melancholy conception of life. Theodor Gomperz in his *Greek Thinkers*, Osler's favorite book, quotes the line "not to be born is the best fate of all" from the *Oedipus at Colonus* of Sophocles, line 1225. Osler has misattributed the line to Euripides.

13. Edwin Charles Markham, "The Man with the Hoe," in *The Man with the Hoe and Other Poems*, stanza 1, lines 1–7. This poem was inspired by Millet's painting.

14. Deuteronomy 28:66–67.

15. *Hopeful, Christian, and Giant Despair:* Characters in *The Pilgrim's Progress* by John Bunyan (1628–1688).

16. John Bunyan, *The Pilgrim's Progress*, (1678; London: George Routledge and Sons, n.d.), p. 173.

17. Thomas Browne, *Hydriotaphia, Urn-Burial* (1658), chap. 5, Keynes' edition, vol. 1, p. 170. The exact quotation is: "The Chaos of pre-ordination, and night of their fore-beings."

is one of the out-standing facts of history. As Sir Henry Maine says: "To one small people . . . it was given to create the principle of progress. That people was the Greek. Except the blind forces of Nature nothing moves in this world which is not Greek in its origin."[18] Though not always recognized, the controlling principles of our art, literature and philosophy, as well as those of science, are Hellenic. We still think in certain levels only with the help of Plato, and there is not a lecture room of this university[19] in which the trained ear may not catch echoes of the Lyceum.[20] In his introductory chapter of his *Rise of the Greek Epic*, Professor Murray[21] dwells on the keen desire of the Greeks to make life a better thing than it is, and to help in the service of man, a thought that pervades Greek life like an aroma. From Homer[22] to Lucian[23] there is one refrain—the pride in the body as a whole; and in the strong conviction that "our soul in its rose-mesh"[24] is quite as much helped by flesh as flesh is by soul, the Greek sang his song "For pleasant is this flesh."[25] The beautiful soul harmonizing with a beautiful body is as much the glorious ideal of Plato as it is the end of the education of Aristotle. What a splendid picture in Book III of the *Republic*, of the day when "our youth will dwell in a land of health, amid fair sights and sounds and receive the good in everything; and beauty, the effluence of fair works, shall flow into the eye and ear like a health-giving breeze from a purer region, and insensibly draw the soul from earliest years into likeness and sympathy with the beauty of reason."[26] The glory of this zeal for the enrichment of the present life was revealed to the Greeks as to no other people, but in respect to care for the body of the common man, we have only seen its fulfilment in our own day, but as a direct result of methods of research initiated by them.

Philosophy, as Plato tells us, begins with wonder;[27] and, staring open-eyed at the starry heavens on the plains of Mesopotamia, man took a first step in

---

18. Henry James Sumner *Maine* (1822–1888): English jurist and author of *Village-Communities in the East and West* (New York: Henry Holt, 1876), p. 238.

19. The University of Edinburgh.

20. *Lyceum:* Gymnasium and garden with covered walks (exercise ground) of ancient Athens where Aristotle taught and where he and his disciples used to philosophize while walking. It derived its name from the temple of Apollo.

21. George Gilbert *Murray* (1866–1957): English classical scholar. See "The Old Humanities and the New Science," p. 97, n. 242.

22. *Homer* (fl. before 700 B.C.): Author of Greek epic poems *The Iliad* and *The Odyssey*.

23. *Lucian* (c.125–c.200 A.D.): Greek writer, sophist, and rhetorician, known for his satirical dialogues against prejudice and superstition.

24. Robert Browning, "Rabbi Ben Ezra," line 60.

25. Ibid., line 61.

26. Plato (427–347 B.C.), *Republic*, book 3, 401c–d.

27. Plato (427–347 B.C.), *Theaetetus*, 155d.

the careful observation of Nature, which carried him a long way in his career. But he was very slow to learn the second step—how to interrogate Nature, to search out her secrets, as Harvey puts it, by way of experiment.[28] The Chaldeans, who invented gnomons,[29] and predicted eclipses, made a good beginning. The Greeks did not get much beyond trained observation, though Pythagoras[30] made one fundamental experiment when he determined the dependence of the pitch of sound on the length of the vibrating cord. So far did unaided observation and brilliant generalization carry Greek thinkers, that there is scarcely a modern discovery which by anticipation cannot be found in their writings. Indeed one is staggered at their grasp of great principles. Man can do a great deal by observation and thinking, but with them alone he cannot unravel the mysteries of Nature. Had it been possible the Greeks would have done it; and could Plato and Aristotle have grasped the value of experiment in the progress of human knowledge, the course of European history might have been very different.

This organon[31] was absent, and even in the art of medicine Hippocrates with all his genius did not get beyond highly trained observation, and a conception of disease as a process of Nature. The great Pergamite, Galen,[32] did indeed realize that the bare fact was only preliminary to the scientific study of disease by experiment, and to the collecting of data, from which principles and laws could be derived. On the dark horizon of the ancient world shone the brightness of the Grecian dawn so clearly that the emancipated mind had an open way. Then something happened—how, who can tell? The light failed or flickered almost to extinction: Greece died into a mediaevalism that for centuries enthralled man in chains, the weary length of which still hampers his progress. The revival of learning awakened at first a suspicion and then a conviction that salvation lay in a return to the old Greek fathers who had set man's feet in the right path, and so it came about that in the study of chemistry, and in the inventions of Copernicus, Kepler and Galileo,[33] modern science took its origin. The growth of the

28. William Harvey, *Anatomical Exercises on the Generation of Animals* (1651). "Epistle Dedicatory," by George Ent, trans. Robert Willis (London: The Sydenham Society, 1847), p. 146. Dr. Ent, a friend of Harvey's, defended his doctrine of the circulation.

29. *gnomon:* An astronomical instrument for measuring the altitudes and declinations of the heavenly bodies.

30. *Pythagoras* (c.582–c.500 B.C.): Greek philosopher and mathematician. See "Physic and Physicians as Depicted in Plato," p. 127, n. 3.

31. *organon:* An instrument of thought or knowledge, a body of principles of scientific or philosophic investigation.

32. Claudius *Galen* (c.130–c.200 A.D.): Greek physician and philosophical writer. See "Teaching and Thinking," p. 181, n. 27.

33. Nicolaus *Copernicus* (1473–1543): Polish astronomer who was a founder of modern astronomy. He

experimental method changed the outlook of mankind, and led directly to the development of the physical and biological sciences by which the modern world has been transformed.

A slow, painful progress, through three centuries, science crept on from point to point, with many mistakes and many failures, a progress often marked and flecked with the stains of human effort, but all the same the most revolutionary and far-reaching advance ever made by man's intellect. We are too close to the events to appreciate fully the changes which it has wrought in man's relation to the world; and the marvellous thing is that the most important of these changes have been effected within the memory of those living. Three stand out as of the first importance.

My generation was brought up in the belief that "Man was in his original state a very noble and exalted creature, being placed as the head and lord of this world, having all the creatures in subjection to him. The powers and operations of his mind were extensive, capacious and perfect"[34]—to quote the words of one of my old Sunday-school lessons. It is not too much to say that Charles Darwin[35] has so turned man right-about-face that, no longer looking back with regret upon a Paradise Lost, he feels already within the gates of a Paradise Regained.[36]

Secondly, Chemistry and Physics have at last given him control of the four elements, and he has harnessed the forces of Nature. As usual Kipling[37] touches

---

also studied medicine. In 1530, after careful observation of the solar system for many years, he put forward the theory that the earth and the other planets revolved around the sun. His theory was widely rejected as contrary to common sense and to the text of the Bible, and it gained acceptance only slowly and after his death.

Johannes *Kepler* (1571–1630): German astronomer who was also a founder of modern astronomy. He compiled astronomical tables and improved the telescope. His laws of motion helped Newton determine the laws of gravity.

Galilei *Galileo* (1564–1642): Italian mathematician, physicist, and astronomer. He invented the first thermometer in 1597 and the telescope in 1609, with which he described many formerly unseen things. He was denounced by the Inquisition and in 1616 was forbidden by the pope to teach that the earth moved. He was later again persecuted and forced to renounce his teachings.

34. The passage is in part a reference to Genesis 1:28–29. Because Osler attributes the quote to "one of my old Sunday-school lessons," he may be quoting his own old notebooks, representing oral instruction by his father or Father Johnson or at the Barrie Grammar School. This line of theological teaching goes back to St. Augustine of Hippo (354–430).

35. Charles Robert *Darwin* (1809–1882): English naturalist. His book *On the Origin of Species by Means of Natural Selection* (1859) aroused a storm of controversy. "Right-about-face" is a marching-maneuver that changes direction by 180 degrees.

36. Osler refers to John Milton's works *Paradise Lost* (1667) and *Paradise Regained* (1671), which are based on the Old and New Testaments of the Bible.

37. Rudyard *Kipling*, "The Four Angels," lines 1–7. The exact quotation is:

the very heart of the matter in his poem on "The Four Angels," who in succession offered to Adam fire, air, earth and water. Happy in the garden, watching the apple tree in bud, in leaf, in blossom and in fruit, he had no use for them; but when the apple tree was cut down, and he had to work outside of Eden wall,—then—

> out of black disaster
> He arose to be the master
> Of Earth and Water, Air and Fire.[38]

And this mastery, won in our day, has made the man with the hoe look up.

But the third and greatest glory is that the leaves of the tree of science have availed for the healing of the nations.[39] Measure as we may the progress of the world—intellectually in the growth and spread of education, materially in the application to life of all mechanical appliances, and morally in a higher standard of ethics between nation and nation, and between individuals, there is no one measure which can compare with the decrease of disease and suffering in man, woman and child. The Psalmist will have it that no man may redeem his brother,[40] but this redemption of his body has been bought at a price of the lives of those who have sought out Nature's processes by study and experiment. Silent workers, often unknown and neglected by their generation, these men have kept alive the fires on the altars of science, and have so opened the doors of knowledge that we now know the laws of health and disease. Time will only permit me to refer to a few of the more important of the measures of man's physical redemption.

Within the life-time of some of us a strange and wonderful thing happened on the earth—something of which no prophet foretold, of which no seer dreamt, nor is it among the beatitudes of Christ Himself;[41] only St. John seems to have had an inkling of it in that splendid chapter in which he describes the new heaven

---

As Adam lay a-dreaming beneath the Apple tree
The Angel of the Earth came down, and offered Earth in fee.

38. Ibid., 12–14.

39. *the leaves of the tree of science have availed for the healing of the nations:* The phrase comes from St. John's vision of the New Jerusalem (Revelation 22:2). The original reads: "In the midst of the street of it, and on either side of the river, *was there* the tree of life . . . and the leaves of the tree *were* for the healing of the nations."

40. Psalm 49–47. Osler is partly remembering the translation in the *Book of Common Prayer* rather than the King James Bible: "no man" comes from the *Book of Common Prayer* but "redeem" from the King James version.

41. *the beatitudes of Christ Himself:* The declarations made in the Sermon on the Mount, which begins with "Blessed are the poor in spirit." Matthew 5:3–12 and Luke 6:20–23.

and the new earth, when the former things should pass away, when all tears should be wiped away, and there should be no more crying nor sorrow.[42] On October 16, 1846, in the amphitheatre of the Massachusetts General Hospital, Boston, a new Prometheus[43] gave a gift as rich as that of fire, the greatest single gift ever made to suffering humanity. The prophecy was fulfilled—*neither shall there be any more pain;*[44] a mystery of the ages had been solved by a daring experiment by man on man in the introduction of anæsthesia. As Weir Mitchell[45] sings in his poem, "The Death of Pain"—

> Whatever triumphs still shall hold the mind,
> Whatever gifts shall yet enrich mankind,
> Ah! here, no hour shall strike through all the years,
> No hour so sweet as when hope, doubt and fears,
> 'Mid deepening silence watched one eager brain
> With Godlike will decree the Death of Pain.[46]

At a stroke the curse of Eve was removed, that multiplied sorrow of sorrows, representing in all ages the very apotheosis[47] of pain. The knife has been robbed of its terrors, and the hospitals are no longer the scenes of those appalling tragedies that made the stoutest quail. To-day we take for granted the silence of the operating-room, but to reach this Elysium[48] we had to travel the slow road of laborious research, which gave us first the chemical agents; and then brave hearts had to risk reputation, and even life itself in experiments, the issue of which was for long doubtful.

More widespread in its benediction, as embracing all races and all classes of society, is the relief of suffering, and the prevention of disease through the

42. *that splendid chapter in which he describes the new heaven and the new earth, when the former things should pass away, when all tears should be wiped away, and there should be no more crying nor sorrow:* Revelation 21:1–4.

43. *Prometheus:* (Greek myth.) He was said to have brought fire down to earth and to have given humanity the knowledge of many other arts. He is celebrated as the benefactor of the human race. Osler here refers to William Thomas Green Morton (1819–1868), American dentist, the first to use anesthesia (ether) during surgery.

44. *neither shall there be any more pain:* Revelation 21:4.

45. Silas Weir *Mitchell* (1829–1914): See "L'Envoi," p. 351, n. 8.

46. Silas Weir Mitchell, "The Birth and Death of Pain," in *The Complete Poems of S. Weir Mitchell* (New York: The Century, 1914), p. 416.

47. *apotheosis:* Deification. Osler means that Genesis 3:16 was interpreted to mean that human pain, and particularly women's pain in childbirth, had been decreed by God as punishment for the disobedience of Adam and Eve.

48. *Elysium:* (Greek myth.) The abode of the blessed after death and of heroes exempt from death. Homer's *Odyssey* (book 4, lines 561–570) describes it as a plain at the end of the earth without snow, storm, or rain.

growth of modern sanitary science in which has been fought out the greatest victory in history. I can only refer to three subjects which illustrate and lead up to the question which is in the minds of all of us to-day.

You have in Scotland the merit of the practical introduction of a method which has revolutionized the treatment of wounds, and changed the whole aspect of modern surgery. I am old enough to have been a dresser in a large general hospital in the pre-Listerian days,[49] when it was the rule for wounds to suppurate, and when cases of severe pyæmia and septicæmia were so common that surgeons dreaded to make even a simple amputation. In the wards of the Edinburgh Royal Infirmary and of the Glasgow Royal Infirmary, Lord Lister's experimental work on the healing of wounds led to results of the deepest moment to every individual subject to an accident, or who has to submit to an operation. It is not simply that the prospect of recovery is enormously enhanced, but Listerian surgery has diminished suffering to an extraordinary degree. In the old days every wound which suppurated had to be dressed, and there was the daily distress and pain, felt particularly by young children. Now, even after operations of the first magnitude, the wound may have but a single dressing, and the after-pain is reduced to a minimum. How well the older ones of us realize that anæsthetics and asepsis between them have wrought a complete revolution in hospital life. I asked the Superintendent of Nurses at the Royal Infirmary to let me know how many patients last night in the wards had actual suffering, and she has sent word that about one in eight had pain, not all of them acute pain.

But man's redemption of man is nowhere so well known as in the abolition and prevention of the group of diseases which we speak of as the fevers, or the acute infections. This is the glory of the science of medicine, and nowhere in the world have its lessons been so thoroughly carried out as in this country. It is too old a story to retell in detail, but I may remind you that in this city within fifty years there has been an annual saving of from four to five thousand lives, by measures which have directly prevented and limited the spread of infectious diseases. The man is still alive, Sir Henry Littlejohn,[50] who made the first sanitary survey of the city. When one reads the account of the condition of the densely crowded districts on the south side of the High Street, one is not surprised that the rate of mortality was 40 and over per thousand. That you now enjoy one of the lowest death rates in Europe—15.3 per thousand for last year—is due to the thoroughness with which measures of recognized efficiency

49. *pre-Listerian days:* Before Joseph *Lister* (1827–1912), English surgeon, who founded antiseptic surgery.
50. Henry Duncan *Littlejohn* (1828–1914): Professor of forensic medicine at the University of Edinburgh and also medical officer of health for Edinburgh.

have been carried out. When we learn that last year there were no deaths from small-pox, not one from typhus, and only twenty-one from fevers of the zymotic group, it is scarcely credible that all this has been brought about within the memory of living men. It is not too much to say that the abolition of small-pox, typhus and typhoid fevers have changed the character of the medical practice in our hospitals. In this country typhoid fever is in its last ditch, and though a more subtle and difficult enemy to conquer than typhus, we may confidently hope that before long it will be as rare.

Here I would like to say a word or two upon one of the most terrible of all acute infections, the one of which we first learned the control through the work of Jenner.[51] A great deal of literature has been distributed, casting discredit upon the value of vaccination in the prevention of small-pox. I do not see how any one who has gone through epidemics as I have, or who is familiar with the history of the subject, and who has any capacity left for clear judgment, can doubt its value. Some months ago I was twitted by the Editor of the Journal of the Anti-Vaccination League for maintaining a curious silence on the subject. I would like to issue a Mount Carmel-like challenge[52] to any ten unvaccinated priests of Baal. I will take ten selected vaccinated persons, and help in the next severe epidemic, with ten selected unvaccinated persons (if available!). I should choose three members of Parliament, three anti-vaccination doctors, if they could be found, and four anti-vaccination propagandists. And I will make this promise—neither to jeer nor to jibe[53] when they catch the disease, but to look after them as brothers; and for the three or four who are certain to die I will try to arrange the funerals with all the pomp and ceremony of an anti-vaccination demonstration.

A blundering art until thirty or forty years ago, preventative medicine was made a science by the discovery of the causes of many of the serious epidemic diseases. To any one of you who wishes to know this side of science, what it is, what it has done, what it may do, let me commend Radot's *Life of Pasteur*,[54] which reads like a fairy tale. It is more particularly in connection with the great plagues of the world that man's redemption of man may be in the future effected; I say in the future because we have only touched the fringe of the subject. How little do we appreciate what even a generation has done. The man is only just

51. Edward *Jenner* (1749–1823): See "Chauvinism in Medicine," p. 237, n. 36.

52. *Mount Carmel-like challenge:* Mount Carmel is a sacred mountain in Israel, where the Carmelite church and convent stand. Osler refers to Elijah, who had a confrontation there with the false prophets of Baal, chief god of the Canaanites (1 Kings 18:19–46).

53. *neither to jeer nor to jibe:* The phrase means "Not like Elijah, who mocked the prophets of Baal." Ibid., 27.

54. René Vallery-Radot, *Life of Pasteur*, trans. R. L. Devonshire, foreword by William Osler (1900; London: Constable, 1911).

dead, Robert Koch,[55] who gave to his fellow-men the control of cholera. Read the history of yellow fever in Havana and in Brazil if you wish to get an idea of the powers of experimental medicine; there is nothing to match it in the history of human achievement. Before our eyes to-day the most striking experiment ever made in sanitation is in progress. The digging of the Panama Canal was acknowledged to be a question of the health of the workers. For four centuries the Isthmus[56] had been a white man's grave, and during the French control of the Canal the mortality once reached the appalling figure of 170 per thousand. Even under the most favourable circumstances it was extraordinarily high. Month by month I get the *Reports* which form by far the most interesting sanitary reading of the present day. Of more than 54,000 employees (about 13,000 of whom are white), the death rate per thousand for the month of March was 8.91, a lower percentage, I believe, than any city in the United States. It has been brought about in great part by researches into the life history of the parasite which produces malaria, and by the effectual measures taken for its destruction. Here again is a chapter in human achievement for which it would be hard to find a parallel. But let us not forget that these are but illustrations of widespread possibilities of organization on modern lines. These are sanitary blessings. To make them available in the Tropics is the heaviest burden of the white man; how heavy you may know from the startling figures which have just been issued from British India. Exclusive of the native states for the year 1908, the total deaths from fever and cholera exceeded 5,000,000, out of a population of 226,000,000. The bright spot in the picture is the diminution of the mortality from plague—not fewer than a million fatal cases as compared with 1907.

These are brief indications of the lines along which effective progress is being made in man's redemption by man. And all this has a direct bearing upon the disease, the fight against which brings us together. Tuberculosis is one of the great infections of the world, and it has been one of the triumphs of our generation to determine its cause. With the improvement of sanitation there has been a reduction in its mortality, amounting since 1850 to above 40 per cent. But it still remains the most formidable single foe, killing a larger number of people than any other disease—some 60,000 in Great Britain and Ireland in 1908, and 589 of this city. Practically between 10 and 11 percent. of all deaths are due to it. A plain proposition is before the people. We know the disease—how it is caused, how it is spread, how it should be prevented, how in suitable cases it may be cured.

55. Robert *Koch* (1843–1910): German bacteriologist who led expeditions to Egypt and India (1883) and discovered the cholera bacillus as well as the one that causes tuberculosis. For his biographical information, see "Books and Men," p. 222, n. 20.

56. The Isthmus of Panama in Central America.

How to make this knowledge effective is the prime reason of this conference. It is a campaign for the public; past history shows that it is a campaign of hope. The measures for its stamping out, though simple on paper, present difficulties interwoven with the very fabric of society, but they are not insuperable, and are gradually disappearing. It is for this reason we urge you to join with enthusiasm in the crusade; remembering, however, that only the prolonged and united efforts, carried through several generations, can place the disease in the same category with typhus fever, typhoid and small-pox.

In the comedies and tragedies of life our immutable human nature reacts very much as in the dawn of science, and yet, with a widening of knowledge, the lights and shadows of the landscape have shifted, and the picture is brighter. Nothing can bring back the hour when sin and disease were correlated as confidently as night and day;[57] and how shall we assess the enormous gain of a new criterion, a new estimate of the value of man's life! There are tones in human sentiment to-day which the ancients never heard, which our fathers indeed heard but faintly, and that without recognizing their significance. The human heart by which we live has been touched as with the wand of a Prospero.[58] What availed the sceptred race![59] what the glory that was Greece, or the grandeur that was Rome! of what avail even has been the message of the gospel,[60] while the people at large were haunted by fear and anxiety, stricken by the pestilence of the darkness and the sickness of the noon-day? The new socialism of Science with its definite mission cares not a rap for the theories of Karl Marx,[61] of Ferdinand Las-

57. *sin and disease were correlated as confidently as night and day:* For information on the concept that sickness is punishment for sin, see "Doctor and Nurse," p. 104, n. 28.

58. *Prospero:* In Shakespeare's *The Tempest* (V, i) he is represented as a wise and good magician, and is the rightful duke of Milan living in exile on an island with his daughter, Miranda. He breaks his magic wand at the end of the play. Osler is saying that science has brought happiness, not prosperity, as Prospero used his magic to bring happiness to his daughter, her lover, and the young man's shipwrecked companions.

59. Walter Savage Landor, "Rose Aylmer," line 1. Osler may have been thinking of the opening line of John of Gaunt's deathbed speech in William Shakespeare's *Richard II* (II, i, 40): "This royal throne of kings, this sceptered isle." A scepter is a ceremonial staff symbolic of authority, and the "sceptred race" here is the British race, which from both Britain and America had in Osler's time brought so much of the world under its rule.

60. *what avail even has been the message of the gospel:* Osler here claims "what good are the words of the Bible when people are ill?" It is rather extraordinary for him, a professed Christian, to ask this question, because the orthodox teaching would be St. Paul's: "I reckon that the sufferings of this present time *are* not worthy *to be compared* with the glory which shall be revealed in us" (Romans 8:18). Osler seems here to have adopted the philosophy of humanity advocated by Auguste Compte.

61. Karl *Marx* (1818–1883): German socialist philosopher and politician who engaged in the revolution in Germany in 1848 and was expelled from the country in 1849. He left for Paris and then went on to London, where he lived until his death. He is best known for his book *Das Kapital* (1867).

salle,[62] or of Henry George;[63] still less for the dreams of Plato[64] or of Sir Thomas More[65]—or at least only so far as they help to realize the well-being of the citizen. Nor is there need to fear that in weighing the world in our balance we may drain the sap of its life, so long as we materialize in the service of man those eternal principles on which life rests—moral fervour, liberty and justice.

The outlook for the world as represented by Mary and John, and Jennie and Tom[66] has never been so hopeful. There is no place for despondency or despair. As for the dour dyspeptics in mind and morals who sit idly croaking like ravens,[67]—let them come into the arena, let them wrestle for their flesh and blood against the principalities and powers[68] represented by bad air and worse houses, by drink and disease, by needless pain, and by the loss annually to the state of thousands of valuable lives—let them fight for the day when a man's life shall be more precious than gold. Now, alas! the cheapness of life is every day's tragedy!

If in the memorable phrase of the Greek philosopher Prodicus,[69] "That which benefits human life is God,"[70] we may see in this new gospel a link betwixt us and the crowning race of those who eye to eye shall look on knowledge, and in whose hand Nature shall be an open book, an approach to the glorious day of which Shelley sings so gloriously:

62. Ferdinand *Lassalle* (1825–1864): German socialist spokesman for the workers, and founder of the German Social Democratic Party.

63. Henry *George* (1839–1897): American political economist and land reformer. In 1886 he was nominated as a United Labor Party candidate for mayor of New York, but was defeated. He believed in common property.

64. *Plato* (c.427–347 B.C.): Greek philosopher. His chief extant works are in the form of dialogues, including the *Republic,* where he searches for justice in the construction of an ideal state.

65. Thomas *More* (1478–1535): English humanist and author of *Utopia* (1516), which is an attempt to depict an ideal state.

66. *Mary and John, and Jennie and Tom:* Typical common or ordinary people of the working class.

67. *sit idly croaking like ravens:* Probably Osler had an (anonymous) ballad in mind. It reads:

> There were three ravens sat on a tree,
> They were as black as they might be.
> The one of them said to his make,
> 'Where shall we our breakfast take?'

68. *wrestle for their flesh and blood against the principalities and powers:* The phrase is a reminiscence of Ephesians 6:12: "For we wrestle not against flesh and blood, but against principalities, against powers, against the rulers of the darkness of this world, against spiritual wickedness in high *places.*"

69. *Prodicus* of Ceos (5th cent. B.C.): Greek sophist and rhetorician. For further information, see "Physic and Physicians as Depicted in Plato," p. 143, n. 92.

70. Marcus Tullius Cicero, *De Natura Deorum* (On the Nature of the Gods), trans. H. Rackham (1933; London: Heinemann; Cambridge, Mass: Harvard University Press, 1972), pp. 112–115. "Prodicus of Ceos, who said that the gods were personifications of things beneficial to the life of man."

Happiness

And Science dawn though late upon the earth;
Peace cheers the mind, health renovates the frame;
Disease and pleasure cease to mingle here,
Reason and passion cease to combat there,
Whilst mind unfettered o'er the earth extends
Its all-subduing energies, and wields
The sceptre of a vast dominion there.[71]

71. Percy Bysshe Shelley, "Queen Mab," canto 8, lines 227–234.

BED-SIDE LIBRARY FOR
MEDICAL STUDENTS

A liberal education may be had at a very slight cost of time and money. Well filled though the day be with appointed tasks, to make the best possible use of your one or of your ten talents, rest not satisfied with this professional training, but try to get the education, if not of a scholar, at least of a gentleman. Before going to sleep read for half an hour, and in the morning have a book open on your dressing table. You will be surprised to find how much can be accomplished in the course of a year. I have put down a list of ten books which you may make close friends. There are many others; studied carefully in your student days these will help in the inner education of which I speak.

    I. Old and New Testament.
   II. Shakespeare.
  III. Montaigne.[1]
  IV. Plutarch's *Lives.*[1]
   V. Marcus Aurelius.[2]
  VI. Epictetus.[2]
 VII. *Religio Medici.*[2]
VIII. *Don Quixote.*
  IX. Emerson.
   X. Oliver Wendell Holmes — Breakfast-Table Series.

1. The Temple Classics, J. M. Dent and Co.
2. Golden Treasury Series, Macmillan and Company, Ltd.

ABBREVIATIONS

a. (before a date)	ante (before; not later than)
b.	born
c. (before a date)	circa (about)
cent.	century
chap.	chapter
Cushing	Harvey Cushing, *The Life of Sir William Osler,* Oxford University Press, 1940.
d.	died
DNB	*Dictionary of National Biography*
fig.	figuratively
fl.	flourished
ibid.	ibidem (in the same place)
marg.	marginal note to the text
myth.	mythology
n.d.	no date (of publication given)
n.p.	no place (of publication given)
op. cit.	opere citato (in the work cited)
Obs.	obsolete
OED	*Oxford English Dictionary*
rev., Rev.	revised
sect.	section
sic	thus; exactly so
v.d.	various dates
vol.	Volume

REFERENCES

The list that follows represents only some of the most frequently used reference tools. We have consulted much more for information, which it would be impractical to include in the list. Grateful thanks are due to the compilers of many other reference sources, especially to writings of individual writers and concordances to poems and prose works of poets, essayists, and novelists.

Osler

Osler, William. *Aequanimitas.* 3d ed. New York: McGraw-Hill, 1961.

——. *Bibliotheca Osleriana* (1929). Ed. by W. W. Francis et al. Reprint. Montreal: McGill-Queen's University Press, 1969.

Abbott, Maude E. *Classified and Annotated Bibliography of Sir William Osler's Publications.* 2d ed. Montreal: The Medical Museum, McGill University, 1939.

Bett, W. R. Osler: *The Man and the Legend.* London: William Heinemann, 1951.

Bliss, Michael. *William Osler: A Life in Medicine.* New York: Oxford University Press, 1999.

Cushing, Harvey. *The Life of Sir William Osler* (1925). Reprint. New York: Oxford University Press, 1977.

Golden, Richard L., and Charles G. Roland, eds. *Sir William Osler, An Annotated Bibliography with Illustrations.* San Francisco: Jeremy Norman and Co., 1988.

McGovern, John P., and Charles G. Roland. *Wm. Osler: The Continuing Education.* Springfield, Ill.: Charles C. Thomas, 1969.

——, eds. *The Collected Essays of Sir William Osler, Volume 1, The Philosophical Essays.* Birmingham, Ala.: The Classics of Medicine Library, Gryphon Editions, 1985.

——, eds. *The Collected Essays of Sir William Osler, Volume II, The Educational Essays.* Birmingham, Ala.: The Classics of Medicine Library, Gryphon Editions, 1985.

——, eds. *The Collected Essays of Sir William Osler, Volume III, The Historical and Biographical Essays.* Birmingham, Ala.: The Classics of Medicine Library, Gryphon Editions, 1985.

Nation, Earl F., Charles G. Roland, and John P. McGovern. *An Annotated Checklist of Osleriana.* Kent, Ohio: Kent State University Press, 1976.

Roland, Charles G. *William Osler's "The Master-Word in Medicine": A Study in Rhetoric.* Springfield, Ill.: Charles C. Thomas, 1972.

ENCYCLOPEDIAS AND DICTIONARIES

Benét's Reader's Encyclopedia. 3d ed. New York: Harper and Row, 1987.

Dictionary of Classical Mythology. Ed. by Pierre Grimal. Trans. by A. R. Maxwell-Hyslop. New York: Blackwell, 1986.

Dictionary of Classical Mythology: Symbols, Attributes, and Associations. Ed. by Robert E. Bell. Santa Barbara, Calif.: ABC-Clio, 1982.

Encyclopedia Americana. Danbury, Conn.: Grolier, 1992.

English Dialect Dictionary. Ed. by Joseph Wright. London: Oxford University Press, 1923.

Guide to Reference Books. 11th ed. Ed. by Eugene P. Sheehy. Chicago: American Library Association, 1996.

The New Encyclopaedia Britannica. 15th ed. Chicago: Encyclopaedia Britannica, 1995.

Notes and Queries. 1849–date. London: Oxford University Press, 1850–date.

Oxford English Dictionary. 2d ed. Prepared by J. A. Simpson and E. S. C. Weiner. Oxford: Clarendon Press, 1989.

Oxford Classical Dictionary. 2d ed. Ed. by N. G. L. Hammond and H. H. Scullard. Oxford: Clarendon Press, 1970.

Random House Dictionary of the English Language. 2d ed. Ed. by Stuart B. Flexner. New York: Random House, 1987.

Shakespeare Glossary. Ed. by C. T. Onions. Oxford: Clarendon Press, 1986.

Webster's Third New International Dictionary of the English Language. Ed. by Philip B. Gove and the Merriam-Webster Editorial Staff. Springfield, Mass.: Merriam-Webster, 1986.

BIOGRAPHICAL DICTIONARIES AND INDEXES

American Men and Women of Science: Physical and Biological Sciences. 16th ed. Ed. by Jaques Cattell Press. New York: Bowker, 1986.

Biography and Genealogy Master Index. 2d ed. Detroit: Gale, 1980. Supplements. 1981–1985. 1986, 1987. to date.

Dictionary of American Biography. New York: Scribner, 1928–1937. Supplements 1–7 and Index, 1944–1981.

Dictionary of Canadian Biography. Toronto: University of Toronto Press, 1966–date.

Dictionary of National Biography. Ed. by Leslie Stephen and Sidney Lee. London: Smith, Elder, 1885–1901. (Reissued. London: Oxford University Press, 1921–1922). Supplements and additional volumes.

Macmillan Dictionary of Canadian Biography. 4th ed. Ed. by W. A. McKay. Toronto: Macmillan, 1978.

Webster's New Biographical Dictionary. Rev. ed. Springfield, Mass.: Merriam-Webster, 1983.

Who Was Who, 1897-1980. London: A. and C. Black, 1929–1981.

Who Was Who in America, 1897–1985. Chicago: Marquis, 1942–1985.

Who Was Who in the Greek World. Ed. by Diana Bowden. Ithaca, New York: Cornell University, 1982.

Who Was Who in the Roman World. Ed. by Diana Bowden. Ithaca, New York: Cornell University, 1980.

QUOTATIONS

Bartlett, John. *Familiar Quotations: A Collection of Passages, Phrases, and Proverbs Traced to Their Sources in Ancient and Modern Literature.* 15th ed. Ed. by Emily M. Beck. Boston: Little Brown, 1980.

Evans, Bergen. *Dictionary of Quotations.* New York: Delacorte, 1968.

Great Treasury of Western Thought: A Compendium of Important Statements on Man and His Institutions by the Great Thinkers in Western History. Ed. by Mortimer J. Adler and Charles Van Doren. New York: Bowker, 1977.

King, William Francis Henry. *Classical and Foreign Quotations.* 3d ed. Detroit: Gale Research, 1968.

Macmillan Book of Proverbs, Maxims, and Famous Phrases. Ed. by Burton E. Stevenson. New York: Macmillan, 1965.

Magill, Frank N., ed. *Magill's Quotations in Context.* New York: Salem Press, 1965.

Stevenson, Burton E. *Home Book of Quotations, Classical and Modern.* 10th ed. New York: Dodd, 1967. Reprint. New York: Greenwich House, 1985.

Dictionary of Biographical Quotation of British and American Subjects. Ed. by Richard Kenin and Justin Wintle. New York: Alfred A. Knopf, 1978.

SPECIAL SUBJECTS

Philosophy and Religion

Biblical quotations are from *The King James* ("*Authorised*") *Version* unless otherwise indicated.

The Book of Common Prayer: references are to the 1662 book of the Church of England, unless otherwise indicated.

Analytical Concordance to the Bible. Robert Young. 22d American ed. Rev. by W. B. Stevenson. New York: Funk and Wagnalls, 1955.

A Concordance to the Apocryphal/Deuterocanonical Books of the Revised Standard Version. Grand Rapids, Mich.: Eerdmans, 1983.

Encyclopedia of Philosophy. Ed. by Paul Edwards. New York: Macmillan, 1967. Reprint, 1972. Supplement, 1996.

Encyclopedia of Religion. Ed. by Mircea Eliade. New York: Macmillan, 1987.

The Exhaustive Concordance of the Bible. Ed. by James Strong. Nashville: Abingdon, 1974.

The Interpreter's Bible. New York: Abingdon, 1951–1957.

The Interpreter's Dictionary of the Bible. Ed. by George A. Buttrick et al. New York: Abingdon, 1962. Supplement, 1976.

Nelson's Complete Concordance of the Revised Standard Version Bible. Ed. by John W. Ellison. New York: Nelson, 1957.

Oxford Dictionary of the Christian Church. 2d ed. Reprint. Ed. by F. L. Cross and E. A. Livingstone. New York: Oxford University Press, 1983.

Strong, James. *The New Strong's Exhaustive Concordance of the Bible.* Nashville: T. Nelson, 1990.

Literature

Allibone, Samuel Austin. *A Critical Dictionary of English Literature and British and American Authors, . . .* Philadelphia: Lippincott, 1872–1875.

Cyclopedia of Literary Characters. Ed. by Frank N. Magill. New York: Harper, 1963.

Dictionary of Fictional Characters. William Freeman. Rev. by Fred Urquhart. Boston: Writer, 1974.

Keynes, Geoffrey. *A Bibliography of Sir Thomas Browne.* 2d ed. Oxford: Clarendon Press, 1968.

The New Oxford Companion to Literature in French. Ed. by Peter France. Oxford: Clarendon Press, 1995.

The Oxford Companion to American Literature. 5th ed. Ed. by James D. Hart. New York: Oxford University Press, 1983.

The Oxford Companion to Classical Literature. Ed. by Paul Harvey. Reprint. Oxford: Clarendon Press, 1974.

The Oxford Companion to English Literature. 5th ed. Ed. by Margaret Drabble. New York: Oxford University Press, 1985.

Spevack, Marvin. *A Complete and Systematic Concordance to the Works of Shakespeare*. Hildesheim, Germany: Georg Olms, 1968–1980.

Medicine and Science

Castiglioni, Arturo. *A History of Medicine*. Trans. by E. B. Krumbhaar. New York: A. A. Knopf, 1941.

Dorland's Illustrated Medical Dictionary. 27th ed. Philadelphia: Saundes, 1988.

McGraw-Hill Encyclopedia of Science and Technology. 6th ed. New York: McGraw-Hill, 1987.

Sarton, George. *Introduction to the History of Science*. Baltimore: Williams and Wilkins, 1927–1948. Reprint. Huntington, N.Y.: Krieger, 1975.

Stedman, Thomas Lathrop. *Stedman's Medical Dictionary*. 25th ed. Baltimore: Williams and Wilkins, 1990.

OTHERS

The following list includes only editions which we find it better to specify because of their variant readings:

Browne, Thomas. *The Works of Sir Thomas Browne*. Ed. by Geoffrey Keynes. Chicago: The University of Chicago Press, 1964.

FitzGerald, Edward. *The Rubáiyát of Omar Khayyám*. 3rd ed. (1872). *The Variorum and Definitive Edition of the Poetical and Prose Writings of Edward Fitzgerald*. New York: Doubleday, 1902–1903.

Plato. *The Dialogues of Plato*. Ed. by Benjamin Jowett. 4th ed. Oxford: Clarendon Press, 1953.

Shakespeare, William. *Shakespeare: the Complete Works*. Ed. by G.B. Harrison. New York: Harcourt, Brace, 1968.

Library of Congress Cataloging-in-Publication Data
Osler, William, Sir, 1849–1919.
Osler's "a way of life" and other addresses,
with commentary and annotations.
Includes bibliographical references.
ISBN 0–8223–2682–5 (cloth : alk. paper)
1. Medicine.   2. Medical ethics.   3. Physician and patient.
I. Title: "Way of life" and other addresses, with commentary
and annotations.   II. Title.
R114 .O84   2001   610—dc21   2001023576